AF598040

METHODS IN MOLECULAR BIOLOGY™

Series Editor
John M. Walker
School of Life Sciences
University of Hertfordshire
Hatfield, Hertfordshire, AL10 9AB, UK

For other titles published in this series, go to
www.springer.com/series/7651

Molecular Imaging

Methods and Protocols

Edited by

Khalid Shah

Massachusetts General Hospital,
Harvard Medical School,
Boston, Massachusetts, USA

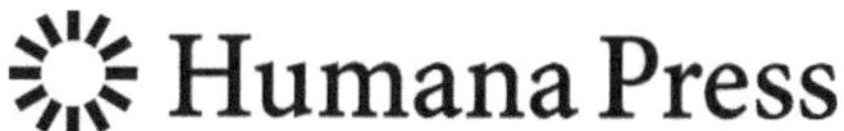

Editor
Dr. Khalid Shah
Molecular Neurotherapy and Imaging Laboratory
Department of Radiology and Neurology
Massachusetts General Hospital
Harvard Medical School
Charlestown, MA, 02129-2060, USA
kshah@helix.mgh.harvard.edu

ISSN 1064-3745 e-ISSN 1940-6029
ISBN 978-1-60761-900-0 e-ISBN 978-1-60761-901-7
DOI 10.1007/978-1-60761-901-7
Springer New York Dordrecht Heidelberg London

Library of Congress Control Number: 2010935924

Printed on acid-free paper

Humana Press is part of Springer Science+Business Media (www.springer.com)

Preface

From the first development of radioactive tracers in the early 1930s, it would take almost seven more decades for molecular imaging to evolve into a mature field of research. Since then, however, molecular imaging techniques have advanced and become invaluable tools for molecular biology research and – to a more modest extent – clinical medicine. Molecular imaging abandons the canonical imaging paradigm of detecting morphological contrasts and aims to explore the dynamics of molecules indicative of physiology and disease in a qualitative and quantitative manner. It allows longitudinal, noninvasive visualization of biological processes at the sub-cellular level, typically but not necessarily through the use of reporters with strong binding affinity to the molecular targets of interest. It follows from this rather unrestrictive definition that molecular imaging is not limited to specific image-capture methods but includes optical (near-infrared and visible spectrum fluorescence, bioluminescence), radio-scintigraphic modalities (PET, SPECT), magnetic resonance imaging (MRI), and magnetic resonance spectroscopy (MRS). All these imaging techniques progressively employ tagged probes with high affinity for molecules of interest, binding-activatable 'smart' probes and genetically engineered stably expressed reporters thus allowing optimized target visualization. Consequently, the list of biological processes that can be investigated is long and continues to expand.

The amount of possibilities offered by different molecular imaging techniques can be puzzling to biologists new to the field. Bearing this in mind, this book sets out to describe a rich variety of practical procedures and methods for diverging imaging technologies. Different sections are devoted to imaging of basic molecular and biochemical events, imaging in pre-clinical and finally in clinical settings and include sufficient practical details for students, established practitioners, and research fellows from different fields to become familiar with molecular imaging and incorporate imaging into their work.

Khalid Shah

Contents

Contributors

DANIEL C. ANTHONY • *Department of Pharmacology, University of Oxford, Oxford OX1 3QX, UK*

AMBROS J. BEER • *Department of Nuclear Medicine, Klinikum rechts der Isar, Technische Universität München, Munich 81675, Germany*

ABDELKADER BENNAGHMOUCH • *Maastricht Molecular Imaging and Therapeutics Laboratory (MMIT Laboratory), Department of Cardiology, Cardiovascular Research Institute Maastricht (CARIM), Maastricht University, Maastricht 6224 ER, The Netherlands*

JEFF W.M. BULTE • *Division of MR Research, Russell H. Morgan Department of Radiology and Radiological Science; Cellular Imaging Section and Vascular Biology Program, Institute for Cell Engineering; Department of Chemical and Biomolecular Engineering; Department of Biomedical Engineering, Whiting School of Engineering, Johns Hopkins University, Baltimore, MD, USA*

ROBIN P. CHOUDHURY • *Department of Cardiovascular Medicine, John Radcliffe Hospital, University of Oxford, Oxford OX3 9DU, UK*

MAARTEN F. CORSTEN • *Maastricht Molecular Imaging and Therapeutics Laboratory (MMIT Laboratory), Department of Cardiology, Cardiovascular Research Institute Maastricht (CARIM), Maastricht University, Maastricht 6224 ER, The Netherlands*

GEORGES EL FAKHRI • *Division of Nuclear Medicine and Molecular Imaging, Department of Radiology, Harvard Medical School, Massachusetts General Hospital, Boston, MA 02114, USA*

LEONARD HOFSTRA • *Maastricht Molecular Imaging and Therapeutics Laboratory (MMIT Laboratory), Department of Cardiology, Cardiovascular Research Institute Maastricht (CARIM), Maastricht University, Maastricht, The Netherlands*

FAROUC A. JAFFER • *Cardiovascular Research Center and Cardiology Division, Center for Molecular Imaging Research, Massachusetts General Hospital, Harvard Medical School, Boston, MA, USA*

CARL HIRSCHIE JOHNSON • *Department of Biological Sciences, Vanderbilt University, Nashville, TN 37235, USA*

DOROTA A. KEDZIOREK • *Division of MR Research, Russell H. Morgan Department of Radiology and Radiological Science, The Johns Hopkins University School of Medicine, Baltimore, MD, USA*

DARA L. KRAITCHMAN • *Division of MR Research, Russell H. Morgan Department of Radiology and Radiological Science, The Johns Hopkins University School of Medicine, Baltimore, MD, USA*

ANAND T.N. KUMAR • *Athinoula A Martinos Center for Biomedical Imaging, Harvard Medical School, Massachusetts General Hospital, Charlestown, MA 02129, USA*

JING LU • *Department of Bioengineering, University of Pennsylvania, Philadelphia, PA 19104, USA*

GARY D. LUKER • *Department of Radiology, University of Michigan, Ann Arbor, MI 48109-2200, USA;Department of Microbiology and Immunology, University of Michigan, Ann Arbor, MI 48109-2200, USA*

KATHRYN E. LUKER • *Department of Radiology, Ann Arbor, MI, USA*

JEREMY J. MAO • *Tissue Engineering and Regenerative Medicine Laboratory, Department of Biomedical Engineering, College of Dental Medicine, Columbia University Medical Center, New York, NY 10032, USA*

MARTINA A. MCATEER • *Department of Cardiovascular Medicine, John Radcliffe Hospital, University of Oxford, Oxford OX3 9DU, UK;Department of Pharmacology, University of Oxford, Oxford OX1 3QX, UK*

RACHEL S. MULLIGAN • *Department of Nuclear Medicine, Centre for PET, Austin Health, Heidelberg, VIC 3084, Australia*

JAGAT NARULA • *Department of Cardiology, University of California, Irvine, CA, USA*

GRAEME O'KEEFE • *Department of Nuclear Medicine, Centre for PET, Austin Health, Heidelberg, VIC 3084, Australia; School of Physics and Department of Medicine, University of Melbourne, Melbourne, VIC, Australia*

CEES OTTO • *Department of Science and Technology, Medical Cell BioPhysics, MIRA Institute for Biomedical Technology and Technical Medicine P.O. Box 217, 7500, AE Enschede, The Netherlands*

JINSONG OUYANG • *Division of Nuclear Medicine and Molecular Imaging, Department of Radiology, Harvard Medical School, Massachusetts General Hospital, Boston, MA 02114, USA*

CHRISTOPHER C. ROWE • *Department of Nuclear Medicine, Centre for PET, Austin Health, Heidelberg, VIC 3084, Australia;Department of Medicine, University of Melbourne, Melbourne, VIC, Australia*

MARKUS SCHWAIGER • *Department of Nuclear Medicine, Klinikum rechts der Isar, Technische Universität München, Munich 81675, Germany*

BHRANTI S. SHAH • *Tissue Engineering and Regenerative Medicine Laboratory, Department of Biomedical Engineering, College of Dental Medicine, Columbia University Medical Center, New York, NY 10032, USA*

KHALID SHAH • *Molecular Neurotherapy and Imaging Laboratory, Department of Radiology and Neurology, Harvard Medical School, Massachusetts General Hospital, Boston, MA 02114, USA*

NICOLA R. SIBSON • *Experimental Neuroimaging Group, Gray Institute for Radiation Oncology and Biology, Churchill Hospital, University of Oxford, Oxford OX3 7LJ, UK*

MOHAMMED SOUTTO • *Department of Biological Sciences, Vanderbilt University, Nashville, TN 37235, USA*

ANDREW TSOURKAS • *Department of Bioengineering, University of Pennsylvania, Philadelphia, PA 19104, USA*

SUSANNE W.M. VAN DE BORNE • *Maastricht Molecular Imaging and Therapeutics Laboratory (MMIT Laboratory), Department of Cardiology, Cardiovascular Research Institute Maastricht (CARIM), Maastricht University, Maastricht, The Netherlands*

HENK-JAN VAN MANEN • *AkzoNobel Research, Development & Innovation Measurement & Analytical Science Molecular Spectroscopy Group, Zutphenseweg 10, 7418 AJ, Deventer, The Netherlands*

JOHAN W.H. VERJANS • *Division of Cardiology, University Medical Center Utrecht, Utrecht, The Netherlands*

VICTOR L. VILLEMAGNE • *Department of Nuclear Medicine, Centre for PET, Austin Health, Heidelberg, VIC 3084, Australia;The Mental Health Research Institute of Victoria, Parkville, VIC, Australia*

CONSTANTIN VON ZUR MUHLEN • *Department of Cardiovascular Medicine, John Radcliffe Hospital, University of Oxford, Oxford OX3 9DU, UK;Department of Pharmacology, University of Oxford, Oxford OX1 3QX, UK*

QIGUANG XIE • *Department of Biological Sciences, Vanderbilt University, Nashville, TN 37235, USA*

XIAODONG XU • *Department of Biological Sciences, Vanderbilt University, Nashville, TN 37235, USA*

YUNFEI ZHANG • *Department of Biological Sciences, Vanderbilt University, Nashville, TN 37235, USA*

Section I

Imaging Biochemical Pathways and Molecular Events

Chapter 1

Bioluminescence Resonance Energy Transfer (BRET) Imaging in Plant Seedlings and Mammalian Cells

Qiguang Xie*, Mohammed Soutto*, Xiaodong Xu*, Yunfei Zhang, and Carl Hirschie Johnson (*equal contributors)

Abstract

Bioluminescence resonance energy transfer (BRET) has become a widely used technique to monitor protein–protein interactions. It involves resonance energy transfer between a bioluminescent donor and a fluorescent acceptor. Because the donor emits photons intrinsically, fluorescence excitation is unnecessary. Therefore, BRET avoids some of the problems inherent in fluorescence resonance energy transfer (FRET) approaches, such as photobleaching, autofluorescence, and undesirable stimulation of photobiological processes. In the past, BRET signals have generally been too dim to be effectively imaged. Newly available cameras that are more sensitive coupled to image splitter now enable BRET imaging in plant and mammalian cells and tissues. In addition, new substrates and enhanced luciferases enable brighter signals that allow even subcellular BRET imaging. Here, we report methods for BRET imaging of (1) localization of COP1 dimerization in plant cells and tissues and (2) subcellular distributions of interactions of the CCAAT/Enhancer Binding Protein α (C/EBPα) in single mammalian cells. We also discuss methods for the correction of BRET images for tissues that absorb light of different spectra. This progress should catalyze further applications of BRET for imaging and high-throughput assays.

Key words: Bioluminescence resonance energy transfer (BRET), imaging assay, protein–protein interaction, *Renilla* luciferase, plant and mammalian cells.

1. Introduction

The complicated network of protein interactions is pivotal to cellular "machinery." Identifying the partners with whom a protein associates is a critical step in the elucidation of underlying mechanisms of action. Various approaches have been used to analyze protein–protein interactions, including the yeast two-hybrid assay, fluorescence resonance energy transfer (FRET), bioluminescence resonance energy transfer (BRET), protein mass spectrometry,

K. Shah (ed.), *Molecular Imaging*, Methods in Molecular Biology 680,
DOI 10.1007/978-1-60761-901-7_1,

and evanescent wave methods (1). FRET and BRET are based on nonradiative energy transfer between a donor and an acceptor. In the case of FRET, two fluorophores with appropriately overlapping emission/absorption spectra (the "donor" and the "acceptor") can transfer excited-state energy from donor to acceptor if they are within ~50 Å of each other (2). The orientation of the donor and acceptor can significantly influence the magnitude of the resonance transfer, as has been dramatically shown in a recent study using BRET fusion proteins (3). In the case of BRET, the donor is a luciferase enzyme that directly emits photons so that fluorescence excitation is unnecessary. This luciferase-catalyzed luminescence utilizes a substrate and can excite an acceptor fluorophore by resonance energy transfer if the luciferase and fluorophore are in close proximity (within a radius of ~50 Å) and have a luminescence emission spectrum for the luciferase that appropriately overlaps the absorption spectrum of the fluorophore. If candidate interacting proteins are fused to the luminescent "donor" and fluorescent "acceptor" molecules, BRET can be used as a gauge of interaction between the candidate proteins (4).

The disadvantages of fluorescence excitation limit the potential applications of FRET. These disadvantages include photobleaching, autofluorescence, direct excitation of the acceptor fluorophore, photoresponsivity of specialized tissues (e.g., retina), and phototoxicity. Because BRET allows the detection of interactions between fusion proteins without direct excitation of the acceptor fluorophore; therefore, it can be used in applications where those potential disadvantages are problematic (5). We initially developed BRET to investigate the oligomerization of circadian clock proteins from cyanobacteria (4). During the past 8 years, the applications of BRET have multiplied (6–10), including new methods of analysis of BRET signals (11, 12), In addition, BRET has recently been coupled with its progenitor technique of FRET for detecting interaction in multi-protein complexes (13). Therefore, BRET has become a widely used technique to identify and monitor protein–protein interactions. BRET is potentially superior to FRET for high-throughput screening (HTS) because luminescence-monitoring HTS instruments are simpler and less expensive if fluorescence excitation is not involved. Moreover, low-resolution BRET imaging has shown in whole-animal analyses that BRET is advantageous for deep penetration of animal tissues (10, 14).

Nevertheless, BRET has not been used for high-resolution imaging of cells and tissues for two major reasons. First, BRET signals are very dim and cannot be increased by "turning up" the excitation, as with FRET (5, 15). Second, a wide range of ancillary techniques has been developed for fluorescence (e.g., FRET, FLIM, etc.) and many laboratories are equipped with microscopic setups that are designed for fluorescence. As we show herein, however, (i) new generation cameras can now detect the dim BRET signals, and (ii) many existing microscopic setups that were designed for FRET could be easily adapted for BRET by simply optimizing photon throughput and using the new cameras. We coupled a sensitive EB-CCD camera with a Dual-View™ image splitter to image BRET signals in two challenging applications: (i) subcellular imaging in single mammalian cells and (ii) tissue and cellular imaging in highly autofluorescent plant material (15, 16). The BRET fusion partners we used were the CCAAT/Enhancer Binding Protein α (C/EBPα) in isolated mammalian cells and COP1 (a regulator of the light signaling pathway) in plant tissues/cells.

This is an exciting time to use BRET technology for studying protein interactions because the application of (i) improved detection devices and (ii) new substrates that allow BRET signals to be easily detected now extends considerably the range of experiments that are feasible. This chapter discusses the use of an EB-CCD camera and Dual-View™ image splitter in addition to the first utilization of the ViviRen™ substrate for enhancing the luminescence intensity. Another publication has used a different but related substrate (EnduRen™) that extends the lifetime of the luminescence signal so that BRET signals can be measured over a long time course (17). In addition, mutagenesis of the luciferase from *Renilla* (RLUC) has resulted in new versions of RLUC that can be of potential benefit, both in terms of brighter signals and in terms of the spectra of luminescence output (14, 18, 19). Finally, the crystal structure of RLUC has been determined (20), and this information can be used to make fusion proteins with RLUC in which the candidate proteins are fused into internal loops of RLUC rather than being limited to merely N- or C-terminal fusions of RLUC to the candidate interactors. We hope that the recent advances in detection devices, luciferase substrates, and luciferase structure will stimulate further applications of BRET for imaging and high-throughput assays.

2. Materials

2.1. Plant and Mammalian Cell Lines

1. *Arabidopsis* seedlings *(Arabidopsis thaliana,* ecotype Col-0).
2. *Arabidopsis* cell suspension culture line (derived from *A. thaliana* seedlings, ecotype Col-0).
3. Tobacco seedlings (*Nicotiana tabacum cv. Xanthi*).
4. Human embryonic kidney 293 (HEK293) cell lines.
5. Mouse pituitary GHFT1 cell lines.

2.2. Plasmids, Vectors, and Strains

2.2.1. For Plants

1. 35 S::Rluc (pBIN19 binary vector with kanamycin marker) (Promega), which contains the *Renilla* luciferase (RLUC) coding region under the control of the 35 S promoter.
2. 35 S::Rluc-Eyfp (pBIN19 binary vector with kanamycin marker), which encodes a fusion protein of RLUC and EYFP (EYFP = enhanced yellow fluorescence protein, which is a red-shifted mutant of the *Aequorea victoria* green fluorescent protein).
3. 35 S::Rluc-COP1(N) (pPZP222 binary vector with gentamycin marker), which encodes a fusion protein of COP1 to N-terminus of RLUC.
4. 35 S::Eyfp-COP1(N) (pBIN19 binary vector with Kanamycin marker), which encodes a fusion protein of COP1 to N-terminus of EYFP.
5. *Agrobacterium tumefaciens* strain GV3101, which is used for transformation of tobacco leaf discs and *Arabidopsis* suspension cell culture lines. *Escherichia coli* DH5α is the host cloning strain.

2.2.2. For Mammalian Cells

1. hRlucC1 (= codon "humanized" pRlucC1 from Perkin-Elmer).
2. Venus, which is a yellow fluorescence protein variant inserted in the PCS2 vector under the control of the CMV promoter.
3. C/EBPalpha244, which is a nuclear transcription factor inserted in the EYFPC1r vector (this vector includes EYFP, but we replaced it with Venus as described below).
4. pcDNA 3.1 + vector (Invitrogen).
5. *E. coli* DH5α is the host cloning strain.

2.3. Media, Buffers, and Reagents

1. Dulbecco's Modified Eagle's Medium (DMEM).
2. Dulbecco's Modified Eagle's phenol-red free Medium (DMEM).
3. Phosphate buffered saline (PBS).
4. Opti-MEM: a reduced serum medium.
5. Fetal bovine serum (FBS).
6. Solution of trypsin (0.25%) and ethylenediamine tetraacetic acid (EDTA) (1 mM).
7. Lipofectamine 2000.
8. LB medium: 10 g/l bacto-tryptone, 5 g/l bacto-yeast extract, 10 g/l NaCl (pH 7.0).

9. Plant seedling growth medium: 1/2 MS salts with vitamins, 30 g/l sucrose, pH 5.8. Solid medium is the same except including 8 g/l agar.
10. *Arabidopsis* calli induction medium: MS medium with 0.5 mg/l 2,4-D (2,4-dichloro-phenoxyacetic acid), 2.0 mg/l NAA (α-naphthaleneacetic acid), 0.5 mg/l 6-BAP (6-benzylamino-purine), pH 5.8.
11. BRET assay buffer for plant seedlings: 1/2 MS salts with 2.5 μM coelenterazine (*see* **Note 1**).
12. BRET assay buffer for *Arabidopsis* suspension cell cultures: MS salts, 30 g/l sucrose, with 2.5 μM coelenterazine.
13. Coelenterazine (Native): 100 μM stock solution preparations dissolved in 95% EtOH. Prepare a fresh working solution before each use. Proper preparation and handling of coelenterazine stock and working solutions is critical (*see* **Note 1**).
14. Deep Blue C™ (BioSignal/PE): 100 μM stock solution, store desiccated and protected from light in deep freeze (–70°C). Deep Blue C™ was prepared the same as for native coelenterazine.
15. ViviRen™ (Promega): diluted in DMSO as a 10 mM stock solution, protected from light and stored at –20°C (*see* **Note 2**). From this 10 mM stock solution, a working solution of 10 μM was prepared on the day of the experiment.
16. PBI 1419 (Promega): diluted in DMSO to a 10 mM stock solution and stored at –20°C. From this 10 mM stock solution, a working solution of 30 μM was prepared on the day of the experiment.

2.4. Apparatus

1. EB-CCD Camera, a modified electron bombardment-charge coupled device camera (Hamamatsu Photonic Systems, Bridgewater NJ, USA) (*see* **Note 3**).
2. Dual-View™ micro-imager (Optical Insights, Tucson AZ, USA) (*see* **Note 4**).
3. Inverted microscope (IX-71, Olympus America Inc., Melville NY, USA), with Macro XLFLuor 2× objective, NA 0.14 (Olympus), UPlanFl 40× objective, NA 1.30 (oil immersion, Olympus), or a Plan Apo 60× objective, NA 1.45 (oil immersion, Olympus # 1-U2B616) (*see* **Note 5**). For measurement of fluorescence, an epifluorescence attachment (EX 500/20 nm, EM 520LP) was connected to the IX-71 inverted microscope.
4. Temperature controlled (22–37°C) light-tight box (*see* **Note 6**).

5. Spectrofluorimeter: QuantaMaster QM-7/SE (Photon Technology International, Birmingham NJ, USA) (*see* **Note 7**).
6. FB12 Luminometer (Zylux Corp., Maryville, TN).

3. Methods

The BRET technique has been widely used for bulk measurement of protein interaction and various methods have been described for bacterial cultures (4, 21), plant tissue (6, 9), and mammalian cell suspensions (7, 10, 22, 23). Nevertheless, BRET imaging of single cells has lagged behind fluorescence imaging because of the dim BRET signals. On the other hand, BRET is preferable to FRET for high-throughput screening because of its ease of measurement, exquisite sensitivity, and independence from excitation. We describe here our application of a modified EB-CCD camera coupled with a microimager to image BRET signals at tissue, cellular, and even subcellular levels. We used BRET imaging to monitor the protein interaction of COP1 in plant seedlings; these plant tissues absorb light of different colors differentially, but quantitative measurements of BRET are allowed by a simple correction using RLUC-EYFP emission profiles. Moreover, we detected CCAAT/Enhancer Binding Protein α (C/EBPα) interactions in the nuclei of isolated mammalian cells.

3.1. Construction of BRET Vectors

3.1.1. Constructs Used for Plants

The following constructs were made to express the fusion proteins under the control of the 35 S promoter:

1. Positive control: $P_{35\,S}$::Rluc-Eyfp for expression of the fusion protein RLUC-EYFP.
2. Negative control: $P_{35\,S}$::Rluc for expression of RLUC.
3. $P_{35\,S}$::Rluc-COP1(N) for expression of COP1 fusions to the N-terminus of RLUC.
4. $P_{35\,S}$::Eyfp-COP1(N) for expression of COP1 fusions to the N-terminus of EYFP.

3.1.2. Constructs Used for Mammalian Cells

The following constructs were made to express the fusion proteins under the control of the CMV promoter:

1. Positive control BRET construct P_{CMV}::hRluc-Venus for expression of fusion protein hRLUC-Venus in cytoplasm (excluded from nucleus) (*see* **Note 8** and **Fig. 1.1f–j**).
2. Negative-control BRET construct P_{CMV}::hRluc.

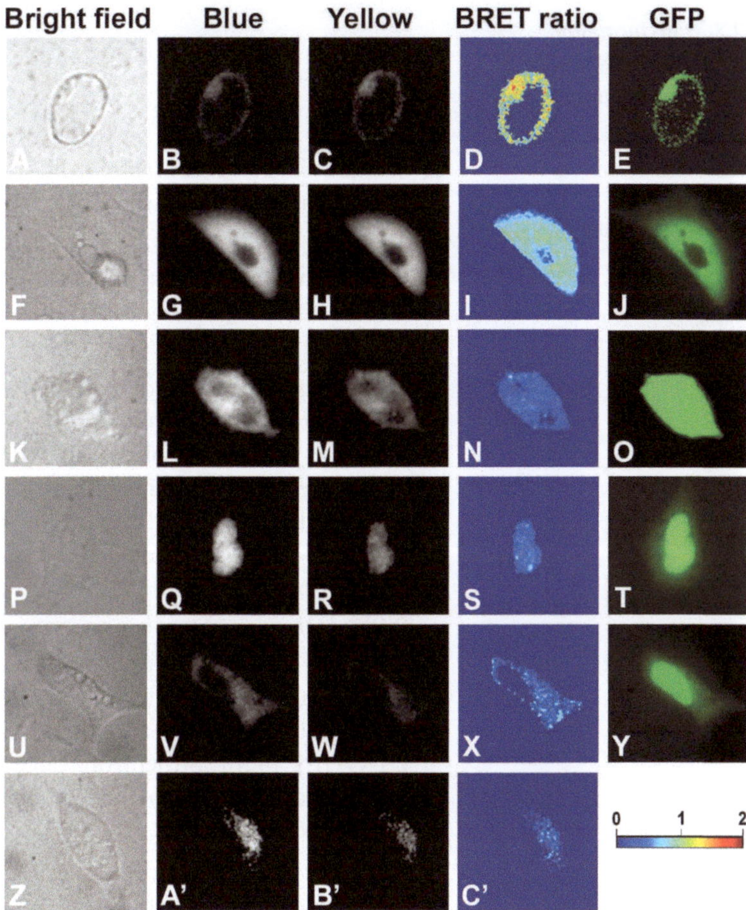

Fig. 1.1. Subcellular imaging of BRET in single plant and animal cells. *Arabidopsis* suspension culture, HEK293, and mouse GHFT1 cells. **a–e** Isolated *Arabidopsis* cell from a suspension culture line that is expressing RLUC-EYFP. **f–j** HEK293 cells expressing hRLUC-Venus; $Y \div B = 0.82 \pm 0.07$ SD over the luminescent portion of the cell. **k–o** HEK293 cell expressing unfused hRLUC and Venus; $Y \div B = 0.36$ over the luminescent portion of this cell. **p–t** Mouse GHFT1 cells expressing hRLUC-C/EBPα + Venus-C/EBPα; $Y \div B = 0.39 \pm 0.04$ SD over the luminescent portion of the cell. **u–y** Mouse GHF1 cells expressing hRLUC + Venus-C/EBPα; $Y \div B = 0.30$ over the luminescent portion of this cell. **z–c'** Mouse GHF1 cells expressing hRLUC-C/EBPα; $Y \div B = 0.24 \pm 0.06$ SD over the luminescent portion of the cell. **Panels a**, **f**, **k**, **p**, **u**, **z** are bright field, **panels b**, **g**, **l**, **q**, **v**, **a'** are *Blue-range luminescence*, **panels c**, **h**, **m**, **r**, **w**, **b'** are Yellow-range luminescence, **panels d**, **i**, **n**, **s**, **x**, **c'** are BRET ratios ($Y \div B$) over the entire images (pseudocolor scale shown below **panel y**), and **panels e**, **j**, **o**, **t**, **y** are fluorescence from EYFP or Venus in the fusion proteins. (Modified from Xu et al. (16).)

3. P_{CMV}::hRluc-C/EBP construct used for expression of the fusion protein hRLUC-C/EBP as a negative control for BRET in the nucleus (*see* **Fig. 1.1z–c'**).
4. P_{CMV}::Venus-C/EBP for expression of the fusion protein Venus-C/EBP in the nucleus (*see* **Note 9** and **Fig. 1.1u–y**).

3.2. Transformation and Cotransfection of BRET Constructs

3.2.1. Induction of Arabidopsis Cell Suspension Culture Lines and Agrobacterium-Mediated Transformation

1. Prepare fresh *Arabidopsis* calli induction medium, 20-ml aliquot in a 100-ml flask.
2. Sterilize *Arabidopsis* seeds: sterilize seeds 30 s in 70% EtOH in a 1.5-ml microcentrifuge tube, followed by rinsing 3× with sterile dH_2O. Then add 20% Clorox bleach for 5 min, rinse 5 times with sterile dH_2O.
3. Transfer sterilized seeds (~100) to a 100-ml volume flask containing 20 ml *Arabidopsis* calli induction medium, and place the flask on a shaker (120 rpm, 22°C, 12-h light/12-h dark cycle). Seeds will germinate in the liquid medium about 4 days later; calli and single cells will be induced from the seedlings directly within 3–4 weeks (24). Subculture every 2 weeks by diluting and adding fresh induction medium (*see* **Note 10**).
4. Inoculate a single clone of *Agrobacterium* carrying the appropriate construct to 5 ml fresh LB medium with appropriate antibiotics and put on a rotating shaker (180 rpm, 28°C) overnight. Subculture once before transformation by transferring 100 μl to 10 ml fresh LB liquid medium and growing overnight.
5. *Agrobacterium*-mediated transformation: inoculate 2 ml *Agrobacterium* culture ($OD_{600} \sim 1.0$) to 20 ml of the cell suspension culture and co-culture for 48 h; rinse collected cells after a gentle centrifugation and replace medium with liquid calli induction medium that includes Cefotaxime (200 μg/ml, Sigma, to kill *Agrobacterium*) and culture for 48 h; after that, rinse the cells and add fresh medium that includes Cefotaxime and appropriate antibiotics (50 μg/ml Kanamycin or 100 μg/ml Gentamycin).

3.2.2. Agrobacterium-Mediated Tobacco Leaf Disk Double-Transformation

1. Take healthy fully expanded leaves from 3- to 4-week-old tissue culture grown tobacco, cut into 0.25 cm^2 leaf disks, and co-culture with the *Agrobacterium* suspension (*see* Section **3.2.1**) for 10 min, then transfer to tobacco culture medium (MS medium with MES 0.59 g/l + NAA 0.1 mg/l + BAP 1 mg/l +Kanamycin 100 mg/l; 10 leaf disks per Petri dishes) for 2–3 days.
2. Rinse leaf disks three times with MS medium that includes Carbenicillin (Sigma; 500 mg/l, to kill *Agrobacterium*), transfer leaf disks to tobacco selective medium (MS medium with MES 0.59 g/l + NAA 0.1 mg/l + BAP 1 mg/l

+Kanamycin 100 mg/l +Carbenicillin 500 mg/l), and subculture with fresh medium every 2 weeks.

3. Shoots should regenerate from the disks – if so, cut the regenerated young shoots from the basal disks, and transfer these shoots to 1/2 MS medium with selective antibiotics for rooting.
4. Prepare leaf disks from the regenerated and resistant seedlings for a second transformation with a second construct (if relevant), and use the same protocol as above, selecting with two antibiotics (e.g., both Gentamycin and Kanamycin added to the selection medium).

3.2.3. Transient Transfection of Mammalian Cells

We have used human HEK293 and mouse pituitary GHFT1 cells for BRET detection. In general, HEK293 transfect well, but for studying the interactions of the C/EBP protein, we have used mouse GHFT1 cells because C/EBP takes up distinctive interaction patterns in the nuclei of GHFT1 cells.

1. Grow cells in DMEM medium supplemented with 10% FBS, 100 U/ml of penicillin, and 100 U/ml of streptomycin until they reach 80% confluence (*see* **Note 11**).
2. Dilute 4 μg of plasmid DNA in 250 μl OptiMEM medium without serum and mix gently.
3. Dilute 10 μl of Lipofectamine 2000 in 250 μl OptiMEM medium without serum. Mix gently and incubate for 5 min at room temperature (*see* **Note 12**).
4. Combine the diluted Lipofectamine 2000 with the diluted DNA and incubate for 20 min at room temperature (*see* **Note 13**).
5. Add the 500 μl of DNA-lipofectamine solution to cells in 35 mm dishes. Mix gently by rocking the dish back and forth.
6. Incubate the cells at 37°C in a CO_2 incubator.
7. After 24–48 h, wash cells in PBS and replace the DMEM medium with phenol-red free DMEM supplemented with 10% FBS for imaging (phenol red absorbs light so it needs to be removed so that it does not absorb the luminescence signal).

3.3. Preparation of Plant Seedlings and Cell Suspension Lines

1. Sterilize *Arabidopsis* or tobacco seeds (*see* Section **3.2.1**): for tobacco seeds, 1 min for EtOH and 10 min for bleach.
2. Place seeds on plant seedling growth medium (1/2 MS + agar), and incubate in a 12-h light/12-h dark cycle, 120 μE m^{-2} s^{-1} (cool-white fluorescence lamps), 22°C.
3. 5-day-old tobacco seedlings or 7-day-old *Arabidopsis* seedlings were used for BRET spectra acquisition and imaging analysis.

4. Newly grown *Arabidopsis* cell suspension lines (7 days after subculture, *see* Section **3.2.1** and **Note 10**) in appropriate selective liquid medium were used for single-cell imaging analysis.

3.4. BRET Luminescence Spectra Acquisition In Vivo

3.4.1. Plant Seedlings

1. Start spectrofluorimeter (QuantaMaster QM-7/SE) before luminescence measurement (*see* **Note 7**).
2. Transfer the transgenic plant seedlings (5-day-old *Arabidopsis* or 7-day-old tobacco) from solid medium directly to a 2-ml fluorescence cuvette containing 0.5 ml plant seedling BRET assay buffer without coelenterazine.
3. Add fresh coelenterazine to the assay buffer to a final concentration of 2.5 μM.
4. With the spectrofluorimeter's fluorescence excitation turned off, measure the luminescence emission spectrum between the wavelengths 440 and 580 nm in 2-nm steps with a 5-s integration for each step (*see* **Note 14**).
5. Analyze the BRET ratio by evaluating the emission spectra, especially the magnitude of the second peak at ~530 nm. Normalization of values is needed before analysis (*see* Section **3.8.2**). Emission spectra of RLUC (negative control) and RLUC-EYFP (positive control) from whole *Arabidopsis* seedlings are shown in **Fig. 1.2a**. Spectra of RLUC-COP1 and RLUC-COP1 + EYFP-COP1 emission from whole *Arabidopsis* seedlings are shown in **Fig. 1.2b**.

3.4.2. Mammalian Cells

1. Wash cells twice with phosphate buffered saline (PBS).
2. Trypsinize the adherent cells with 0.05% trypsin-EDTA solution at 37°C for 5~10 min.
3. Add 900 μl of serum-containing DMEM to inactivate the trypsin. Transfer the cells to a 1.5-Ml microcentrifuge tube.
4. Centrifuge the cells at 300×*g* for 5 min and wash twice with PBS.
5. Resuspend cells with phenol-red free DMEM supplemented with 10% FBS.
6. Add ViviRen^{TM} to the assay buffer to a final concentration of 10 μM.
7. Check the total luminescence using the F12 Luminometer.

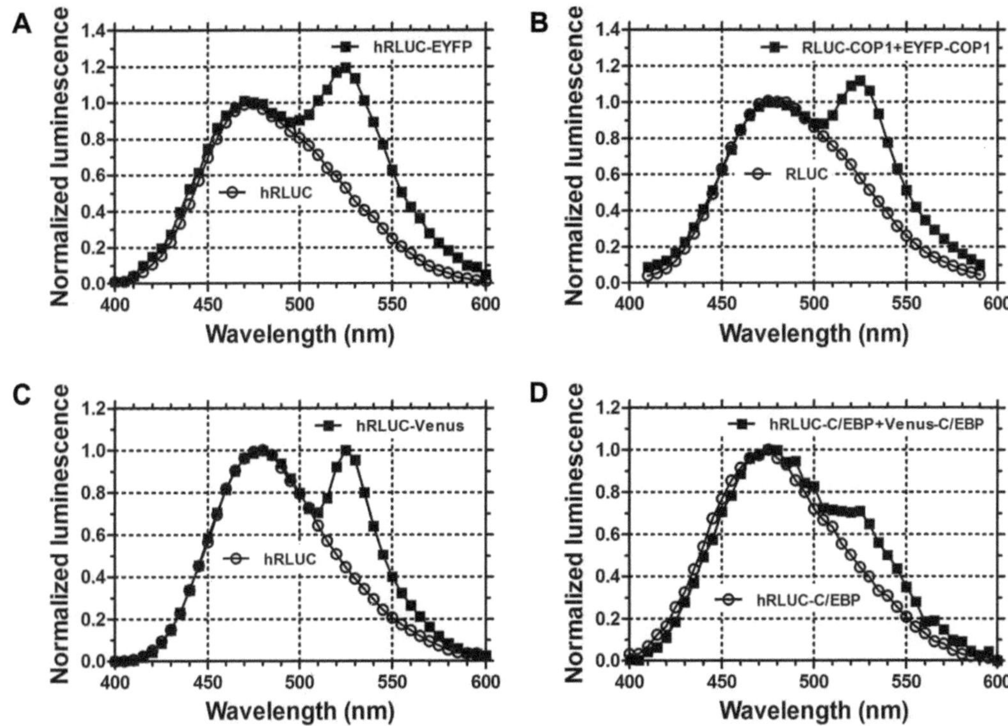

Fig. 1.2. Luminescence emission spectra from whole plant seedlings and mammalian cells. **a** The hRLUC vs. hRLUC-EYFP emission spectra from 7-day-old transgenic *Arabidopsis* seedlings. **b** The spectra of RLUC vs. RLUC-COP1+EYFP-COP1 emission from 5-day-old transgenic tobacco seedlings. **c** Luminescence spectra of hRLUC and hRLUC-Venus emission from HEK 293 cells. **d** The spectra of hRLUC-C/EBPα vs. hRLUC-C/EBPα + Venus-C/EBPα emission from single mouse GHFT1 cells. Luminescence spectra were normalized to the emission at 480 nm. (Modified from Xu et al. (16).)

8. With the spectrofluorimeter's (QuantaMaster QM-7/SE) fluorescence excitation turned off, record the luminescence emission spectrum between the wavelengths 440 and 580 nm in 2-nm steps with a 5-s integration for each step (*see* **Fig. 2c, d**).

3.5. Comparison of Substrates for BRET Imaging (Native Coelenterazine, Deep Blue C^{TM}, and ViviRen^{TM})

3.5.1. Autoluminescence, Brightness, and Stability

For assessing autoluminescence, we tested different substrates in DMEM phenol-red free medium with or without 10% FBS. For assessing enzyme-catalyzed brightness and stability, we used transfected HEK293 cells in DMEM with or without serum (*see* **Note 15**).

1. 24–48 h after transfection, cells were washed twice with phosphate buffered saline (PBS).
2. Release adherent cells by adding trypsin to a final concentration of 0.05% trypsin-EDTA (incubate at 37°C for 5∼10 min).
3. Add 900 μl DMEM supplemented with 10% FBS to inactivate the trypsin and collect the cells in a 1.5-ml microcentrifuge tube.
4. Gently spin down the cells and wash them twice with PBS.
5. Gently resuspend the cell pellet in 1 ml of phenol-red free DMEM with or without 10%FBS.
6. Add substrate solution (100 μl) to cells to reach a final concentration of 5–10 μM. For the stability assay, add 30 μM of stabilizer to the ViviRen™-treated samples (*see* **Note 15**).
7. Record the time dependence of total luminescence in the FB12 luminometer (*see* **Fig. 1.3a–c**).

3.5.2. Cell Viability Assay

Cell viability was assayed to test the possibility of toxicity of the different substrates.

1. Grow HEK293cells in 24-well plates overnight until they reach 80% confluence.
2. Wash cells with PBS.
3. Add medium with or without serum to the cells.
4. Incubate cells for 1 h or 6 h with the different substrates to a final concentration of 5 μM (native coelenterazine and coelenterazine-h) or 10 μM (ViviRen™).
5. Count viable cells by using 0.4% (w/v) Trypan Blue in a hemacytometer under the microscope (*see* **Note 16, Fig. 1.3d**). Viable cells exclude the Trypan Blue whereas the dye stains dead cells.

3.6. BRET Imaging

3.6.1. Apparatus for Whole Organism and Microscopic Imaging

1. Microscope setup: for plant cell and mammalian cell imaging, the EB-CCD camera was coupled to the Dual-View™ image splitter, which was connected to the bottom port of the IX-71 microscope. The inverted microscope (but not the EB-CCD camera or Dual-View™) resided inside a temperature controlled light-tight box (*see* **Note 6**).
2. "Box" setup for whole organism imaging: non-infinity-corrected objectives were attached directly to the Dual-View™ inside a light-tight box (at room temperature ∼ 22°C). The EB-CCD camera was coupled to the Dual-View™, but the camera resided outside the box (*see* **Note 17**). Dual-View™ requires precise alignment before use (*see* **Note 18**).

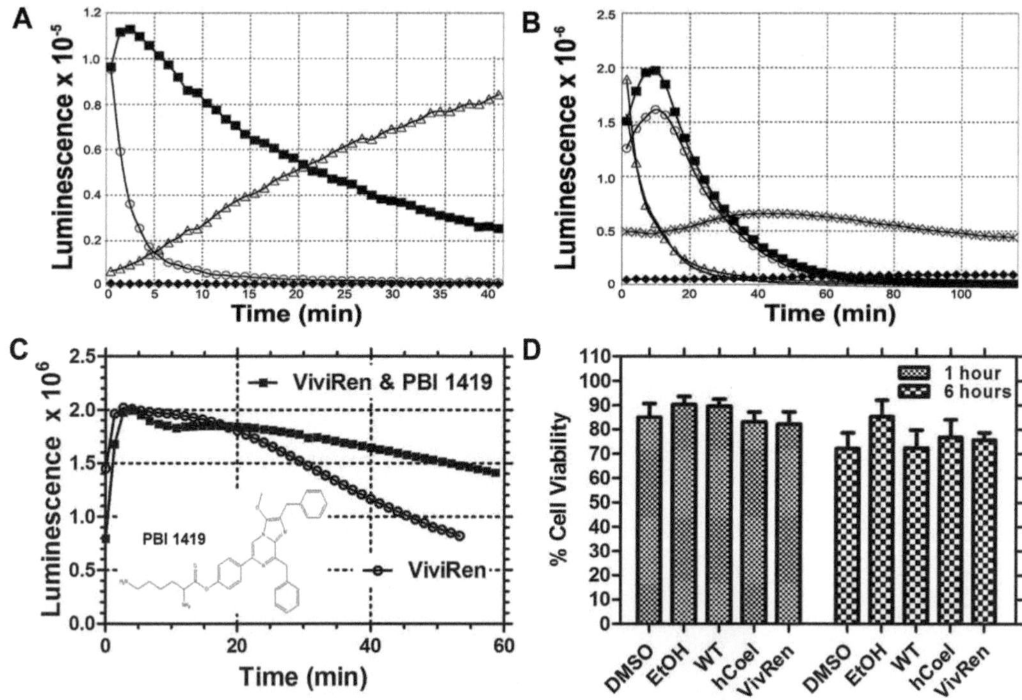

Fig. 1.3. Comparison of coelenterazine substrates. **a** Autoluminescence of substrates in DMEM with and without 10% FBS (no cells present): for 10 μM native coelenterazine, *closed squares* = DMEM + 10% FBS and *open circles* = DMEM without FBS; for 10 μM ViviRen^{TM}, *open triangles* = DMEM + 10% FBS and *closed diamonds* = DMEM without FBS. **b** Brightness of enzyme-catalyzed luminescence with native vs. ViviRen^{TM} coelenterazine. For HEK293 cells in DMEM + 10% FBS and transfected with P_{CMV}::hRLUC-Venus: *line without symbols* = 5 μM native coelenterazine, *open triangles* = 10 μM native coelenterazine, *open circles* = 5 μM ViviRen^{TM}, *closed squares* = 10 μM ViviRen^{TM}. For tobacco seedlings transfected with P_{35S}::RLUC-EYFP in 1/2 MS medium: "x" = 10 μM native coelenterazine, *closed diamonds* = 10 μM ViviRen^{TM}. **c** Stability of enzyme-catalyzed luminescence with ViviRen^{TM} vs. ViviRen^{TM} and the stabilizer PBI 1419. For HEK293 cells in DMEM + 10% FBS and transfected with P_{CMV}::hRluc-Venus: *open circles* = 10 μM ViviRen^{TM}, *closed squares* = 10 μM ViviRen^{TM} + 30 μM PBI 1419. Inset: structure of PBI 1419, a stabilizer molecule for ViviRen^{TM} (obtainable from Promega by special request). **d** HEK293 cell viability after exposure to three different substrates. Cell viability was assayed by Trypan Blue exclusion after exposure to substrates and/or solvents for 1 or 6 h. HEK293 cells were in DMEM + 10% FBS. Data are shown as % viability (± S.E.M.) as compared with untreated cells. Treatments were as follows: 0.1% DMSO, 0.1% ethanol, 10 μM native coelenterazine (0.1% ethanol final concentration), 10 μM coelenterazine-h (0.1% ethanol final concentration), and 10 μM ViviRen^{TM} (0.1% DMSO final concentration).

3.6.2. Plant Seedlings Imaged in the "Box" Setup

1. Plant seedlings were placed into a drop of BRET assay buffer on a slide without coelenterazine, room temperature 22°C.
2. Put the slide onto a support jack to fine-tune and focus using the non-infinity-corrected objectives (e.g., Plan 4×, NA=0.13 DL, 160/–; and Plan 10×, NA=0.30 DL, 160/0.17; Nikon).
3. Gently add the coelenterazine to the samples (final concentration of 10 μM).
4. Fine-tune and focus the samples precisely in brightfield with the Dual-View^{TM} in "Bypass Mode." Then turn the

Dual-View^{TM} off "Bypass Mode" and push the filter holder inside the tube. Close the light-tight box carefully (*see* **Note 19**).

5. Capture the BRET images of short-pass ("Blue") and long-pass ("Yellow") emission simultaneously from the whole seedlings (~7- to 10-min exposure time) (*see* **Fig. 1.4**).
6. Take a brightfield image of the above same sample with the door of the light-tight box opened (*see* **Note 19, Fig. 1.4, panels a, f, k**).

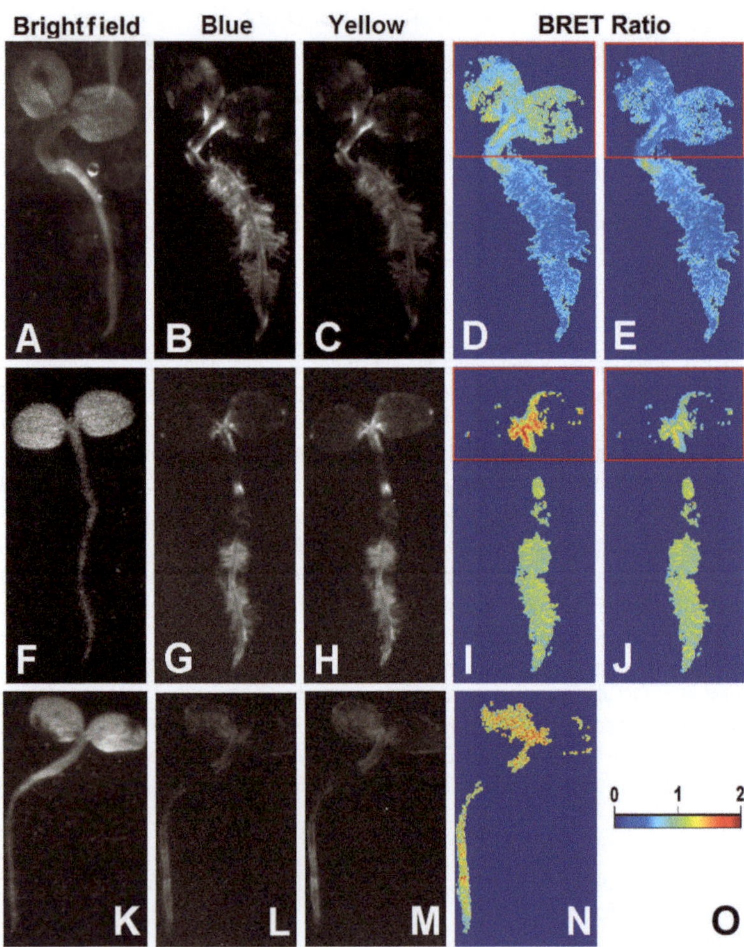

Fig. 1.4. BRET macro-imaging of tobacco seedlings. Seven-day-old tobacco seedlings were transformed with (i) $P_{35\,S}$::Rluc (**a–e**), (ii) $P_{35\,S}$::Rluc-EYFP (**f–j**), or (iii) $P_{35\,S}$::Rluc-COP1+ $P_{35\,S}$::Eyfp-COP1 (**k–n**). **Panels a**, **f**, **k** are *bright field* images, **panels b**, **g**, **l** are images of short-pass luminescence (*Blue*), **panels c**, **h**, **m** are images of long-pass luminescence (*Yellow*), **panels d**, **i**, **n** are BRET ratios (Y÷B) over the entire luminescent portion of the image (pseudocolor scale shown in **panel o**), **panels e** and **j** are corrected images of **panel d** and **i**, respectively, shown with a *red box* encasing the pigmented (cotyledon) portion of the seedlings (correction factor for boxed regions of **panels e** and **j** was 1.27). (Modified from Xu et al. (16).)

3.6.3. Plant Cell Cultures Imaged in the Microscope Setup

1. Let the flask of cell culture stand for several seconds, then remove suspension cells from the middle of the flask gently and quickly place a drop onto the slide.
2. Mix the sample with the coelenterazine working solution (for *Arabidopsis* suspension cell use, *see* Section **2.3**) and place a cover glass atop the sample.
3. In brightfield, focus on a single cell using the inverted microscope with the 40× oil immersion objective (NA 1.30). Close the box for imaging (exclude ALL incidental light by using a light-tight box!).
4. Capture the BRET images of short-pass ("Blue") and long-pass ("Yellow") simultaneously using the Dual-View^{TM} and EB-CCD (~5- 15-min exposure time).
5. Take fluorescence images (EX 500/20 nm, EM 520LP) and/or brightfield images (*see* **Fig. 1.1a–e**). It is usually better to take the luminescence image first while the substrate is active and before fluorescence or brightfield excitation causes any photobleaching and/or phototoxicity of the sample.

3.6.4. Mammalian Cells Imaged in the Microscope Setup

1. Wash cells with PBS that have been transfected and grown in 35-mm petri dishes with cover-glass bottoms (MatTek Corporation).
2. Add 1 ml of phenol-red free DMEM supplemented with 10%FBS.
3. Add ViviRen^{TM} substrate directly to the medium to a final concentration of 10 μM.
4. Gently agitate the petri dish by hand to mix the substrate and medium.
5. Check the total luminescence in the FB12 luminometer before looking at the sample in the microscope. The brightness of luminescence as measured by the luminometer gives an approximation of the transfection efficiency of the luminescence constructs.
6. In brightfield, focus on a single cell using the inverted microscope with the Plan Apo 60× objective, NA 1.45 (oil immersion, Olympus # 1-U2B616) using the Dual-View^{TM} in "Bypass Mode."
7. After focusing in brightfield, turn off the brightfield excitation and switch the Dual-View^{TM} out of "Bypass Mode" by pushing the filter holder inside the Dual-View^{TM}. Close the box for imaging (exclude ALL incidental light by using a light-tight box!).
8. Capture the BRET images of short-pass ("Blue") and long-pass ("Yellow") simultaneously for sequential exposures of

100 ms (*see* **Note 20**). *See* **Fig. 1.1, panels g–i, l–n, q–S, v–x, a'–c'**.

9. Take fluorescence images (EX 500/20 nm, EM 520LP, *see* **Fig. 1.1, panels j, o, t, y**), and/or brightfield images (*see* **Fig. 1.1, panels f, k, p, u, z**). It is usually better to take the luminescence image first while the substrate is active and before fluorescence or brightfield excitation causes any photobleaching and/or phototoxicity of the sample.

3.7. Set Up Appropriate "Controls"

1. "Negative control": RLUC alone. It is used for normalization (*see* **Fig. 1.1a**)
2. "Positive control": RLUC-EYFP or hRLUC-Venus fusion proteins. These are commonly used to test the whole system, e.g., the setup of the spectrofluorimeter or imaging apparatus, especially since they tend to be the brightest construct in our experience with plant and mammalian cells. The RLUC-EYFP (or hRLUC-Venus) spectrum can also be used to calculate the absorption ratio for differentially absorbing tissues, and for other image corrections (*see* **Fig. 1.1a** and **Note 21**). For examples of images using these positive control fusion proteins, *see* **Figs. 1.1f–j** and **1.4f–j**.
3. Unfused luciferase + unfused yellow fluorescent protein: this combination is to confirm that the luciferase and yellow fluorescent protein will not spuriously interact by themselves, as shown in **Fig. 1.1 k–o** for unfused hRLUC + unfused Venus (in bacterial, plant, and mammalian cells, we have found that these proteins do not interact, but this should be tested for any new cell type).
4. Measure the spectra of relevant fusion proteins alone (e.g., RLUC vs. RLUC-COP1; or EYFP vs. EYFP-COP1) to make sure that the fusion proteins do not alter the spectra of RLUC emission or EYFP fluorescence. For an example of an image with hRLUC-C/EBPα, *see* **Fig. 1.1z–c'**.
5. Control for RLUC and EYFP concentrations: This kind of control is important to confirm that the BRET ratio is independent of the concentration of RLUC/EYFP molecules. In some cases, energy transfer can arise from random interactions of the luciferase and fluorophore in a cellular compartment (e.g., the membrane), and testing a range of concentrations of the RLUC and EYFP fusion proteins to assess which concentrations of those proteins lead to a constant BRET ratio is an important control (8). Also, in situations where RLUC and EYFP fusion protein are produced independently or expressed at different concentrations, this control is important for quantitative measurement of protein interaction (25). In the case of transient transfections, the

experimenter can vary the intracellular concentration of the BRET proteins by using different amounts of plasmids in the transfection reaction.

6. Make sure your imaging setup totally excludes all incidental light. BRET signals are very dim and any incidental light will ruin image quality and/or generate misleading images.

3.8. Calculation of BRET Ratio

3.8.1. Correction of BRET Signal in Differentially Absorbing Tissues

Many types of tissue contain pigments that differentially absorb light, and this property can interfere with an accurate measurement of BRET or FRET spectra. An example of this problem is green plant tissue, which contains many pigments that differentially absorb luminescence of different wavelengths. Green plant tissue absorbs more strongly at 480 nm than at 530 nm (*see* **Fig. 1.5a**), and this can be visualized by the difference in RLUC-EYFP spectrum from green plant tissue as compared with etiolated (= non-pigmented) plant tissue (*see* **Fig. 1.5b, c**). Therefore, to obtain an accurate BRET spectrum from pigmented tissue, the BRET signal should be corrected for differential absorption (*see* **Note 21**).

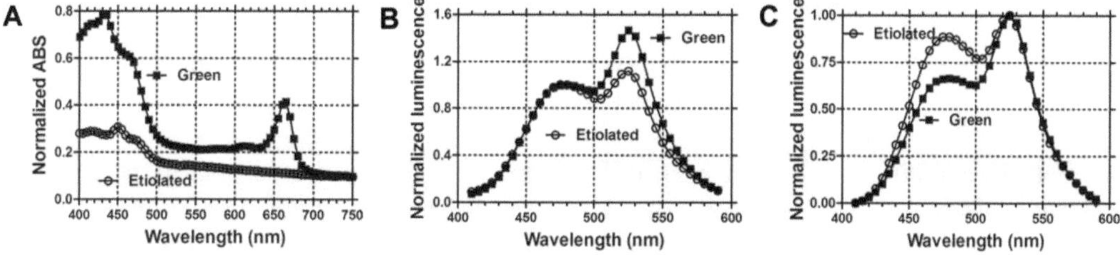

Fig. 1.5. Correction of BRET signals from tobacco seedlings for differential absorption of luminescence. **a** Absorption spectra of an ethanol extraction of pigments from light-grown (*"green," filled squares*) and dark-grown ("etiolated," *open circles*) seedlings. **b** RLUC-EYFP emission spectra for *green* and etiolated seedlings, normalized to the emission at 480 nm. **c** RLUC-EYFP emission spectra for *green* and etiolated seedlings, normalized to the emission at 530 nm. (Modified from Xu et al. (16).)

1. Prepare light-grown ("green") and dark-grown ("etiolated") seedlings (e.g., 5-day-old tobacco seedlings). Measure the emission spectrum of RLUC-EYFP in etiolated and green seedlings using the spectrofluorimeter.
2. Extract the total pigments from tobacco cotyledons (both green and etiolated seedlings) using ethanol.
3. Measure the absorption of above two kinds of ethanol extracts with spectrophotometer. Calculate the absorption ratio 480:530 for green seedlings (e.g., 2.07) and etiolated seedlings (e.g., 1.64) to get the correction factor, 1.27 (e.g., $1.27 = 2.07 \div 1.64$) (*see* **Fig. 1.5a**).

4. The factor can be used to correct the image for the differential absorption using the image calculation function of ImageJ (or an equivalent function in other imaging software) (*compare* **Fig. 1.4d** with **1.4e and 1.4i** with **1.4j**). In the case of the plant seedlings, the areas which are to be corrected in the "Blue image" are multiplied by the correction factor to produce a "corrected Blue image," then the BRET ratio image can be produced by re-calculating the ratio between the "Yellow image" and the "corrected Blue image."
5. We describe the correction process for plant tissue here, but this correction could be applied to any kind of tissue, plant, or animal, by simply assuming the spectrum of RLUC-EYFP emission from the tissue in question should have roughly equivalent peaks at 480 nm and at 530 nm. Deviations from equal 480/530 nm peaks can be assumed to be due to differential tissue absorption (as in **Fig. 1.5b, c**) and a correction factor can be derived from those deviations.

3.8.2. Normalization and Ratio Calculation

1. To compare the BRET luminescence spectra traces between RLUC-EYFP and RLUC (negative control), we normalized the first peak (480 nm) to 1.0 (as in all panels of **Fig. 1.2**).
2. Calculate BRET ratio (530 nm ÷ 480 nm) of individual traces.
3. Take the average of replicate samples and calculate standard deviations (*see* **Note 22**).

3.9. Methods of BRET Imaging Analysis

1. Background subtraction: first, select a region to serve as background and calculate the average optical density, then use the image calculator function to subtract the background (ImageJ has a plug-in for background subtraction).
2. Image alignment: In some situations where the two images from the Dual-View™ (i.e., the short-pass "Blue" and the long-pass "Yellow") do not align well (e.g., which might be caused by poor alignment within the Dual-View™), imaging alignment should be processed before image ratio calculation. (ImageJ and some other software packages have this function and can align two images automatically by calculating an optimal alignment. Image alignment can also be accomplished by manual translation, rotation, and scaling.)
3. Derivation of BRET ratio image: divide "Yellow" by "Blue" ({Yellow range}÷{Blue range}= Y÷B), to produce a ratiometric image with pseudo-color (as in **Figs. 1.1, panels d, i, n, s, x, c' and 1.4, panels d, e, i, j, n**).
4. Using ImageJ's ROI (Region Of Interest) and measurement functions, select the same ROI in both Blue and Yellow

images; calculate the densities inside the ROIs that have been selected.

5. Calculate the ratio of density of objects between images (Y÷B). Take the average and standard deviation on parallel experiments (*see* **Note 23**).

4. Notes

1. Coelenterazine is sensitive to light, so store the powder and stock solutions in the dark at –70°C with desiccant. For preparation of stock solutions (e.g., 250 μM), dissolve powder with 95% EtOH, distribute 40–120 μl aliquots to a set of microcentrifuge tubes, and dry down in a Speed-Vac. After the samples are dried into the bottom of the microcentrifuge tubes, replace the air in the tubes with gaseous N_2 or Ar (Gently! Don't blow off the coelenterazine! We place all the tubes in a box and flow N_2 gas into the box for 20 min to replace all the air. Argon gas is helpful because it is heavier than air and will settle in the tubes, but it is more expensive). The tubes are then capped and returned to –70°C for long-term storage. To make a working solution, dissolve the dried coelenterazine in one or more tubes with a minimal amount of 95% EtOH, and then dilute to 10 μM with distilled water or medium. Be sure to prepare a fresh working solution before each experiment – keep the working solution on ice and in the dark (we wrap the tubes with aluminum foil).
2. ViviRen™ (Promega) is a modified version of the coelenterazine analog, coelenterazine-h, to which ester groups have been attached. The design intention of ViviRen™ was to develop an inactive RLUC substrate that would not release oxidation-induced autoluminescence in a serum-containing extracellular medium, but that would permeate into cells where intracellular esterases cleave the ester groups to generate active coelenterazine-h intracellularly. EnduRen™ (Promega) is a related substrate that is very stable and can be used for longer term measurement of luminescence and therefore BRET (17). In our experience, the luminescence intensity with EnduRen™ is much lower than with ViviRen™, but this limitation can potentially be counteracted by a very sensitive detection system.
3. We used a modified electron bombardment-charge coupled device (EB-CCD) camera (Hamamatsu Photonic Systems, Bridgewater NJ, USA); the modifications were a GaAsP

photocathode with low ion feedback and increased photocathode cooling to –25°C. The low ion feedback was achieved by a special modification to the EB-CCD camera by Hamamatsu to remove the aluminum mask from the sensor that is normally included to avoid the "double focus phenomenon." In the case of low light imaging, this problem is negligible. In addition, the camera is using full frame transfer CCD, so it is possible to remove the mask. As a result, the sensor gets the same gain at a lower acceleration voltage. This low acceleration voltage reduces the ion feedback phenomenon drastically, improving performance for very low light level imaging. Finally, the cooling of the photocathode to –25°C reduces the dark current of the photocathode. The acquisition software was Photonics-WASABI (Hamamatsu).

4. The Dual-View^{TM} micro-imager (Optical Insights, LLC) is an image splitter that is coupled to the EB-CCD camera to allow the simultaneous acquisition of luminescence images at two wavelengths. It consists of a dichroic mirror (in our case, to split the emission at 505 nm using Q505LPxr) and interference filters to refine wavelengths (i) below 505 nm (HQ505SP, short-pass filter; "Blue") and (ii) above 505 nm (HQ505LP, long-pass filter; "Yellow"). For BRET imaging, the ratio of emission in the two wavelength ranges can be calculated without the complications due to possible changes in the total luminescence signal over the time course of the exposure (this kind of problem could occur with long exposure time if we exposed the camera to one wavelength and subsequently to a second wavelength – if the total luminescence).
5. An epifluorescence attachment (EX 500/20 nm, EM 520LP) is connected to the IX-71 inverted microscope to allow the measurement of fluorescence images. For low-power imaging (e.g., *Arabidopsis* cotyledons, roots etc.), we used an Olympus Macro XLFLuor 2× objective, NA 0.14 (working distance of 16.3 mm). For higher magnification imaging, an Olympus UPlanFl 40× objective, NA 1.30 (oil immersion) was used for *Arabidopsis* suspension culture cells, or an Olympus Plan Apo 60× objective, NA 1.45 (oil immersion) was used for mammalian cells.
6. Light-tight boxes for imaging: #1. For imaging larger samples, e.g., plant seedlings that are 1- to 3-cm long, we used a light-tight "box setup." For plant tissues, like tobacco or *Arabidopsis* seedlings, non-infinity-corrected objectives (Plan 4×, NA=0.13 DL, 160/–; or Plan 10×, NA=0.30 DL, 160/0.17; both manufactured by Nikon) were attached directly to the Dual-View^{TM} image splitter, which was

placed through a hole in the box (the hole was sealed with black felt to prevent light leaks). The EB-CCD was coupled to the Dual-View^{TM} outside the box. The box was in a room whose temperature was set at 22°C. Under these conditions, spontaneous YFP fluorescence or auto-fluorescence in the absence of coelenterazine (as might occur if there was a light leak into the box) could not be detected for 10- to 30-min exposures – therefore, the box setup was confirmed to be light-tight. After treating the transgenic seedlings with coelenterazine, images could be detected by the EB-CCD camera for exposures of 5 min or less. *See* images in **Fig. 1.4**.

#2. For microscopic imaging of mammalian cells (36°C) or plant cells (22°C), the IX-71 microscope was encased in a temperature-controlled (22–37°C) light-tight box with the Dual-View^{TM} and EB-CCD attached to the bottom port of the microscope (Dual-View^{TM} and EB-CCD camera were outside of the box). *See* images in **Fig. 1.1**.

7. A spectrofluorimeter (QuantaMaster QM-7/SE) was used for spectral measurements of BRET emission. For luminescence spectrum acquisition, the excitation beam was blocked and the slit width was set to 16 nm.

8. BRET experiments should always include a positive control – in our experiments, we used either RLUC-EYFP (for the plant studies) or hRLUC-Venus (for the mammalian cell studies). *See* **Figs. 1.1f–j** and **1.4f–j**. The production of the hRLUC-Venus construct is described in the next note (*see* **Note 9**).

9. CCAAT/Enhancer Binding Protein α (C/EBPα) is a transcriptional factor that localizes to heterochromatin in the nucleus and dimerizes. To test BRET signal detection in the nucleus, we made two fusion proteins with the nuclear transcriptional factor C/EBPα, one with hRluc and another with Venus. C/EBP was amplified from the EYFPC1r-C/EBPalpha244 plasmid (obtained from Dr. R.N. Day) using *Xho*I and *Hind*III linkers. The PCR product was fused to the C-terminus of hRluc by insertion into the *Xho*I/*Hind*III site of P_{CMV}::hRluc to give P_{CMV}::hRluc-C/EBP. For the other fusion protein (Venus-C/EBP), Venus (YFP) was amplified from its original plasmid Venus/pCS2 (obtained from Dr. Roger Tsien). The amplicon with *Nhe*I and *Hind*III linkers was inserted into the *Xho*I/*Hind*III site of the EYFPC1r-C/EBPalpha244 plasmid by replacing the EYFP with Venus at the N-terminus of C/EBP forming a Venus-C/EBP fusion construct. For an image of GHFT1 cells expressing hRLUC-C/EBPα + Venus-C/EBPα, *see* **Fig. 1.1p–t**.

10. After germination in calli induction medium, the young seedlings grow with two normal cotyledons (= embryonic "leaves"), a short hypocotyl (= embryonic stem), and tiny roots. Calli and single cells could be easily detected with the microscope. For subculturing, material that floats in the flask (enriched single cells and small calli) was transferred to fresh liquid medium. The green color of newly induced suspension lines turns to light brown after several subculture passages. To isolate single *Arabidopsis* suspension cells, the cell culture solution can be passed through a sterilized Nylon mesh filter.
11. Cells were grown in two different types of 35-mm dishes. We used normal 35 mm dishes (Nunclon^{R}, InterMed) for cell viability and spectral assays. We used 35-mm dishes with cover-glass bottoms (MatTek Corporation) for BRET imaging.
12. Longer incubation times may decrease the activity of lipofectamine.
13. The 20 min incubation is to allow DNA-lipofectamine 2000 complexes to form; this complex is stable for 6 h at room temperature.
14. After adding coelenterazine to the assay buffer, start measurements immediately. Our measurements were manually controlled for exposure duration and frequency.
15. For autoluminescence in phenol-red free DMEM only: we added substrate to 100 μl medium ± serum to a final concentration of 10 μM. The total luminescence was measured using the FB12 luminometer. In our tests, we found that ViviRen^{TM} has less autoluminescence than native coelenterazine in serum-containing medium for the first 15–20 min, but that its autoluminescence level steadily increases so that after 20 min, it has more autoluminescence than native coelenterazine (*see* **Fig. 1.3a**). In serum-free medium, native coelenterazine has a brief burst of autoluminescence upon addition but thereafter both native and ViviRen^{TM} coelenterazine have low autoluminescence. The autoluminescence of native and ViviRen^{TM} coelenterazines in the simple salt medium (1/2 MS) was comparable to that of serum-free DMEM (*see* **Fig. 1.3a**). For brightness tests, we used HEK293 cells transfected with P_{CMV}::hRluc-Venus and tobacco seedlings transfected with $P_{35\ S}$::RLUC-EYFP. HEK293 cells transfected with BRET constructs have brighter luminescence when using ViviRen^{TM} than when using native coelenterazine in serum-containing medium during the interval 5–50 min after addition (*see* **Fig. 1.3b**). Therefore, for mammalian cells in

serum-containing medium, ViviRen^{TM} has a better trade-off of brightness vs. autoluminescene than native coelenterazine (compare **Fig. 1.3a** with **3b**). On the other hand, ViviRen^{TM} does not appear to be useful for BRET in plant seedlings – native coelenterazine has very low autoluminescence in simple salt medium (1/2 MS), and the brightness signal for native coelenterazine is higher than for ViviRen^{TM} in plant seedlings, in addition to being well sustained for over 100 min (*see* **Fig. 1.3b**). For improving the stability of ViviRen^{TM} in serum-containing medium, we used PBI 1419 (obtained from Erika Hawkins at Promega) along with ViviRen^{TM}. PBI 1419 stabilizes the signal of ViviRen^{TM}-dependent luminescence (*see* **Fig. 1.3c**; the structure of PBI 1419 is shown in the inset). Note that PBI 1419 is not commercially available as of this printing, but Dr. Erika Hawkins at Promega says that Promega will provide PBI 1419 to interested users (Dr. Erika Hawkins, personal communication).

16. The cells were incubated for one or 6 h with different substrates: native coelenterazine, coelenterazine-h, or ViviRen^{TM}. Coelenterazine and coelenterazine-h were dissolved in ethanol and ViviRen^{TM} was dissolved in DMSO. Final concentrations were 5 μM for coelenterazine and coelenterazine-h and 10 μM for ViviRen^{TM}. After the incubation, the cells were harvested and 0.1 ml 0.4% (w/v) Trypan Blue was added to 0.1 ml of the cell suspension from each sample. The stained and unstained cells were counted using a hemacytometer. Viable cells exclude the Trypan Blue dye. Therefore, blue-stained cells were scored as nonviable and unstained cells were scored as viable. Therefore, "Percent Viability" = number of viable cells ÷ total number of cells. The viability of cells was not significantly affected by treatment for 1–6 h with either native coelenterazine or ViviRen^{TM} as compared with the solvent controls (*see* **Fig. 1.3d**)
17. For focusing the samples in the "box setup," a scissors-jack was used to support the sample under the non-infinity-corrected objective (e.g., Plan 4×, NA=0.13 DL, 160/–; or Plan 10×, NA=0.30 DL, 160/0.17; Nikon) that was attached to the Dual-View^{TM} and EB-CCD. Therefore this scissors-jack provided a moveable stage which was moved up and down to focus the sample. The sample was placed on the jack on top of a white paper background.
18. The Dual-View^{TM} micro-imager needs to be precisely aligned before use. To set up "Full View" (Bypass Mode), pull the filter holder half-way out of the Dual-View^{TM} tube to image normal brightfield.

19. Float the plant seedling on a drop of assay buffer and do a preliminary focusing. Then, aspirate the extra buffer while keeping the seedling surrounded by a thin film of buffer. Fine-focus and acquire the BRET image in darkness. Bright-field (and fluorescence) images can be acquired after the BRET image is taken. Plant seedling images can be acquired in the "box setup" to capture the entire seedling's image (as in **Fig. 1.4**) or by using the inverted microscope setup with the Macro XLFLuor 2× objective (NA 0.14, working distance of 16.3 mm).
20. For mammalian cells, 20 sequential 100-ms exposures were acquired and then placed into a "stack" in ImageJ (version WCIF). These stacks were integrated to improve signal:noise by choosing the median value for each pixel over the sequence of 20 exposures and generating an integrated image that was used for subsequent analyses.
21. When RLUC-EYFP is expressed in *E. coli* and mammalian cells, the emission peaks at 480 nm vs. 530 nm are approximately equal (as in **Fig. 1.2c**), while the BRET ratio of RLUC-EYFP expressed in green plant tissue was usually greater than 1.0 (as in **Fig. 1.5b**). When we measured the emission spectrum of RLUC-EYFP in etiolated tobacco seedlings, we indeed found the emission spectrum was closer to 1:1 for 480 nm: 530 nm (*see* **Fig. 1.5b, c**). This is probably due to the greater absorption of plant pigments at 480 nm than that at 530 nm in green tissue, which can be visualized by the normalization of luminescence spectra to 530 nm and by absorption spectra of extracted plant tissue (*see* **Fig. 1.5a**). The correction factor can be used to correct the image for the differential absorption (compare **Fig. 1.4d** with **4e** and **1.4i** with **4j**).
22. We determined the average ratio over the entire sample along with standard deviation calculation between samples to demonstrate the reproducibility of replicate samples. In the case of RLUC being directly fused to EYFP, the expected BRET ratio is quantifiable (e.g., for RLUC-EYFP, the 530:480 ratio should be ~1:1). In situations where RLUC and EYFP are fused to interacting proteins (e.g., RLUC-COP1, YFP-COP1 or C/EBP fusions) and are expressed from independent promoters, it is better to show the averaged BRET ratio (or ratio in a given region). When using the same promoter to drive the expression of both constructs, the estimated relative amount of RLUC and EYFP fusion proteins varied by less than 10% in our plant and mammalian cell studies.

23. Several programs or software can be used to analyze BRET images. We prefer to use the open architecture "ImageJ" program. There are also other commercially available programs that work well, such as "Image Pro Plus" or "Autoquant."

Acknowledgments

We thank Dr. R.N. Day for mouse GHFT1 cells and C/EBP244 fused to EYFP, Dr. Roger Tsien for Venus YFP, Stein Servick for technical assistance, Drs. Yao Xu, Michael Geusz, David Piston & Shin Yamazaki for advice concerning BRET techniques, imaging techniques, and image analysis, and Drs. Keith Wood & Erika Hawkins of Promega for making ViviRenTM and PBI 1419 available to us prior to its commercial release. This work was supported by NSF grant MCB-0114653 to Drs. Albrecht von Arnim and Carl Johnson as part of the *Arabidopsis* 2010 project, and the following grants to Dr. Carl Johnson: NSF SGER grant # IOS-0854942, National Institutes of General Medical Science R01 GM065467, and National Institute of Mental Health R21 MH 080035.

References

1. Mendelsohn, A. R. and Brent, G. (1999) Protein biochemistry: protein interaction methods-toward an endgame. *Science* **284**, 1948–50.
2. Periasamy, A. and Day, R. N. (2005) Molecular imaging: FRET microscopy and spectroscopy. Oxford University Press, New York, NY, p. 321.
3. Hoshino, H., Nakajima, Y., and Ohmiya, Y. (2007) Luciferase-YFP fusion tag with enhanced emission for single-cell luminescence imaging. *Nat. Methods* **4**, 637–9.
4. Xu, Y., Piston, D. W., and Johnson, C. H. (1999) A bioluminescence resonance energy transfer (BRET) system: application to interacting circadian clock proteins. *Proc. Natl. Acad. Sci. USA* **96**, 151–6.
5. Pfleger, K. D. G. and Eidne, K. A. (2006) Illuminating insights into protein–protein interactions using bioluminescence resonance energy transfer (BRET). *Nat. Methods* **3**, 165–74.
6. Subramanian, C., Kim, B. H., Lyssenko, N. N., Xu, X. D., Johnson, C. H., and von Arnim, A. G. (2004) The Arabidopsis repressor of light signaling, COP1, is regulated by nuclear exclusion: mutational analysis by bioluminescence resonance energy transfer. *Proc. Natl. Acad. Sci. USA* **101**, 6798–802.
7. Gales, C., Rebois, R. V., Hogue, M., Trieu, P., Breit, A., Hebert, T. E., and Bouvier, M. (2005) Real-time monitoring of receptor and G-protein interactions in living cells. *Nat. Methods* **2**, 177–84.
8. James, J. R., Oliveira, M. I., Carmo, A. M., Iaboni, A., and Davis, S. J. (2006) A rigorous experimental framework for detecting protein oligomerization using bioluminescence resonance energy transfer. *Nat. Methods* **3**, 1001–6.
9. Subramanian, C., Woo, J., Cai, X., Xu, X. D., Servick, S., Johnson, C. H., Nebenfuhr, A., and von Arnim, A. G. (2006) A suite of tools and application notes for in vivo protein interaction assays using bioluminescence resonance energy transfer (BRET). *Plant J.* **48**, 138–52.
10. De, A. and Gambhir, S. S. (2005) Noninvasive imaging of protein–protein interactions from live cells and living subjects using

bioluminescence resonance energy transfer. *FASEB J.* **19**, 2017–9.

11. Pfleger, K. D., Seeber, R. M., and Eidne, K. A. (2006) bioluminescence resonance energy transfer (BRET) for the real-time detection of protein–protein interactions. *Nat. Protoc.* **1**, 337–45.
12. James, J. R., Oliveira, M. I., Carmo, A. M., Iaboni, A., and Davis, S. J. (2006) A rigorous experimental framework for detecting protein oligomerization using bioluminescence resonance energy transfer. *Nat. Methods* **3**, 1001–6.
13. Carriba, P., Navarro, G., Ciruela, F., Ferre, S., Casado, V., Agnati, L., Cortes, A., Mallol, J., Fuxe, K., Canela, E. I., Lluis, C., and Franco, R. (2008) Detection of heteromerization of more than two proteins by sequential BRET-FRET. *Nat. Methods* **5**, 727–33.
14. De, A., Loening, A. M., and Gambhir, S. S. (2007) An improved bioluminescence resonance energy transfer strategy for imaging intracellular events in single cells and living subjects. *Cancer Res.* **67**, 7175–83.
15. Dixit, R., Cyr, R., and Gilroy, S. (2006) Using intrinsically fluorescent proteins for plant cell imaging. *Plant J.* **45**, 599–615.
16. Xu, X. D., Soutto, M., Xie, Q. G., Servick, S., Subramanian, C., von Arnim, A., and Johnson, C. H. (2007) Imaging protein interactions with BRET in plant and mammalian cells and tissues. *Proc. Natl. Acad. Sci. USA* **104**, 10264–9.
17. Pfleger, K. D., Dromey, J. R., Dalrymple, M. B., Lim, E. M., Thomas, W. G., and Eidne, K. A. (2006) Extended bioluminescence resonance energy transfer (eBRET) for monitoring prolonged protein–protein interactions in live cells. *Cell Signal.* **18**, 1664–70.
18. Loening, A. M., Fenn, T. D., Wu, A. M., and Gambhir, S. S. (2006) Consensus guided mutagenesis of Renilla luciferase yields enhanced stability and light output. *Protein Eng. Des. Sel.* **19**, 391–400.
19. Loening, A. M., Wu, A. M., and Gambhir, S. S. (2007) Red-shifted Renilla reniformis luciferase variants for imaging in living subjects. *Nat. Methods* **4**, 641–3.
20. Loening, A. M., Fenn, T. D., and Gambhir, S. S. (2007) Crystal structures of the luciferase and green fluorescent protein from Renilla reniformis. *J. Mol. Biol.* **374**, 1017–28.
21. Xu, Y., Piston, D., and Johnson, C. H. (2002) BRET assays for protein–protein interactions in living cells. In Green fluorescent protein: applications and protocols (methods in molecular biology series). Humana Press, Totowa, NJ, pp. 121–33.
22. Angers, S., Salahpour, A., Joly, E., Hilairet, S., Chelsky, D., Dennis, M., and Bouvier, M. (2000) Detection of beta 2-adrenergic receptor dimerization in living cells using bioluminescence resonance energy transfer (BRET). *Proc. Natl. Acad. Sci. USA* **97**, 3684–9.
23. Soutto, M., Xu, Y., and Johnson, C. H. (2005) Bioluminescence RET (BRET): techniques and potential. In Molecular imaging: FRET microscopy and spectroscopy. Oxford University Press, New York, NY, pp. 260–71.
24. Mathur, J. and Koncz, C. (1998) Establishment and maintenance of cell suspension cultures. In Arabidopsis protocols. Humana Press, Totowa, NJ, pp. 27–30.
25. Siegel, R. M., Chan, F. K.-M., Zacharias, D. A., Swofford, R., Holmes, K. L., Tsien, R. Y., and Lenardo, M. J. (2000) Measurement of molecular interactions in living cells by fluorescence resonance energy transfer between variants of the green fluorescent protein. *Sci. STKE* **2000**, PL1.

Chapter 2

Luciferase Protein Complementation Assays for Bioluminescence Imaging of Cells and Mice

Gary D. Luker and Kathryn E. Luker

Abstract

Protein fragment complementation assays (PCAs) with luciferase reporters currently are the preferred method for detecting and quantifying protein–protein interactions in living animals. At the most basic level, PCAs involve fusion of two proteins of interest to enzymatically inactive fragments of luciferase. Upon association of the proteins of interest, the luciferase fragments are capable of reconstituting enzymatic activity to generate luminescence in vivo. In addition to bi-molecular luciferase PCAs, unimolecular biosensors for hormones, kinases, and proteases also have been developed using target peptides inserted between inactive luciferase fragments. Luciferase PCAs offer unprecedented opportunities to quantify dynamics of protein–protein interactions in intact cells and living animals, but successful use of luciferase PCAs in cells and mice involves careful consideration of many technical factors. This chapter discusses the design of luciferase PCAs appropriate for animal imaging, including construction of reporters, incorporation of reporters into cells and mice, imaging techniques, and data analysis.

Key words: Molecular imaging, optical imaging, split luciferase, bioluminescence, protein complementation assay, PCA.

1. Introduction

Bioluminescence imaging of intact animals is a powerful technology for detecting and quantifying the spatial and temporal occurrence of cellular and molecular events using luminescent enzyme reporters. Traditionally, luciferase enzymes have been used as reporters of promoter activity and, in the case of firefly luciferase, as an assay for ATP. In contrast to these methods, luciferase protein complementation assays (PCAs) were developed to measure post-translational events such as protein interactions,

K. Shah (ed.), *Molecular Imaging*, Methods in Molecular Biology 680,
DOI 10.1007/978-1-60761-901-7_2, © Springer Science+Business Media, LLC 2011

phosphorylation, and enzymatic cleavage of substrates. Luciferase PCAs have been developed for three major luciferases from firefly (1, 2), sea pansy (*Renilla reniformis*) (3, 4), and the copepod *Gaussia* (*Gaussia princeps*) (5). Several firefly and *Renilla* luciferase PCAs have been published for use in animals. Although in vivo *Gaussia* luciferase PCAs have been published only for live cells, this technology should be easily translatable to animal work. This chapter details the steps in developing an in vivo assay based on luciferase protein complementation, including reporter vector design, introduction of reporters into cells and animals, and bioluminescence imaging of the luciferase PCA in live cells and mice, with an emphasis on firefly luciferase.

2. Materials

2.1. Molecular Biology Reagents

1. Plasmids with open reading frames coding for proteins of interest and luciferases
2. Expression vectors suitable for PCA expression
3. Molecular biology reagents and equipment for PCR, restriction digests, and ligations.

2.2. Cells Culture Reagents

1. HEK-293 or other cell line with high transfection efficiency
2. Tumor cell line or other biologically relevant cell lines of interest
3. General cell culture reagents and plasticware.

2.3. Reagents for Cell Imaging

1. 96-well plates, black plate, clear bottom with lid, tissue culture treated (Costar #3603)
2. Multichannel pipettes suitable for delivering 1–10 and 20–200 μl
3. Low adherence sterile pipette tips (Maxymum Recovery from Axygen, or similar)
4. Sterile commercial 1 × phosphate buffered saline (PBS) solution
5. Luciferin solution 15 mg/ml in PBS (sterile filtered, store at –20°C) (firefly luciferase substrate)
6. Coelenterazine 1 mg/ml stock in acidified MeOH (0.5% HCL (v/v)), store at –20°C (substrate for *Renilla* and *Gaussia* luciferases)
7. IVIS-200 or IVIS-100 (Caliper) or similar bioluminescence imaging system with software for region of interest analysis.

2.4. Animal Imaging Materials

In addition to the items listed above in **Section 2.3**, the following items are required or suggested for animal imaging.

1. Mice for construction of animal models (nude or SCID for xenografts)
2. Coelenterazine, 10 mg/ml stock in acidified MeOH (0.5% HCL (v/v)), store at –20°C, dilute to desired concentration immediately before imaging in 40% DMSO/PBS for animal imaging (needed only for *Renilla* and *Gaussia* luciferases)
3. Small animal shaver (Wahl compact cordless trimmer recommended) (optional)
4. Depiliatory lotion such as Nair or Neet (optional).

3. Methods

3.1. Constructing a Luciferase PCA

1. Select a suitable target for the luciferase PCA. *See* **Note 1** for suggestions regarding PCA target selection.
2. Plan relevant orientation of fusion constructs. It is best to test all reasonable orientations of the fusions, keeping in mind the cellular location of the fusion. *See* **Note 2** for examples of bimolecular protein interaction assays and *see* **Note 3** for unimolecular luciferase PCAs.
3. Select an appropriate luciferase for your assay. Several properties of firefly *Renilla*, and *Gaussia* luciferases should be considered in choosing a luciferase enzyme for the PCA (*see* **Table 2.1** and **Note 4**).
4. Design a linker to insert between protein folding domains. Linkers may be used to control the spacing and freedom of motion for the enzyme fragments relative to the proteins of interests. *See* **Note 5** on linker design.
5. Design control constructs. Control constructs that are identical to experimental constructs with the exception of the control feature, such as mutation of a phosphorylation or cleavage site, or substitution of a non-interacting protein should be prepared.
6. Choose a vector to express the constructs. Fusion constructs should be inserted in a mammalian expression vector consistent with the selection method for producing stable cell lines. For pairs of vectors, orthogonal selection methods will be required. *See* **Note 7** for additional information related to generating stable cell lines.
7. Verify constructs. Engineered open reading frames should be fully sequenced. To efficiently choose clones to sequence,

Table 2.1
Properties of intact luciferases

Luciferase	Amino acids	Cofactors	λ max (nm) (in solution)	λ range (nm)	Relative intensity (intracellular)[a]	Relative intensity (mouse tissue)[a]
Firefly	550	ATP, Mg^+, O_2	578 at 37°C[b]	520–740 at 37°C[b]	1	1
Renilla	311	O_2	475[a]	420–580[a]	1	ND[c]
Gaussia	185 (secreted form)	O_2	480[a]	440–590[a]	Approx 100	2

Sources: [a]Tannous et al. (15).
[b]Zhao et al. (23).
[c]Reference (1) includes data for secreted *Gaussia* luciferase in mice compared with *Renilla* luciferase, but this data is not applicable to intracellular *Gaussia* complementation assays.

it is sometimes helpful to test plasmid minipreps in transient transfections (*see* **Section 2.1**) to identify clones that produce luminescence signals.

3.2. Introduction of PCA Constructs into Cells

1. Test reporters in transient transfections. Seed HEK-293 cells in 6-well plates at 150,000 per well. Transfect cells the next day with 1 μg plasmid DNA for each PCA or control construct (0.5 μg, each for pairs of constructs). On the day after transfection, split cells into black 96-well plates (1×10^5 cells/well) to be used the next day for imaging. *See* **Section 3.3** for cell imaging. Prepare parallel sets of transfected cells for western blotting or other relevant biochemical assays. These assays are important assure that the bioluminescence output reflects relevant biochemical events. *See* **Note 6** for suggested controls for cell assays.
2. Produce stable reporter cell lines. In a relevant tumor cell line, prepare a batch of stable transfectants using standard methods and isolate clonal sublines expressing the PCA reporters. *See* **Note 7** for suggested strategies.
3. Test clonal lines. Test tumor cell PCA sublines in culture to identify a small number of lines that exhibit a good signal-to-background ratio and produce relatively bright bioluminescence in the PCA. *See* **Section 3.3** for cell imaging.

3.3. Bioluminescence Imaging of Cells

1. Seed cells in black-walled, clear bottom 96-well tissue culture plates at a density of 10,000–20,000 cells per well. Permit cells to adhere overnight.

2. Remove media next day and treat as needed in a minimum volume of fresh media (e.g., 50 μl). To construct a time course of drug treatments, it may be helpful to replace the media then add treatments at 10× to the cells on a single plate in reverse time order. The plate may then be imaged at the completion of the course.
3. For imaging firefly luciferase, add luciferin (for firefly luciferase) to the medium in 1/10 volume at a final concentration of 0.15 mg/ml using a multichannel pipette and low adherence tips. A low volume multichannel reservoir is helpful for reducing luciferin waste. Tip the plate and insert the pipette tip under the fluid level before expelling the luciferin to assure full delivery of the substrate. Rock the plate in a figure-8 motion.
4. For *Gaussia* or *Renilla* luciferase imaging in cells, albumin in media will cause considerable background luminescence with coelenterazine. To eliminate albumin background with native coelenterazine, short-term treatments may be performed in media lacking albumin, or media may be removed and cells washed with PBS prior to imaging. Add coelenterazine (1:1,000 of 1 mg/ml MeOH stock) in 50 μl PBS per well.
5. After addition of luciferase substrate, take a brief test image of 1–10 s on the IVIS. Use this image to estimate the exposure and binning needed for subsequent images. Typical settings for luciferase complementation imaging would be 0.5- to 1-min exposure at maximum binning. Take subsequent images with the appropriate exposure and binning in serial mode to assure capture of the peak luminescence signal. For firefly luciferase, peak light production from intact cells occurs approximately 5–10 min after substrate addition. Peak bioluminescence from *Gaussia* or *Renilla* luciferases occurs rapidly within the first minute after adding coelenterazine. *See* **Section 3.6** for data analysis.

3.4. Construction of Mouse Tumor Model

Tumor cells ($\approx 1 \times 10^6$) stably expressing the PCA reporter or control reporter are injected in contralateral flanks of the mouse. Tumor cells may be injected subcutaneously or orthotopically, such as in the mammary fat pad. After palpable tumors form, mice should be imaged as below. For alternative approaches to construction of mouse models, *see* **Note 8**.

3.5. Mouse Imaging

For firefly luciferase imaging, mice should be injected intraperitoneally with luciferin (15 mg/ml stock in PBS, 150 μg/g mouse) 10 min before imaging is to begin. Mice are placed in the isoflurane induction chamber 5 min before imaging, then transferred to the IVIS imaging chamber after they are fully anesthetized. Imaging is performed essentially as for cells (**Section 3.3**). For *Renilla* or *Gaussia* luciferase PCAs, we recommend injection of coelenterazine (2.5 mg/kg dissolved in 40% DMSO in PBS, 50 μl) by tail vein, followed by immediate imaging for 1–5 min (*see* **Note 9**).

3.6. Region of Interest Analysis

Quantify luminescence (photons/s) in a region of interest (ROI) which encompasses the area of luminescence, keeping a standard ROI for all the mice in the experiment (*see* **Note 10**).

4. Notes

1. Luciferase PCAs could be designed for almost any biochemical event that involves a change in the conformation or association of proteins. Luciferase PCAs can be designed to measure either association or dissociation of the luciferase fragments. (In contrast, only association can be measured with PCAs based on fluorescent proteins such as GFP (6), since this method traps the fragments irreversibly in the bound state.) One important consideration is the availability of agents targeting the pathway of interest, or other strategies (such as mutant forms of the proteins of interest) that will result in an "on" and an "off" state for the PCA. For investigation of new biochemical targets, it is also helpful to prepare a control PCA with related, well-studied proteins that can be used to help validate the PCA for the new target. PCAs may be more easily designed for proteins that have been demonstrated to permit fusions, such as GFP fusions, without significant perturbation of function.

   One very useful application of the luciferase PCA is to adapt a FRET or BRET assay for bioluminescence imaging in mice. The user should note that luciferase PCAs differ from FRET and BRET in that PCAs depend on direct contact of the luciferase fragments to reconstitute enzymatic activity. FRET and BRET, in contrast, generate signals based on proximity of fusion proteins. Consequently, some adjustment of the design of the fusion constructs, such as length of linkers, may be required to convert a FRET or BRET assay to a luciferase PCA.

   Our experience with luciferase PCAs indicates that they perform optimally at moderate expression levels, such as those typically achieved in stable cell lines. PCAs necessarily require expression of non-native proteins and should be designed to minimize any impact of the reporter on cell function. Gross over-expression of PCA constructs could, in principle, induce artificially high protein–protein association or enzyme-substrate interactions, for example. As with any fusion protein or transgene, the user should validate by methods other than bioluminescence that the luciferase PCA constructs perform as intended.

2. Two separate open reading frames are used to express the two fusion proteins in a bimolecular PCA. These may be incorporated into two vectors (which facilitates a mix-and-match strategy for co-transfections with other PCA reporters) or in a single plasmid construct (to more closely link expression of the two reporters). **Figure 2.1** illustrates features of bimolecular luciferase reporters. Both rational design and empiric experience govern the construction of luciferase PCA constructs. In many cases, a review of the literature will reveal previous fusions, such as those to fluorescent proteins, which provide valuable insight into the impact of fusions on protein localization and function. Sites

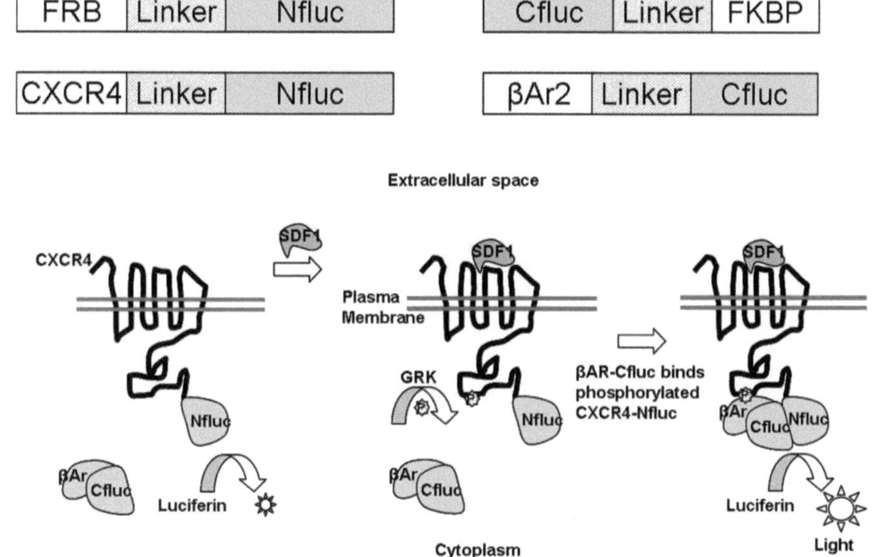

Fig. 2.1. Bimolecular constructs for luciferase PCAs. The *upper pair* of constructs shows two interacting cytoplasmic proteins (FRB domain from the mammalian target of rapaymycin (mTOR) and FK506 binding protein (FKBP)), which associate upon binding of the compound rapamycin. This association brings Nfluc and Cfluc into close proximity, reconstituting firefly luciferase activity. In this case, the linkers are 16 amino acids long and contain the motif GGGSSSGGG with restriction sites (2). The *lower pair* of constructs shows the 7-transmembrane receptor CXCR4 fused as above to Nfluc, while its cytoplasmic binding partner, β-arrestin 2, is fused to Cfluc with a similar linker consisting of 14 amino acids (20). Note that the optimal construct orientation for this PCA was with the interacting protein at the N-terminus of Cfluc (20). The schematic diagram illustrates the concept of bimolecular luciferase complementation for CXCR4-Nfluc and β-arrestin 2-Cfluc. CXCR4-Nfluc binds the chemokine SDF-1, resulting in phosphorylation of the intracellular C-terminal domain of CXCR4 by a G-protein receptor kinase (GRK) and subsequent recruitment of β-arrestin2-Cfluc to reconstitute luciferase activity.

of post-translational modification and important interactions with other binding partners should also be considered. Finally, it is advisable to attempt more than one orientation for fusions identify an optimal design.

3. Luciferase PCAs constructed as a single open reading frame have been used to image of several kinds of biochemical events, including ligand binding, phosphorylation, and proteolytic cleavage events (**Fig. 2.2**). *See* **Note 2** for additional advice regarding general construction of PCAs.

4. We generally prefer firefly luciferase PCA for intracellular protein interactions and biosensors because for reasons related to mouse imaging in particular. The more red-shifted light of firefly luciferase (**Table 2.1**) penetrates mouse tissues better, improving signal detection, and

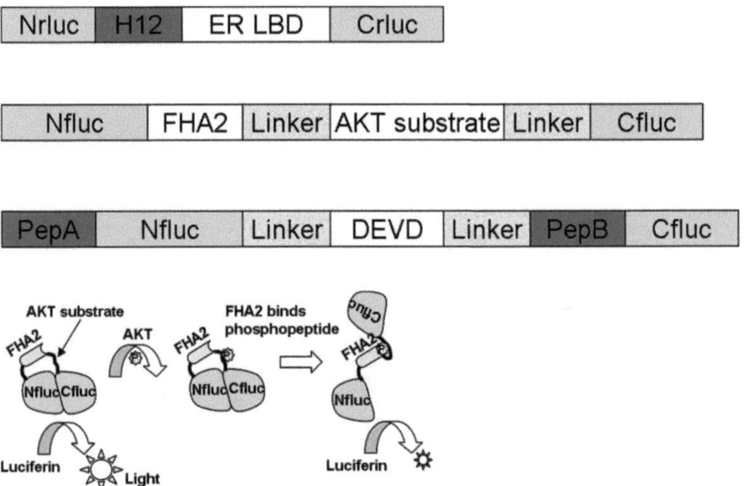

Fig. 2.2. Unimolecular constructs for luciferase PCAs. The *upper* construct contains a single protein fragment for the human estrogen receptor with amino acids 281–549 encompassing helix 12 (H12) and the ligand binding domain (LBD) of the receptor, flanked by inactive fragments of *Renilla* luciferase (Nrluc and Crluc) (3). This sensor for estrogen agonists and antagonists produces strong luminescence activity upon ligand-induced interaction of H12 with the LBD. The *middle* construct contains two interacting protein/peptide regions, an FHA2 phosphopeptide binding domain, and an AKT substrate peptide, separated by short linkers and flanked by inactive fragments of firefly luciferase. This sensor for active (21) produces luminescence upon AKT phosphorylation of the substrate peptide, which binds to the FHA2 region of the protein and disrupts complementation of the luciferase fragments. (*See* diagram.) The *third* construct codes for a single protein which is cleaved to form a bimolecular product. The construct includes three functional regions: PepA and PepB are proteins with a strong constitutive interaction which is disrupted in the intact fusion protein, and DEVD is a substrate for Caspase-3, an enzyme which is activated early in apoptosis. This apoptosis sensor produces increased luminescence upon cleavage of the DEVD peptide by Caspase-3 and subsequent complementation of the luciferase fragments driven by association of PepA and PepB (22).

bioluminescence from this luciferase is more stable over the course of imaging. Luciferin, the substrate for firefly luciferase, has more favorable biodistribution than coelenterazine. In addition, i.p. injection of luciferin is much more reproducible for many investigators than tail vein or intracardiac injection required for coelenterazine.

Nevertheless, there are several applications that might benefit from other bioluminescent PCAs. For example, in situations where the firefly luciferase cofactors Mg^+ and ATP may be limiting, *Renilla* or *Gaussia* luciferase may be used successfully, although as yet no specific examples of this exist in the literature. Steric bulk can also be reduced by employing *Renilla* and especially *Gaussia* PCAs due to their smaller sizes. Finally, it should be noted that luciferase PCAs are not the only bioluminescent imaging approach to PCAs. β-galactosidase PCAs have been adapted for bioluminescence imaging by using intact firefly luciferase as a secondary reporter for β-galactosidase activity (7, 8).

Several different strategies have emerged for bisecting various luciferase enzymes. For firefly luciferase, we used a library screening approach to identify fragments of NLuc 2–416 and CLuc 398–550 as the best overall combination of low background and high signal, and we continue to find that this pair is optimal for our assays (2). Recently, Paulmurugan et al. reported alternative firefly luciferase PCA fragments NLuc 2–398 and CLuc 394–550 that may provide higher signal-to-background for some protein interactions (9). Two pairs of *Renilla* luciferase enzyme fragments have been recommended for their performance in PCAs: 1–229 and 230–311 (10), and 1–110 and 111–311 (4). A single recommended *Gaussia* PCA pair has been reported (5), consisting of NGluc 1–93, CGluc 94–169. (Because native *Gaussia* luciferase contains a 16 amino acid secretion signal that was removed for the study, the first three amino acids of the Ngluc are MKP, the final three are GIG.) Performance of PCAs is heavily impacted by many factors, so the user should consider testing different pairs of luciferase fragments to optimize signal-to-background for a particular application.

5. Linkers serve to provide points for restriction site in the DNA construct and to control distance and flexibility between protein domains in the reporter. Flexible linkers (such as GGGSSGGG flanked by restriction sites necessary for cloning) may be helpful in reducing the interference between separate folding domains. For more constraint, a short tri-glycine linker, or no linker at all, may produce good results. The user should consider hydrophilicity of

amino acids, steric bulk, and tendency for secondary structure formation in selecting a linker sequence.

6. To distinguish a true PCA signal from effects that impact luciferase enzyme function, the PCA conditions may be tested on full length luciferase in parallel with the PCA. PCA reporter function then can be normalized to function of the intact enzyme to eliminate general effects on enzyme function. In 96-well plate assays, it may also be necessary to include a transfection control, such as β-galactosidase, or to normalize to total protein in a well by an assay such as sulforhodamine B (11), crystal violet, or BCA (Pierce).

7. Our own experience is that lentiviral constructs tagged with fluorescent proteins can be used to rapidly and efficiently obtain batch transductants, from which clonal sublines can be generated if needed for optimal performance. Transductions can be performed with two viral vectors simultaneously to generate stable reporter cell lines more rapidly. Lentiviruses significantly reduce the time required for obtaining stable lines compared with traditional plasmid strategies.

   Use of a selectable marker, linked to the reporter through an IRES, can help assure retention of the reporter in cell culture, as well as provide a means to select for cells expressing the reporter at higher levels. Bimolecular reporters may be introduced with tri-cistronic expression vectors (the third position being occupied by a selection marker), although this strategy commonly results in attenuated expression of mRNA molecules further removed from the promoter. Available drug selection markers include neomycin, hygromycin, blasticidin, and zeocin, among others. Of course, use of selectable markers is not possible in mice, so poorly tolerated constructs may not be retained when these constructs are incorporated into solid tumor models.

   To rapidly isolate clonal reporter lines, a batch of cells stably expressing the PCA reporter is seeded in 15-mm dishes at 100–300 cells/dish. After colonies of 50 or more cells form, a grid is drawn on the bottom of the dish with heavy black marker, and the dish is imaged in the IVIS under basal conditions or conditions that activate the PCA to identify luminescent colonies. Placing a layer of aluminum foil, nitrocellulose, or other non-bioluminescent material under the dish in the IVIS enables the grid on the dish to be seen, so that colonies are easily located. Using the grid system, locate the luminescent colony and mark it on the underside of the dish with a colored marker. Clones can be harvested from the dish using cloning rings and trypsin, or by direct "picking" of colonies. A second round of colony selection is helpful to insure stability of the clonal line.

8. For short-term testing of a luciferase PCA, the simplest mouse experiment is to conduct treatment tests within minutes or hours after implanting PCA-expressing cells. This approach depends only on the short-term survival of cells in the animal, so that non-tumorigenic cell lines and transient transfectants can be employed. For this approach we implant (i.p. or s.q.) 5–10 $\times$ 10^6 cells in PBS. To produce a more confined locus of cell deposition, cells can be injected in a 1:1 mixture of PBS (or DMEM) and matrigel. Cells bearing a relevant control PCA (non-interacting protein, uncleavable peptide, etc.) should be implanted in a parallel set of mice (for i.p.) or in the contralateral flanks of the mice (for s.q.).

   Stable cell lines expressing PCAs can be easily used to construct mouse models by implanting luciferase PCA cell lines to form tumors. Cells may be injected subcutaneously to form flank tumors, or in relevant physiologic sites, such as the mammary fat pad for breast tumor lines. In principle, PCA constructs could also be introduced to mice directly, by construction of transgenic animals or infection with viral vectors, for example, although such assays are not reported in the literature as yet.

   In calculating numbers of cells needed to obtain a detectable signal, the user should consider the depth and optical properties of the tissue through which the light will pass. As a rule of thumb, firefly luciferase light will be attenuated approximately tenfold for each centimeter of tissue, but optically dense tissues such as liver will attenuate light much more than skin, bone, or lung. Best results generally will be obtained by maximizing the number of cells and the perfusion of those cells in the mouse.

9. One of the strengths of luciferase imaging in mice is that a mouse can be imaged repetitively, such as before and after a defined pharmacologic intervention. This strategy allows each mouse to serve as its own control, which reduces experimental variations. To perform repetitive imaging of mice, the user should take into account that luciferase levels in mice peak approximately 10 min after i.p. injection, then decline slowly to background levels by $\approx$ 6 h post injection (12). Luciferin biodistribution for imaging firefly luciferase PCA can be stabilized for hours or days by using an osmotic pump (Alzet) (13). This method has the advantage of producing a relatively constant bioluminescence signal in mice, though i.p. injection of luciferin results in higher tissue concentrations of luciferin and increased signal.

Coelenterazine has a more rapid kinetic course in mice. Therefore, maximum imaging signal for *Renilla* or *Gaussia* luciferases is obtained immediately after injecting coelenterazine through intravenous or intracardiac routes (14–16). In our hands, coelenterazine is not soluble in PBS unless a co-solvent such as DMSO or ethanol is used, though several publications recommend only PBS as a solvent. Injection of a coelenterazine suspension in PBS is not recommended. Biodistribution of coelenterazine in some tissues, such as the intact brain, is limited by drug transport proteins, which can hinder in vivo imaging of *Renilla* or *Gaussia* PCAs in some tissues (17).

Mouse fur attenuates and scatters light, and this effect is most pronounced in black mice. This problem may be overcome by using nude mice or shaving animals over the region(s) of interest for imaging. For black mice, further hair removal with a depiliatory lotion (Nair, Neet) after shaving is helpful. Care should be taken with depiliatories to limit exposure time and abrasion as mouse skin is quite delicate.

10. Software accompanying the imaging equipment is used to perform the region of interest (ROI) analysis. **Figure 2.3** shows an example image and quantified luminescence obtained with a firefly PCA in cell culture. The photons detected by the machine are summed over the

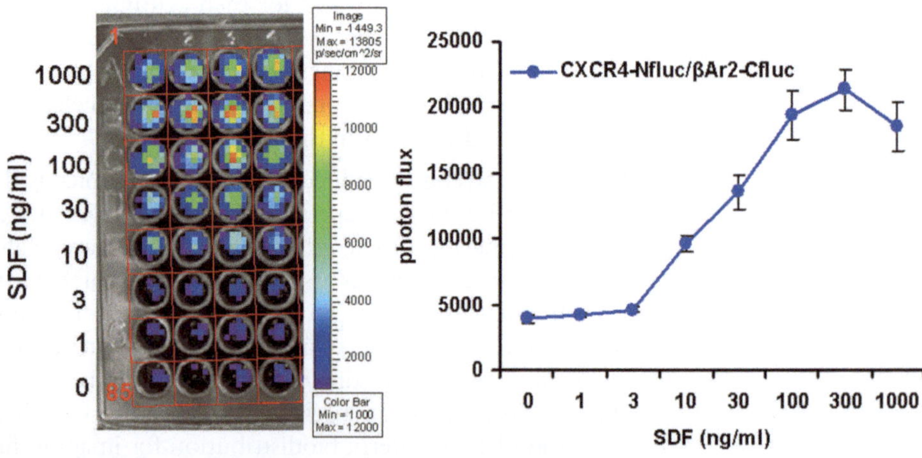

Fig. 2.3. Sample firefly luciferase PCA in cell culture. The assay was prepared as described in **Section 3.3**, using the CXCR4-Nfluc/βAr2-Cfluc pair diagramed in **Fig. 2.1**. In this image, the luminescence data appear as a pseudocolor overlay on the plate photo and is adjusted to illustrate the range of luminescence in the plate. The *red grid* marks superimposed on the image denote the regions of interest, one for each well. Total photons/s are summed over each region and averaged over the quadruplicate samples, to obtain the graphical data on the *right* of the figure. In this case, the data illustrate the association of the PCA pair upon incubation for 10 min with the chemokine SDF.

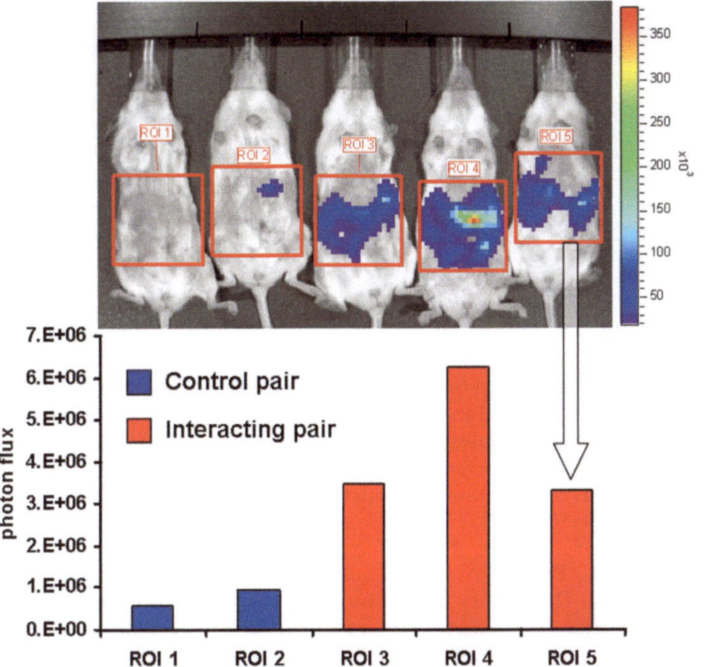

Fig. 2.4. Sample mouse imaging data. These sample data illustrate the region of interest analysis, denoted by the *identical red squares* on each mouse. Photon flux in each area is quantified in the graph below the image. These data illustrate results for a control firefly luciferase PCA, and a constitutively interacting PCA pair in transiently transfected cells (5×10^6) implanted into the peritoneal cavity of the mouse.

area of the ROI to obtain data with units of photons/time (s), or photon flux. Maintaining a standard region of interest within an experiment (or series of experiments) is important to facilitate comparison of mouse imaging data. A simple circular, oval, or square ROI is normally sufficient to be used for all the mice within a set (*see* **Fig. 2.4**). It is helpful to image a "blank" mouse injected with luciferin to obtain a background reading if background subtraction is desired. It is important to note that manipulation of the pseudocolor image display does not alter the quantitative data set for emitted photons. The user should manipulate the display range of pseudocolor image to best highlight the luminescence qualities of their sample.

To control for mouse-to-mouse variations, bioluminescence data may be normalized to one of several markers. For firefly luciferase PCAs, data may be normalized to intact *Renilla* or *Gaussia* luciferase incorporated into PCA cells. Other useful markers could include fluorescent proteins, such as mPlum or tdTomato (18–20), which can be detected using the fluorescence imaging capabilities of the IVIS and appropriate filters. (Care should be taken in fluorescence imaging to account for the red shift imposed by mouse tissue when selecting excitation and emission filters.) Fluorescence imaging is best performed prior to injection of substrates for bioluminescence imaging. Finally, for solid tumors, simple tumor volumes can suffice for normalizing luminescence signals.

References

1. Paulmurugan, R., Umezawa, Y., and Gambhir, S. (2002) Noninvasive imaging of protein–protein interactions in living subjects by using reporter protein complementation and reconstitution strategies. *Proc. Natl. Acad. Sci. USA* **99**, 15608–13.
2. Luker, K., Smith, M., Luker, G., Gammon, S., Piwnica-Worms, H., and Piwnica-Worms, D. (2004) Kinetics of regulated protein-protein interactions revealed with firefly luciferase complementation imaging in cells and living animals. *Proc. Natl. Acad. Sci. USA* **101**, 12288–93.
3. Paulmurugan, R. and Gambhir, S. (2006) An intramolecular folding sensor for imaging estrogen receptor-ligand interactions. *Proc. Natl. Acad. Sci. USA* **103**, 15883–88.
4. Stefan, E., Aquin, S., Berger, N., et al. (2007) Quantification of dynamic protein complexes using Renilla luciferase fragment complementation applied to protein kinase A activities in vivo. *Proc. Natl. Acad. Sci. USA* **104**, 16916–21.
5. Remy, I. and Michnick, S. (2006) A highly sensitive protein–protein interaction assay based on Gaussia luciferase. *Nat. Methods* **3**, 977–9.
6. Hu, C., Chinenov, Y., and Kerppola, T. (2002) Visualization of interactions among bZIP and Rel family proteins in living cells using bimolecular fluorescence complementation. *Mol. Cell.* **9**, 789–98.
7. Wehrman, T., Kleaveland, B., Her, J., Balint, R., and Blau, H. (2002) Protein–protein interactions monitored in mammalian cells via complementation of beta -lactamase enzyme fragments. *Proc. Natl. Acad. Sci. USA* **99**, 3469–74.
8. von Degenfeld, G., Wehrman, T., Hammer, M., and Blau, H. (2007) A universal technology for monitoring G-protein-coupled receptor activation in vitro and noninvasively in live animals. *FASEB J.* **21**, 3819–26.
9. Paulmurugan, R. and Gambhir, S. (2007) Combinatorial library screening for developing an improved split-firefly luciferase fragment-assisted complementation system for studying protein-protein interactions. *Anal. Chem.* **79**, 2346–53.
10. Paulmurugan, R. and Gambhir, S. (2003) Monitoring protein-protein interactions using split synthetic renilla luciferase protein-fragment-assisted complementation. *Anal. Chem.* **75**, 1584–89.
11. Sharma, V., Crankshaw, C., and Piwnica-Worms, D. (1996) Effects of multidrug resistance (MDR1) P-glycoprotein expression levels and coordination metal on the cytotoxic potency of multidentate (N_4O_2) (ethylenediamine)bis[propyl (R-benzylimino)]metal(III) cations. *J. Med. Chem.* **39**, 3483–90.
12. Paroo, Z., Bollinger, R., Braasch, D., et al. (2004) Validating bioluminescence imaging as a high-throughput, quantitative modality for assessing tumor burden. *Mol. Imaging* **3**, 117–24.
13. Gross, S., Abraham, U., Prior, J., Herzog, E., and Piwnica-Worms, D. (2007) Continuous delivery of D-luciferin by implanted micro-osmotic pumps enables true real-time bioluminescence imaging of luciferase activity in vivo. *Mol. Imaging* **6**, 121–30.
14. Bhaumik, S. and Gambhir, S. (2002) Optical imaging of Renilla luciferase reporter gene expression in living mice. *Proc. Natl. Acad. Sci. USA* **99**, 377–82.
15. Tannous, B., Kim, D., Fernandez, J., Weissleder, R., and Breakefield, X. (2005) Codon-optimized Gaussia luciferase cDNA for mammalian gene expression in culture and in vivo. *Mol. Ther.* **11**, 435–43.
16. Venisnik, K., Olafsen, T., Gambhir, S., and Wu, A. (2007) Fusion of Gaussia luciferase to an engineered anti-carcinoembryonic antigen (CEA) antibody for in vivo optical imaging. *Mol. Imaging Biol.* **9**, 267–77.
17. Pichler, A., Prior, J., and Piwnica-Worms, D. (2004) Imaging reversal of multidrug

resistance in living mice with bioluminescence: MDR1 P-glycoprotein transports coelenterazine. *Proc. Natl. Acad. Sci. USA* **101**, 1702–7.

18. Wang, L., Jackson, W., Steinbach, P., and Tsien, R. (2004) Evolution of new nonantibody proteins via iterative somatic hypermutation. *Proc. Natl. Acad. Sci. USA* **101**, 16745–9.
19. Winnard, P. J., Kluth, J., and Raman, V. (2006) Noninvasive optical tracking of red fluorescent protein-expressing cancer cells in a model of metastatic breast cancer. *Neoplasia* **8**, 796–806.
20. Luker, K. E., Gupta, M., and Luker, G. D. (2008) Imaging CXCR4 signaling with firefly luciferase complementation. *Anal Chem.* **80**, 5565–73.
21. Zhang, L., Lee, K., Bhojani, M., et al. (2007) Molecular imaging of Akt kinase activity. *Nat. Med.* **13**, 1114–9.
22. Coppola, J., Ross, B., and Rehemtulla, A. (2008) Noninvasive imaging of apoptosis and its application in cancer therapeutics. *Clin. Cancer Res.* **14**, 2492–501.
23. Zhao, H., Doyle, T., Coquoz, O., Kalish, F., Rice, B., and Contag, C. (2005) Emission spectra of bioluminescent reporters and interaction with mammalian tissue determine the sensitivity of detection in vivo. *J. Biomed. Opt.* **10**, 41210.

Chapter 3

Hybrid Raman-Fluorescence Microscopy on Single Cells Using Quantum Dots

Henk-Jan van Manen and Cees Otto

Abstract

Raman spectral imaging is a label-free, noninvasive optical technique to visualize the spatial distribution of biomolecules such as DNA, RNA, proteins, and lipids in cells and tissues. Although Raman imaging has been successfully used in the last 5 years on single cells, an important drawback of this technique is that it is traditionally regarded as incompatible with fluorescence microscopy. This is because fluorescence signals from fluorophore-labeled cells usually overwhelm the orders of magnitude weaker Raman signals from cellular biomolecules. However, we have recently shown that both nonresonance and resonance Raman microscopy can be combined with fluorescence microscopy on the same cells by spectrally separating fluorescence emission from Raman scattering. The fluorophores that are used in this case are semiconductor quantum dots (QDs), which have suitable properties in hybrid Raman-fluorescence experiments, in particular a large separation between absorption and emission wavelengths. We envisage that the combination of fluorescence microscopy with Raman spectroscopy or imaging on cells will lead to new application in cell biology. Here, we will describe detailed protocols for performing hybrid Raman-fluorescence experiments on single QD-labeled cells.

Key words: Quantum dots, Raman microscopy, resonance Raman, two-photon fluorescence microscopy, flavocytochrome b_{558}, neutrophils, macrophages.

1. Introduction

The use of label-free vibrational spectroscopies such as infrared and Raman spectroscopy in cell and tissue biology has increased in recent years because vibrational spectra provide detailed information about the biochemical composition of small intracellular volumes or tissues. Examples of single-cell Raman spectroscopy studies include the visualization of DNA/RNA, proteins, and lipid droplets in apoptotic HeLa cells (1) or phagocytosing neutrophils

K. Shah (ed.), *Molecular Imaging*, Methods in Molecular Biology 680,
DOI 10.1007/978-1-60761-901-7_3, © Springer Science+Business Media, LLC 2011

(2), the differentiation of embryonic murine stem cells (3), the study of stress-induced changes in lung fibroblasts (4), and the identification of individual leukemia cells (5). In our group, we have also employed resonant Raman spectroscopy and imaging to selectively visualize changes in the activation and distribution of flavocytochrome b_{558} in single neutrophils (reviewed in (6, 7)). This cytochrome is the catalytic subunit of the NADPH oxidase enzyme that is critical in the innate immune response against invading microorganisms.

Raman spectroscopy and microscopy have traditionally been regarded as incompatible with fluorescence microscopy on fluorophore-labeled or autofluorescent cells because the Raman scattering cross-section of cellular biomolecules is orders of magnitude lower than the product of absorption cross-section and quantum yield of common fluorophores, which results in a fluorescence signal that overwhelms the Raman signals. This is an unfortunate situation because the enhanced information content of a hybrid Raman-fluorescence method would provide new multiplexing possibilities for single-cell optical microscopy and intracellular chemical analysis. We have previously demonstrated the feasibility of such a hybrid experiment by combining nonresonant Raman imaging with continuous-wave two-photon excitation (cw-TPE) fluorescence microscopy of the organic fluorophore Hoechst 33,342 in the nucleus of HeLa cells (8). A large spectral separation between fluorescence and Raman scattering was obtained in this case because the fluorescence emission occurs at the anti-Stokes side of the laser excitation wavelength, whereas the Raman scattering is detected on the Stokes side. More recently, we have extended this strategy (9) by using semiconductor quantum dot (QD) nanocrystals, which are gaining popularity because of their excellent fluorescence properties in live-cell microscopy and in vivo imaging of organisms (10–12). QDs display a large Stokes shift, a high absorption cross-section, and a narrow emission bandwidth compared to conventional fluorophores. We have shown (9) that resonant Raman spectroscopy and imaging on single cells can be combined with one-photon excitation (OPE) fluorescence microscopy on QD-labeled cells. Moreover, we demonstrated that cw-TPE microscopy on QD-labeled cells is fully compatible with single-cell nonresonant Raman microscopy. Both cw-TPE fluorescence microscopy and Raman spectroscopy and imaging are performed with the same laser beam in these experiments. Two-photon excitation microscopy would be even more efficient with a pulsed light source. An advantage of using QDs is that they can be targeted to selective intracellular locations by conjugating them to ligands, antibodies, or peptide localization sequences, which will enable the correlation of QD fluorescence to the Raman signal from cellular biomolecules.

2. Materials

2.1. QD-Labeled Polystyrene Microspheres

1. Streptavidin-conjugated quantum dots (QDs) with a fluorescence emission maximum of 605 nm are used for hybrid *r*esonance *R*aman/*o*ne-*p*hoton *e*xcitation (RR/OPE) fluorescence microscopy, while similar QDs with a fluorescence emission maximum of 585 nm are used for hybrid *n*onresonance *R*aman/*t*wo-*p*hoton *e*xcitation (NR/TPE) fluorescence microscopy. Both types of QDs, and also QDs with other emission properties, are sold as 1 μM solutions by Invitrogen (Carlsbad, CA) (*see* **Note 1**). Before use, these QD solutions should be kept at 4°C (*see* **Note 2**).
2. Biotin-conjugated polystyrene microspheres (diameter 2.2 μm) are obtained as a 1.25% solids suspension in water (cat. no. 24172; Polysciences, Inc., Warrington, PA) and kept at 4°C.
3. Phosphate-buffered saline (PBS) is prepared as a 10× aqueous stock solution with 1.37 M NaCl, 27 mM KCl, 100 mM Na_2HPO_4, and 18 mM KH_2PO_4 and autoclaved before storage at 4°C. Working solutions are prepared by 10× dilution with water (*see* **Note 3**).
4. Binding buffer: 1% (w/v) bovine serum albumin in PBS.

2.2. QD-Labeled RAW 264.7 Cells

1. The RAW 264.7 macrophage cell line (obtained from the European Collection of Cell Cultures) is used to exemplify NR/TPE microscopy on QD-labeled cells because we have found that these macrophages efficiently internalize QDs by endocytosis. The QDs are therefore easily observed as bright punctate features (endosomes) in these cells (*see* **Note 4**).
2. RAW 264. 7 cell culture medium is prepared by supplementing RPMI-1640 medium (Gibco/Invitrogen) with 10% (v/v) fetal calf serum, 2 mM glutamine, 100 U/ml penicillin, and 50 μg/ml streptomycin.
3. Substrate for hybrid Raman-fluorescence microscopy experiments: CaF_2 slides (diameter 25 mm, thickness 2 mm) (*see* **Note 5**).
4. Poly-L-lysine: A 0.4% (w/v) stock solution is prepared in water, filtered (0.2 μm), and kept at 4°C. For each new experiment, a working solution of 0.01% (w/v) in water is prepared.
5. Paraformaldehyde: 1,000 ml of PBS is heated to 60°C and 40 g of paraformaldehyde is added. The turbid solution is stirred until cleared, cooled, and filtered (0.2 μm). Aliquots of 10 ml are kept at −20°C and warmed to room temperature before use.

2.3. QD-Labeled Granulocytes

1. To demonstrate RR/OPE microscopy on cells, granulocytes isolated from venous blood of a healthy volunteer are used. Neutrophilic granulocytes have a high concentration of flavocytochrome b_{558} in specific granules. The heme groups in this flavocytochrome provide a large Raman signal in experiments performed under resonance conditions at an excitation wavelength of 413 nm (reviewed in (6, 7)).
2. Granulocyte buffer: PBS with 0.5% (w/v) BSA and 0.38% (w/v) trisodium citrate.
3. Labeling buffer: PBS with 1% (w/v) BSA, 1 mM $CaCl_2$, 0.5 mM $MgSO_4$, and 5 mM glucose.

2.4. The Combined Raman-Fluorescence Microscope

To combine confocal Raman microscopy with fluorescence microscopy on the same cells, we added a fluorescence branch in the detection part of an existing, home-built confocal Raman microspectrometer. The combined setup is schematically depicted in **Fig. 3.1**. The following is a detailed description of the equipment that is used for hybrid Raman-fluorescence experiments:

1. A Kr^+ gas laser (Innova 90-K; Coherent, Santa Clara, CA) is used as excitation source in both RR/OPE and NR/TPE experiments because this laser can be switched between 413 nm (for RR/OPE microscopy) and 647 nm (for NR/TPE microscopy) output. The output power of the laser is ~30 mW for 413 nm and ~800 mW for 647 nm.
2. The laser beam is guided with mirrors to a beamsplitter positioned at an angle of 45° with respect to the incoming beam. For experiments at 413 nm, a silver-coated beamsplitter with 30%/70% reflection/transmission is used, while a dichroic beamsplitter with >90% reflection at 647 nm and >90% transmission at 673 nm (= 600 cm^{-1}) and higher is used for experiments at 647 nm (660DCLP; Chroma Technology, Rockingham, VT).
3. From the beamsplitter the laser beam is guided to a biaxial scanning mirror (Leica Lasertechnique, Heidelberg, Germany) positioned at an angle of 45° with respect to the incoming beam in neutral position. The maximum scan area of the scanning mirror in this work is 15 × 15 μm^2.
4. After passing a lens (focal distance 100 mm), the laser beam enters the back aperture of a water-dipping objective (Plan Neofluar; Carl Zeiss, Jena, Germany) placed in an upright microscope (Olympus). The objective has a magnification of 63× and a numerical aperture of 1.2, which brings the excitation light to a focus in a diffraction-limited spot of 0.32 μm (at 413 nm) or 0.49 μm (at 647 nm) ($1/e^2$) diameter of the laser beam waist under the objective, according to a Gaussian beam approximation (13).

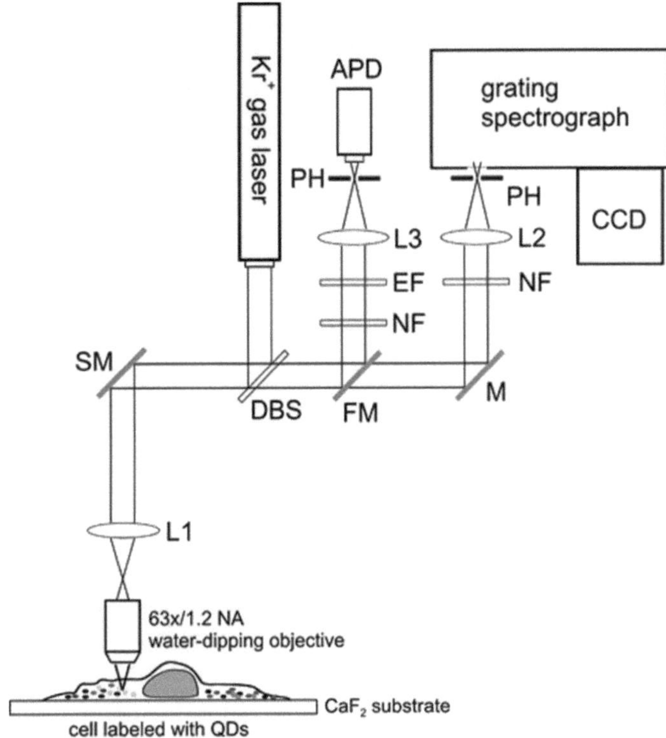

Fig. 3.1. Schematic representation of the combined Raman-fluorescence microscopy setup. Abbreviations: DBS, dichroic beamsplitter; SM, scanning mirror; L1, lens 1 (focal length 100 mm); FM, mirror on foldable mount; M, mirror; NF, notch filter; EF, emission filter; L2 and L3, lens 2 and 3 (focal length 35 mm); PH, pinhole; APD, avalanche photodiode; CCD, charge-coupled device. The individual components are further described in the text.

Before entering the objective, the laser beam diameter was adjusted to 6.3 mm, which was truncated to $(1/e^2)$-points by the back aperture of the objective.

5. The scattered Raman light and emitted fluorescence is collected by the same objective, reflected again by the scanning mirror, transmitted through the beamsplitter, and directed to either the fluorescence or Raman detection branch by a mirror in a foldable mount. In this way, Raman and fluorescence images are collected sequentially (*see* **Note 6**).
6. In the Raman detection branch, a holographic notch filter for 413 or 647 nm (both from Kaiser Optical Systems, Ann Arbor, MI) is used to filter reflected and Rayleigh-scattered laser light, and a lens with a focal length of 35 mm brings the Raman scattering to a focus on a pinhole (diameter 25 μm) placed at the entrance of a spectrograph. The pinhole reduces out-of-focus contributions to the Raman

signal and limits the detection volume to <0.5 μm^3. The axial resolution provided by the objective/pinhole is ~2.5 μm (FWHM).

7. The spectrograph (HR460; Jobin Yvon, Villeneuve d'Ascq, France) contains a blazed holographic grating (1,200 lines/mm for 413 nm, 600 lines/mm for 647 nm) for dispersion of the Raman signal, which is subsequently detected by a liquid nitrogen-cooled CCD (1,100 PB/VISAR; Princeton Instruments, Trenton, NJ) with 1,100 × 330 pixels of 24 × 24 μm^2. The spectrograph/CCD combination provides spectral resolutions of 2.1 cm^{-1}/pixel and 1.7 cm^{-1}/pixel for experiments at 413- and 647-nm excitation, respectively.
8. In the fluorescence branch, a holographic notch filter for 413 or 647 nm (both from Kaiser Optical Systems, Ann Arbor, MI) is used to filter reflected and Rayleigh-scattered laser light, and a bandpass emission filter (590–650 nm; Chroma Technology, Rockingham, VT) to detect Qdot® 605 fluorescence in RR/OPE experiments and 577.5–632.5 nm (Chroma Technology) to detect Qdot® 585 fluorescence in NR/TPE experiments) is used for the selective detection of QD fluorescence.
9. A lens with a focal length of 35 mm brings the fluorescence light to a focus on a pinhole (diameter 25 μm) placed before an avalanche photodiode (APD) detector (SPCM-200; PerkinElmer Optoelectronics, Fremont, CA).
10. The scanning mirror and APD acquisition of fluorescence is controlled by home-written routines in LabVIEW (National Instruments, Austin, TX). Acquisition of Raman data is controlled by WinSpec software (Princeton Instruments, Trenton, NJ).
11. Accessories that are convenient to use and indispensable for successful hybrid Raman-fluorescence microscopy experiments:
    (a) A collection of grey filters to decrease the laser excitation power. This is especially important for fluorescence detection at 413-nm excitation because photobleaching of QDs occurs at too high excitation powers.
    (b) A power meter to measure the laser excitation power under the microscope objective and elsewhere in the set up.
    (c) Fluorescent plastic slides (*see* **Note 7**) to optimize the optical alignment of the fluorescence branch. Alternatively, 10 μl of a dilute QD solution may be sandwiched between glass coverslips and used for optimization of the fluorescence signal.

(d) Polystyrene Petri dishes to optimize the optical alignment of the Raman branch. Polystyrene gives sharp and strong Raman signals both in the fingerprint region (500–1,800 cm^{-1}) and high-frequency region (2,800–3,100 cm^{-1}).

(e) Capillaries filled with toluene for calibration of the Raman wavenumber axis. To calibrate the fingerprint region, toluene Raman bands at 521, 785, 1,004, 1,210, and 1,604 cm^{-1} are used and a third-order polynomial is used for fitting. A toluene-filled capillary may also be used to optimize the optical alignment of the Raman branch.

(f) A tungsten halogen light source (AvaLight-HAL; Avantes BV, Eerbeek, The Netherlands) with a known emission spectrum to correct the acquired Raman spectra for the frequency-dependent optical detection efficiency of the setup.

3. Methods

3.1. Preparation of QD-Coated Polystyrene Microspheres

1. Biotin-conjugated polystyrene microspheres (10 μl of the suspension obtained from Polysciences) are suspended in 500 μl of binding buffer.
2. The suspension is briefly vortexed, sonicated for 5 min (to break up microsphere aggregates), and centrifuged at 5,000×g for 3 min in a microcentrifuge.
3. The supernatant is carefully aspirated and the microspheres are resuspended in 500 μl of binding buffer and centrifuged again.
4. The supernatant is carefully aspirated and the microspheres are resuspended in 200 μl of binding buffer. Next, 2 μl of QD stock solution (Qdot® 605 streptavidin conjugate or Qdot® 585 streptavidin conjugate) are added to the microsphere suspension. This mixture is incubated for 30 min at room temperature while gently shaking the microtube.
5. Excess QDs are removed by two washing and centrifugation steps in binding buffer.
6. The QD-labeled microspheres are finally resuspended in 200 μl of PBS and used within 2 days.
7. To check for a homogeneous distribution of QDs on the microspheres, aliquots (~10 μl) of the suspension are sandwiched between two coverslips (thickness 170 μm) and examined by confocal laser scanning microscopy on

a Zeiss LSM510 microscope (Carl Zeiss, Göttingen, Germany) (*see* **Note 8**). Confocal fluorescence imaging is performed with Zeiss LSM acquisition software, using a C-Apochromat 63×/1.2 numerical-aperture water-immersion objective, 488-nm excitation (from an Ar^+ laser), and a Hamamatsu R6357 photomultiplier tube to detect the QD fluorescence after spectral filtering through a 560-nm long-pass filter. A representative confocal fluorescence image of QD-labeled microspheres is shown in **Fig. 3.2**.

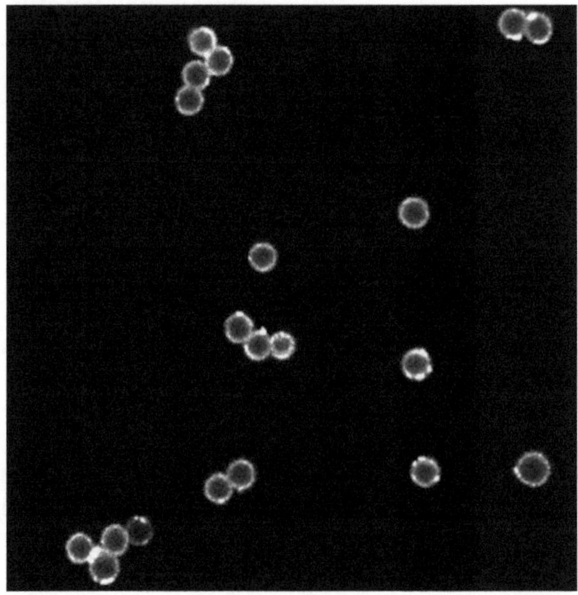

Fig. 3.2. Confocal fluorescence image (100 × 100 μm^2) of Qdot® 585-coated polystyrene microspheres (diameter 4.3 μm). Excitation 488 nm, emission >560 nm.

3.2. Preparation of QD-Labeled RAW 264.7 Cells

1. RAW 264.7 macrophages are maintained at 37°C in a 5% CO_2 atmosphere and passaged twice a week by gently scraping them off the tissue culture flask surface and diluting them 1:6 (v/v) with fresh culture medium into a new tissue culture flask.
2. To prepare CaF_2 slides coated with poly-L-lysine, clean CaF_2 slides are thoroughly rinsed with ethanol and water and subsequently incubated with a poly-L-lysine solution for 1 h at 60°C. The slides are washed 3× with water and kept in PBS until use (*see* **Note 9**).
3. Samples for NR/TPE hybrid Raman-fluorescence experiments are prepared by first pipetting 250 μl of a RAW 264.7 cell suspension (~10^6 cells/ml) in culture medium onto poly-L-lysine-coated CaF_2 slides and incubating the slides overnight at 37°C in a 5% CO_2 atmosphere. Next,

cell-coated CaF_2 slides are immersed in 20 nM of QDs (Qdot® 585 streptavidin conjugate) in culture medium and incubated for 2 h at 37°C to allow internalization of QDs by the macrophages.

4. After two wash steps with PBS, the QD-containing cells are fixed by immersing the slides in 4% paraformaldehyde for 1 h at room temperature.
5. The slides are washed 2× with PBS and kept in PBS during hybrid NR/TPE microscopy experiments.

3.3. Preparation of QD-Labeled Neutrophilic Granulocytes

1. Peripheral blood from a healthy donor is obtained by venipuncture and collected in a 10-ml heparinized tube. Granulocytes are freshly isolated from this blood according to a published procedure (*see* **Note 10**) and suspended at $\sim 2 \times 10^6$ cells/ml in granulocyte buffer (*see* **Note 8**).
2. A 250-μl aliquot of granulocytes is pipetted onto a poly-L-lysine-coated CaF_2 slide (*see* **Section 3.2, Step 2**) and incubated for 30 min at 37°C.
3. Unbound granulocytes are removed by washing with granulocyte buffer.
4. Granulocyte-coated CaF_2 slides are immersed in 20 nM of QDs (Qdot® 605 streptavidin conjugate) in labeling buffer and incubated for 30 min at 37°C to allow internalization of QDs by the granulocytes.
5. After two wash steps with PBS, the QD-containing cells are fixed by immersing the slides in 2% paraformaldehyde for 1 h at room temperature.
6. The slides are washed 2× with PBS and kept in PBS during hybrid RR/OPE microscopy experiments.
7. To verify that the granulocytes have internalized QDs, a similar procedure as described in this section is performed using freshly isolated granulocytes adhered to LabTek 8-well glass chamber slides (Nalge Nunc, Rochester, NY) and incubated with 20 nM QDs for 30 min. The slides are examined on a Zeiss LSM510 microscope. Confocal fluorescence imaging is performed with Zeiss LSM acquisition software, using a C-Apochromat 63×/1.2 numerical-aperture water-immersion objective, 488-nm excitation (from an Ar^+ laser), and a Hamamatsu R6357 photomultiplier tube to detect the QD fluorescence after spectral filtering through a 560-nm longpass filter. A representative confocal fluorescence image of QD-labeled neutrophilic granulocytes is shown in **Fig. 3.3a**. The corresponding brightfield image is shown in **Fig. 3.3b**. The accumulation of QDs in intracellular vesicles is clearly visible in the fluorescence image.

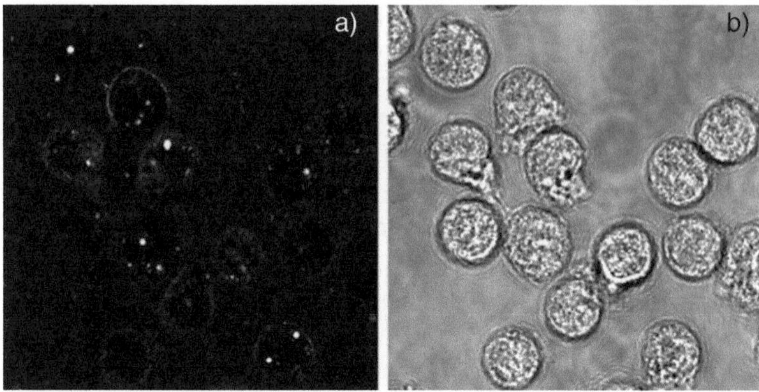

Fig. 3.3. Confocal fluorescence image (**a**) and corresponding brightfield image (**b**) of neutrophils incubated with QDs. The accumulation of QDs into vesicles is clearly shown in the fluorescence image.

3.4. Hybrid Raman-Fluorescence Microscopy

3.4.1. General Guidelines

In combined Raman-fluorescence experiments on QD-labeled samples, it is recommended to perform fluorescence microscopy before Raman microscopy because a fluorescence image is acquired in a few seconds while a Raman image may take up to 15 min. Therefore, fluorescence imaging allows one to quickly select cells with a level of QD-labeling that is suitable for hybrid imaging. Moreover, in experiments at 413 nm the laser power that is necessary for obtaining a high-quality resonance Raman signal of flavocytochrome b_{558} in granulocytes (~0.5–1 mW) will destroy QD fluorescence by photobleaching. In that case, acquiring the fluorescence image before the RR image is the only successful hybrid Raman-fluorescence procedure. For NR/TPE experiments at 647-nm excitation, both images are acquired at the same laser power (~25–50 mW) and photobleaching of QDs is less of a problem. However, we have observed that the use of too high laser powers at 647 nm may result in disruption of the cell morphology and a large increase in background in the Raman signal, presumably due to photothermal cell ablation caused by excessive absorption of energy by QDs. The effect of the high laser powers that are used in Raman microspectroscopy on cells is always an important issue, as we have previously discussed (7).

The Raman setup allows three types of Raman microspectroscopy experiments:

- *Point spectroscopy*, where the laser beam is positioned into the sample and a Raman spectrum is obtained from that position;
- *Scanning spectroscopy*, where the laser beam is scanned over a region of interest and one Raman spectrum is recorded, which is representative for the whole region;

- *Spectral imaging*, where the laser beam is scanned over a region of interest and a Raman spectrum is recorded at every image position. From the resulting 3D data set (one spectral and two spatial dimensions), Raman images are constructed by plotting the integrated intensity of a Raman band of interest as a function of position. In addition, multivariate data analysis techniques such as principal component analysis (PCA) and hierarchical cluster analysis (HCA) may be used to investigate in more detail the major variances in the spectral imaging data set.

Each of these three spectroscopy modes is fully compatible with fluorescence microscopy. For example, a fluorescence image may reveal an interesting location in the cell, after which the laser beam is positioned in that location to record a Raman spectrum containing a wealth of chemically specific information.

In the next section we discuss the general start-up procedure for hybrid Raman-fluorescence microscopy. The subsequent sections will provide protocols for performing hybrid experiments on QD-coated microspheres and QD-labeled cells.

3.4.2. Start-Up Procedure

1. The CCD camera is filled with liquid nitrogen to cool the CCD chip. It takes ~1 h to reach the operating temperature.
2. All of the equipment is switched on. The laser is allowed to stabilize its output power for ~0.5 h.
3. A polystyrene Petri dish is mounted on the microscope stage and the laser is focused just inside the dish. The sensitivity of the Raman detection branch is checked by using a known amount of excitation light (for example, 1 mW of 413 nm or 100 mW (could be (significantly) less) of 647 nm) and recording the number of counts detected for the polystyrene Raman band at 1,000 cm^{-1}. If the number of detected counts is too low (with respect to previous experience), an optical alignment of the excitation and/or Raman detection branch should be performed. If the number of detected counts is as expected, then the Raman wavenumber axis is calibrated with a toluene-filled capillary (*see* **Section 2.4 Step 11e**). Subsequently, record a white-light spectrum using the tungsten halogen light source (*see* **Section 2.4 Step 11f**).
4. A mirror is flipped into the detection branch by using the foldable mount (*see* **Fig. 3.1**).
5. A green fluorescent plastic slide is mounted on the microscope stage and the laser power is decreased to ~10 μW of 413 nm (*see* **Note 11**) by using a grey filter. The laser is focused just inside the slide. The sensitivity of the fluorescence detection branch is checked by recording the number of counts detected on the APD for the fluorescent slide.

If the number of detected counts is too low (with respect to previous experience), an optical alignment of the excitation and/or fluorescence detection branch should be performed.

6. The setup is now ready for hybrid NR/TPE or RR/OPE microscopy experiments.

3.4.3. Hybrid Raman-Fluorescence Microscopy on QD-Coated Microspheres

1. An aliquot (~100 μl) of QD-coated microspheres is pipetted onto a clean and dry CaF_2 slide and incubated for 30 min at room temperature. Most microspheres will stick to the surface and remain fixed during a hybrid Raman-fluorescence experiment.
2. The microscope start-up procedure described in **Section 3.4.2** is performed.
3. The CaF_2 slide is mounted on the microscope stage and the microspheres are brought into focus by using brightfield illumination. A few microspheres are positioned in the $15 \times 15\ \mu m^2$ field of view of the scanning mirror. The brightfield illumination is turned off.
4. The mirror is inserted into the detection branch with the foldable mount.
5. The laser power is adjusted to ~10 μW for 413-nm excitation or ~100 mW (could be (significantly) less) for 647-nm excitation.
6. A fluorescence image of the microspheres is acquired. Typical acquisition parameters on our setup are 128 × 128 pixels and 0.25 ms/pixel.
7. The mirror from the detection branch is flipped away with the foldable mount.
8. The laser power is adjusted to ~1 mW for 413-nm excitation or left at ~100 mW for 647-nm excitation (*see* **Note 12**).
9. A Raman image of the microspheres is acquired. Typical acquisition parameters on our setup are 32 × 32 pixels and 1 s/pixel.
10. A Raman image is constructed by plotting the 1,000 cm^{-1} Raman band of polystyrene as a function of image pixel position.

3.4.4. Hybrid NR/TPE Raman-Fluorescence Microscopy on QD-Labeled Cells

1. The start-up procedure described in **Section 3.4.2** is performed.
2. The CaF_2 slide with QD-labeled RAW 264.7 cells is mounted on the microscope stage and the cells are brought in focus using brightfield illumination. A cell is positioned in the $15 \times 15\ \mu m^2$ field of view of the scanning mirror. The brightfield illumination is turned off.

3. The mirror is inserted into the detection branch with the foldable mount.
4. The laser power is adjusted to ~25 mW for 647-nm excitation.
5. A TPE fluorescence image of the QDs located inside the cell is acquired. Typical acquisition parameters on our setup are 128 × 128 pixels and 0.25 ms/pixel.
6. The mirror from the detection branch is flipped away with the foldable mount.
7. A Raman image of the cell is acquired. Typical acquisition parameters on our setup are 32 × 32 pixels and 1 s/pixel. Alternatively, if the QD fluorescence image shows a cellular location that is interesting for further study by Raman microspectroscopy, the laser beam can be positioned in that location and a Raman spectrum can be acquired at only that location. This saves time in comparison with the acquisition of a full Raman image of the cell.
8. **Steps 3–7** are repeated for other cells.
9. Raman images of the cells are constructed by plotting Raman bands of known origin (for example, the phenylalanine band at 1,004 cm^{-1} or the DNA band at 785 cm^{-1}) as a function of image pixel position.
10. **Figure 3.4** shows a NR image (a) and a TPE image (b) of a QD-labeled RAW 264.7 cell. The accumulation of QDs into vesicular organelles is clearly shown in the TPE image. The NR image shows areas rich in lipids, for example, the lipid droplets (LDs) marked with arrows.

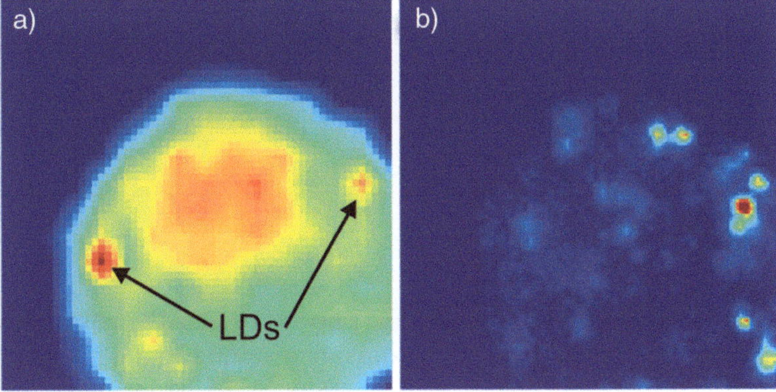

Fig. 3.4. Hybrid Raman-fluorescence microscopy on a single cell. Nonresonant Raman image (**a**) constructed from the high-frequency region (2,800–3,050 cm^{-1}) and corresponding two-photon excitation fluorescence image (**b**) of a RAW 264.7 cell incubated with QDs. The colors range from blue (lowest intensity) to red (highest intensity). Lipid droplets in (**a**) are marked with *arrows*.

3.4.5. Hybrid RR/OPE Raman-Fluorescence Microscopy on QD-Labeled Cells

1. The start-up procedure described in **Section 3.4.2** is performed.
2. The CaF_2 slide with QD-labeled granulocytes is mounted on the microscope stage and the cells are brought in focus using brightfield illumination. A cell is positioned in the $15 \times 15\ \mu m^2$ field of view of the scanning mirror. The brightfield illumination is turned off.
3. The mirror is inserted into the detection branch with the foldable mount.
4. The laser power is adjusted to ~25 μW for 413-nm excitation.
5. A OPE fluorescence image of the QDs located inside the cell is acquired. Typical acquisition parameters on our setup are 128 × 128 pixels and 0.25 ms/pixel.
6. The mirror from the detection branch is flipped away with the foldable mount.
7. The laser power is adjusted to ~0.5–1 mW.
8. A Raman image of the cell is acquired. Typical acquisition parameters on our setup are 32 × 32 pixels and 1 s/pixel. Alternatively, if the QD fluorescence image shows a cellular location that is interesting for further study by Raman microspectroscopy, the laser beam can be positioned in that location and a Raman spectrum can be acquired at only that location. This saves a lot of time in comparison with recording a full Raman image of the cell.
9. **Steps 3–7** are repeated for other cells.
10. Raman images of the cells are constructed by plotting the flavocytochrome b_{558} RR band at 1,375 cm^{-1} as a function of image pixel position.

4. Notes

1. Cat. no. Q10151MP from Invitrogen is a sampler kit containing streptavidin conjugates of Qdot® 525, Qdot® 565, Qdot® 585, Qdot® 605, and Qdot® 655.
2. The QD solutions supplied by Invitrogen should never be stored at −20°C because this will induce aggregation of the QDs.

3. All solutions and buffers are prepared in water with a resistivity of 18.2 MΩ·cm.
4. In principle, any cell type or tissue that can be labeled with QDs is amenable to hybrid Raman-fluorescence microscopy. For example, QDs functionalized with antibodies or receptor ligands might be employed to label specific cells or subcellular sites such as the plasma membrane. Demonstrations of such use of QDs abound in the literature. Recent reviews are available (10–12).
5. CaF_2 slides are used because glass and quartz cover slips cause a large background signal in Raman experiments. Besides a relatively strong Raman band at 323 cm^{-1}, CaF_2 slides from different vendors may also show large Raman signals at other frequencies due to impurities, which may obscure the observation of Raman bands from cellular components. It is therefore recommended to investigate the quality of CaF_2 slides with Raman spectroscopy before Raman experiments on cells are undertaken.
6. Using a dichroic beamsplitter instead of a foldable mirror, it will be possible to collect Raman and fluorescence images simultaneously, if the pixel dwell times were identical.
7. Different fluorescent plastic slides suitable for common excitation wavelengths (for example, 488, 543, 568, and 633 nm) are available from Chroma Technology, Rockingham, VT. These slides are sometimes handed out at conference exhibition booths.
8. Other confocal laser scanning microscopes or widefield fluorescent microscopes may be used to check the distribution of QDs on the microspheres.
9. CaF_2 slides freshly coated with poly-L-lysine are used immediately to prepare cell samples for combined Raman-fluorescence microscopy. Since CaF_2 slides can be reused, they are cleaned after microscopy experiments with detergent, rinsed copiously with water and ethanol, and allowed to dry. The commercial value of CaF_2 is appreciable and re-use is economic for that reason.
10. A step-by-step protocol describing the isolation of granulocytes from peripheral blood is beyond the scope of this chapter. A detailed protocol has been published (14).
11. Granulocytes should be used within 4 h from isolation in order to avoid extensive cell death.
12. In case of 647-nm excitation, the laser power can be kept at ~100 mW because continuous-wave two-photon excitation fluorescence requires high laser powers (8, 15).

References

1. Uzunbajakava, N., Lenferink, A., Kraan, Y., Volokhina, E., Vrensen, G., Greve, J., and Otto, C. (2003) Nonresonant confocal Raman imaging of DNA and protein distribution in apoptotic cells. *Biophys. J.* **84**, 3968–81.
2. Van Manen, H.-J., Kraan, Y. M., Roos, D., and Otto, C. (2005) Single-cell Raman and fluorescence microscopy reveal the association of lipid bodies with phagosomes in leukocytes. *Proc. Natl. Acad. Sci. USA* **102**, 10159–64.
3. Notingher, I., Bisson, I., Bishop, A. E., Randle, W. L., Polak, J. M. P., and Hench, L. L. (2004) In situ spectral monitoring of mRNA translation in embryonic stem cells during differentiation in vitro. *Anal. Chem.* **76**, 3185–93.
4. Krafft, C., Knetschke, T., Funk, R. H., and Salzer, R. (2006) Studies on stress-induced changes at the subcellular level by Raman microspectroscopic mapping. *Anal. Chem.* **78**, 4424–9.
5. Chan, J. W., Taylor, D. S., Lane, S. M., Zwerdling, T., Tuscano, J., and Huser, T. (2008) Nondestructive identification of individual leukemia cells by laser trapping Raman spectroscopy. *Anal. Chem.* **80**, 2180–7.
6. Van Manen, H.-J., Van Bruggen, R., Roos, D., and Otto, C. (2006) Single-cell optical imaging of the phagocyte NADPH oxidase. *Antioxid. Redox Signal.* **8**, 1509–22.
7. Van Manen, H.-J., Morin, C., Roos, D., and Otto, C. (2008) Resonance Raman microspectroscopy and imaging of hemoproteins in single leukocytes. In Biomedical vibrational spectroscopy, Lasch, P. and Kneipp, J., (Eds.). Wiley, Hoboken, pp. 153–179.
8. Uzunbajakava, N. and Otto, C. (2003) Combined Raman and continuous-wave-excited two-photon fluorescence cell imaging. *Opt. Lett.* **28**, 2073–5.
9. Van Manen, H.-J. and Otto, C. (2007) Hybrid confocal Raman fluorescence microscopy on single cells using semiconductor quantum dots. *Nano Lett.* 7, 1631–36.
10. Michalet, X., Pinaud, F. F., Bentolila, L. A., Tsay, J. M., Doose, S., Li, J. J., Sundaresan, G., Wu, A. M., Gambhir, S. S., and Weiss, S. (2005) Quantum dots for live cells, in vivo imaging, and diagnostics. *Science* **307**, 538–44.
11. Medintz, I. L., Uyeda, H. T., Goldman, E. R., and Mattoussi, H. (2005) Quantum dot bioconjugates for imaging, labelling, and sensing. *Nat. Mater.* **4**, 435–46.
12. Alivisatos, A. P., Gu, W., and Larabell, C. (2005) Quantum dots as cellular probes. *Annu. Rev. Biomed. Eng.* 7, 55–76.
13. De Grauw, C. J., Sijtsema, N. M., Otto, C., and Greve, J. (1997) Axial resolution of confocal Raman microscopes: Gaussian beam theory and practice. *J. Microsc.* **188**, 273–9.
14. Roos, D. and De Boer, M. (1986) Purification and cryopreservation of phagocytes from human blood. *Methods Enzymol.* **132**, 225–43.
15. Booth, M. J. and Hell, S. W. (1998) Continuous wave excitation two-photon fluorescence microscopy exemplified with the 647-nm ArKr laser line. *J. Microsc.* **190**, 298–304.

Chapter 4

Labeling of Mesenchymal Stem Cells with Bioconjugated Quantum Dots

Bhranti S. Shah and Jeremy J. Mao

Abstract

Quantum dots (QDs) are semiconductor nanocrystals, and recently they have been shown as effective probes for cell labeling. Due to their unique spectral, physical, and chemical properties, QDs can concurrently tag multiple intercellular and intracellular components of live cells for time ranging from seconds to months. Different color QDs can label different cell components that can be visualized with fluorescent microscopy or in vivo. Here, we provide a detailed protocol for labeling postnatal and differentiated stem/progenitor cells with bioconjugated quantum dots. For example, peptide CGGGRGD is immobilized on CdSe-ZnS QDs with free carboxyl groups. These bioconjugates label selected integrins on cell membrane of human mesenchymal stem cells (hMSCs). QD concentration and incubation time to effectively label hMSCs is optimized. We discovered that bioconjugated QDs effectively label hMSCs not only during population doubling, but also during multi-lineage differentiation into osteoblasts, chondrocytes, and adipocytes. Undifferentiated and differentiated stem cells labeled with bioconjugated QDs can be readily imaged by fluorescent microscopy. Thus, quantum dots represent an effective cell labeling probe and an alternative to organic dyes and fluorescent proteins for cell labeling and cell tracking.

Key words: Quantum dots, mesenchymal stem cells, cell differentiation, cell labeling, peptide, fluorescent.

1. Introduction

Our understanding of cell biology originated from anatomical and histological observations. Cells that are morphologically alike and reside in a given tissue are specifically named, such as cardiomyocytes in the heart, hepatocytes in the liver, and osteoblasts in bone. Developmental biology studies later identified that the end-stage differentiated cells such as cardiomyocytes, hepatocytes, and osteoblasts derive from progenitor cells or stem cells.

K. Shah (ed.), *Molecular Imaging*, Methods in Molecular Biology 680,
DOI 10.1007/978-1-60761-901-7_4, © Springer Science+Business Media, LLC 2011

In multicellular organisms, each tissue consists of multiple cell types. For example, bone consists of osteoblasts or bone forming cells, osteoclasts or bone-breaking cells, and osteocytes that are mature osteoblasts entrapped in mineralized matrix. There has been a long-lasting aspiration to effectively label cells and track their fate in developmental biology, preferably in vivo and in real time (1). Under the same token, there is an acute need to track the fate of stem cells in tissue engineereing and regenerative medicine (2, 3). There are broadly three types of cell labeling probes: organic dyes, fluorescent proteins, and quantum dots (**Table 4.1**).

Organic dyes have been widely utilized in cell biology and developmental biology such as dapi, rhodamine phalloidin, Di-I (4–7). Organic dyes are capable of labeling cells in culture for short time and can be observed under fluorescent microscope. However, organic dyes readily photobleach and lose fluorescence, and therefore are only useful for short-term cell labeling. Additionally, organic dyes have broad emission spectrum, but narrow excitation spectrum, causing an overlap of different emission spectrum, which is undesirable. Organic dyes are sensitive to changes in local pH, and accordingly may readily disintegrate and lose fluorescence. Organic dyes are virtually impossible for long-term in vivo cell tracking. On the plus side, organic dyes are easy to use and inexpensive.

Genetically encoded fluorescent proteins such as green fluorescent protein (GFP) have been widely used for cell labeling (8–10). GFPs are typically transfected into the cells via retrovirus, lentivirus, or non-viral approaches. GFPs have a number of important advantages over organic dyes for cell labeling. For example, GFPs have better photostability and pH tolerance, in

Table 4.1
Comparison of cell labeling and tracking probes

	Organic dyes	Fluorescent proteins (e.g., GFP)	Quantum dots (QDs)
Emission spectrum	Broad	Broad	*Narrow*
Excitation spectrum	Narrow	Narrow	*Broad*
Photostability	Poor	*Good*	*Good*
pH sensitivity	Yes	*No*	*No*
Luminescence time	Minutes to hours	*Months*	*Months*
Fluorescence intensity in vivo	Weak	Moderate	*Strong*
Overlap with autofluorescence	No	Yes	*No*
Multi-color labeling	Cumbersome	Cumbersome	*Readily*
In vivo cell tracking	No	Questionable	*Yes*

Italic texts denote advantageous features, in comparison with non-italic text.

addition to much longer luminescence time. However, GFPs suffer from a number of intrinsic deficiencies such as sensitivities to proteolytic enzymes, difficulty for labeling multiple cell lineages, and overlap with body's autofluorescence signal spectrum, which makes it difficult to use for in vivo cell tracking. Whereas a critical advantage of GFPs over QDs is genetic incorporation of GFPs, QDs nonetheless are several times brighter than GFPs and have excitation and emission spectra that are different from body's autofluorescence.

Quantum dots (QDs) are small light-emitting semiconductor particles, typically in the size range of 2–0 nm (11–14). After years of non-biological applications, two independent communications in *Science* in 1998 showed that highly luminescent QDs could be made water soluble and tethered to biomolecules for cell labeling (15, 16). Subsequently, the fluorescence yield of bioconjugated QDs has been enhanced (17). Currently, QDs are commercially available from several companies. In contrast to organic dyes or fluorescent proteins, QDs have several distinctive advantages, especially for long-term cell labeling and in vivo cell tracking (**Table 4.1**). QDs are photostable and maintain fluorescence intensity in the culture of tumor cells (7, 18). The narrow emission and broad excitation spectrum of QDs enable the viewing of multiple colors at a given wavelength. Both the emission and excitation spectra of QDs can be fine-tuned (19). QDs are internalized primarily by endocytosis and continue to reside in cytoplasm (20, 21). Detailed protocols for QD labeling and the imaging of live cells have been elegantly documented (18, 19).

The primary objective of this chapter is to provide an effective protocol for labeling postnatal stem/progenitor cells with quantum dots. We will discuss the following aspects of QD labeling of stem/progenitor cells: (1) conjugate RGD peptide to quantum dot nanoparticles; (2) label hMSCs during self-replication with QD bioconjugates; (3) determine cytocompatibility of QD-bioconjugates; and (4) explore QD labeling of hMSCs during differentiation into lineage-specific cells.

2. Materials

2.1. Culture and Expansion of Human Mesenchymal Stem Cells

1. Bone marrow samples from healthy human donors (AllCells, Berkeley, CA)
2. RosetteSep™ (Stem Cell Technologies, Vancouver, BC, Canada)
3. 35-mm petri dishes (Falcon, Becton Dickinson Labware, Franklin Lakes, NJ)

4. DMEM: Dulbecco's Modified Eagle's Minimal Essential Medium Low Glucose (DMEM-LG) (Sigma, St. Louis, MO) supplemented with 10% fetal bovine serum (FBS, Atlanta Biologicals, Lawrenceville, GA) and 1% antibiotic-antimycotic (10,000 U/ml penicillin, 10,000 μg/ml streptomycin, and 25 μg/ml amphotericin B) (Atlanta Biologicals, Lawrenceville, GA)
5. Phosphate buffered saline (PBS) (Lonza, Walkersville, MD)
6. Solution of trypsin (0.25%) and ethylenediamine tetraacetic acid (EDTA) (1 mM) (Atlanta Biologicals)
7. 5% DH autoflow CO_2 air-jacketed incubator (Nuaire, Plymouth, MN)
8. Trypan blue solution (Sigma, St. Louis, MO)
9. Tissue culture six-well plate (Becton Dickinson Labware, Franklin Lakes, NJ)
10. Centrifuge 5417R machine (Eppendorf, Westbury, NY).

2.2. Quantum Dot Bioconjugation

1. Zinc sulphide (ZnS) capped cadmium selenium (CdSe) quantum dots with functionalized carboxyl surface groups (0.25 mg/ml) (Evident Technologies, Troy, NY or Invitrogen, Carlsbad, CA) (*see* **Note 2**) and stored at 4°C without exposure to light
2. CGGGRGD peptide: prepare 1 mg/ml solution in water and store it at 4°C (*see* **Note 3**)
3. EDC (1-ethyl-3-(3-dimethylaminopropyl) carbodiimide. HCl) (Pierce, Rockford, IL)
4. MES buffer (1 M) (Sigma, St. Louis, MO)
5. Sulfo NHS (*N*-hydrocylsulfo-succinimide) (Sigma, St. Louis, MO)
6. Sodium borate buffer: 0.1 M borate (Sigma, St. Louis, MO), 0.5 M NaCl (Sigma, St. Louis, MO), pH 8.3, and sterilize before storage at room temperature
7. Distilled water (DI) (Millipore, Billerica, MA)
8. Ultrasonic cleaner (Fisher Scientific, Pittsburgh, PA)
9. Stir Plate (Fisher Scientific, Pittsburgh, PA)

2.3. Human Mesenchymal Stem Cell Differentiation into Osteoblasts

1. Dexamethasone (Sigma, St. Louis, MO) is dissolved in sterile PBS at 100 nM, stored in aliquots at –80°C, and then added to the osteogenic medium as required
2. L-Ascorbic acid (Sigma, St. Louis, MO) is dissolved in sterile PBS at 0.05 mg/ml, stored in aliquots at –80°C, and then added to the osteogenic medium as required

3. Glycerol 2-phosphate disodium salt hydrate (β-glycerophosphate) (Sigma, St. Louis, MO) is dissolved in sterile PBS at 0.01 M, stored in aliquots at –80°C, and then added to the osteogenic medium as required
4. Osteogenic medium: Dulbecco's Modified Eagle's Minimal Essential Medium Low Glucose (DMEM-LG) (Sigma, St. Louis, MO) supplemented with 10% FBS, 1% antibiotic-antimycotic, 100 nM dexamethasone, 0.05 mg/ml ascorbic acid, and 0.01 M β-glycerophosphate (22–24)
5. Alkaline phosphatase reagent (Raichem, San Deigo, CA) (25–28)
6. Calcium content (Raichem, San Deigo, CA) (25–28)

2.4. Human Mesenchymal Stem Cell Differentiation into Chondrocytes

1. Sodium pyruvate (Sigma, St. Louis, MO) is dissolved in sterile PBS at 100 μg/ml, stored in aliquots at –80°C, and then added to the chondrogenic medium as required
2. L-Ascorbic acid (Sigma, St. Louis, MO) is dissolved in sterile PBS at 50 μg/ml, stored in aliquots at –80°C, and then added to the chondrogenic medium as required
3. L-Proline (Sigma, St. Louis, MO) is dissolved in sterile PBS at 40 μg/ml, stored in aliquots at –80°C, and then added to the chondrogenic medium as required
4. Dexamethasone (Sigma, St. Louis, MO) is dissolved in sterile PBS at 0.01 μM, stored in aliquots at –80°C, and then added to the chondrogenic medium as required
5. Albumin from bovine serum (Sigma, St. Louis, MO) is dissolved in sterile distilled water at 2 mg/ml and stored in single aliquots at –80°C
6. TGFβ3 (R&D Systems, Minneapolis, MN) is reconstituted in 50-μl solution of 4 mM HCl (Fisher Scientific, Pittsburgh, PA) and 2 mg/ml BSA, stored in aliquots at –80°C, and then added to the chondrogenic medium as required
7. Chondrogenic medium: Dulbecco's Modified Eagle's Minimal Essential Medium High Glucose (DMEM-HG) supplemented with 1% antibiotic-antimycotic, 1% ITS+1 Liquid Media Supplement (100×) (Sigma, St. Louis, MO), 100 μg/ml sodium pyruvate, 50 μg/ml L-ascorbic acid, 40 μg/ml L-proline, 0.01 μM dexamethasone, 10 ng/ml TGFβ3 (23, 26, 27, 29)
8. Alcian Blue 8X (Sigma, St. Louis, MO)
9. Blyscan glycosaminoglycan assay (Accurate Chemical and Scientific Corp., Westbury, NY) (23, 26, 27, 29)

2.5. Human Mesenchymal Stem Cell Differentiation into Adipocytes

1. Dexamethasone (Sigma, St. Louis, MO) is dissolved in sterile PBS at 50 nM, stored in aliquots at –80°C, and then added to the adipogenic medium as required
2. Insulin (Sigma, St. Louis, MO) is dissolved in sterile DMEM at 10 μg/ml, stored in single use aliquot at –80°C, and then added to the adipogenic medium as required
3. 3-Isobutyl-1-methylxanthine (Sigma, St. Louis, MO) is dissolved in sterile DMSO (Fisher Scientific, Pittsburgh, PA) at 0.5 μM, stored in aliquots at –80°C, and then added to the adipogenic medium as required
4. Indomethacin (Sigma, St. Louis, MO) is dissolved in sterile 100% ethanol (Sigma, St. Louis, MO) at 60 μM, stored in aliquots at –80°C, and then added to the adipogenic medium as required
5. Adipogenic medium: Dulbecco's Modified Eagle's Minimal Essential Medium Low Glucose (DMEM-LG) supplemented with 50 nM dexamethasone, 10 μg/ml insulin, and 5 mM isobutyl-methylxanthine, 10% FBS and 1% antibiotics-antimycotics (26, 30–32)
6. Oil Red O staining (Cambrex, East Rutherford, NJ) (26, 30–32)
7. Free glycerol determination kit (Sigma, St. Louis, MO) (26, 32)

2.6. Brightfield and Fluorescence Microscopy

1. Inverted microscope (Leica, Northvale, NJ) equipped with a mercury arc lamp (100 W) (Chiu Technology Corp., Kings Park, NY) and a 32,007 Qdot 605 with 40-nm emission filter (Chroma, Rockingham, VT).
2. Original images were captured using a microscope mounted camera (Leica, Northvale, NJ) controlled by image acquisition software (Leica 3.0 Suite, Leica, Northvale, NJ).
3. Adobe Photoshop 7.0 (Adobe Systems Incorporated, San Jose, CA).

3. Methods

Short peptides containing a motif such as RGD mimic cell adhesion proteins and serve as ligands for integrin receptors including hMSCs. RGD peptide serves as a ligand for $\alpha_3\beta_1$, $\alpha_v\beta_1$, $\alpha_v\beta_5$, and other integrin receptors. The free carboxyl group on QDs is available for covalent coupling to biomolecules such as proteins, peptides, and nucleic acids by cross-linking to reactive amine groups

(33). The cystine (C) amino acid of the CGGGRGD peptide links to the CdSe-ZnS quantum dot through an amide bond, the GGG sequences of glycine (G) amino acids provide a spacer in the amino acid, and the RGD peptide goes and binds itself to specific integrins present on the cell surface. These QDs absorb light in the near UV spectrum (<450 nm) and emit in the orange spectrum (600 ± 10 nm). The orange emission has prompted Evident Technologies, Inc. to refer to the quantum dots as "Fort Orange quantum dots" (*see* **Note 4**). QDs are conjugated to the CGGGRGD peptide through simple covalent bonding by using a common cross linking reagent EDC.

3.1. Preparation of Bioconjuagted Quantum Dots

1. A solution of 5 mg EDC, 3.75 mg Sulfo-NHS, 0.2 ml MES buffer, and 0.3 ml DI water is sterilized (*see* **Note 4**) and added to 0.5 ml of carboxyl QDs (*see* **Note 2**), stirred, and allowed to react at room temperature for 30 min.
2. This solution is then centrifuged at 4,000 rpm for 60 min to obtain a precipitated QD-Sulfo-NHS pellet.
3. QD-Sulfo-NHS pellet is rinsed twice with DI water to remove unbound particles, and then a solution consisting of 0.5 ml of CGGGRGD peptide solution, 0.3 ml of DI water, and 0.2 ml of sodium borate buffer is sterilized (*see* **Note 3**) and added to the pellet.
4. QD-Sulfo-NHS pellet is then dissolved in the above peptide containing solution using an ultrasonic cleaner.
5. RGD peptide is allowed to react with QDs bound to Sulfo-NHS at 4°C overnight. After the overnight reaction, RGD peptide replaces Sulfo-NHS to get bound to the QD to form a QD-peptide complex.
6. Any excess CGGGRGD peptide is removed via centrifugation at 4,000 rpm for 90 min.
7. Bioconjugated QDs pellet is then dissolved in 2 ml of sterile DI water using an ultrasonic cleaner and wrapped in tin foil before storing at 4°C.
8. Bioconjugated QDs can be further diluted in DMEM to obtain 0.5, 5, 20, and 50 nM concentrations.

3.2. Culture and Expansion of Human Mesenchymal Stem Cells

1. Primary human MSCs are extracted from the human bone marrow using RossetteSep procedure, cultured in DMEM, and maintained at 37°C.
2. When the cells approached confluence, they are serially passaged using trypsin/EDTA.
3. Human MSCs from passage #3–4 are re-plated onto a six-well tissue culture treated dish with 5,000 cells per well and used for cell labeling experiments with bioconjugated QDs.

4. Cultures are kept overnight in 2 ml of DMEM to allow cell attachment.
5. Upon microscopic confirmation of cell attachment, hMSCs are gently washed several times with PBS to remove any cell debris (**Note 5**).

3.3. Incubation of Human Mesenchymal Stem Cells with Bioconjugated Quantum Dots

1. To determine the optimal labeling concentration, hMSCs are incubated with different concentrations of bioconjugated QDs, i.e., 0.5, 5, 20, and 50 nM for 16–20 h (*see* **Note 6**).
2. To determine the optimal labeling time, hMSCs are incubated with bioconjugated QDs at a concentration of 30 nM for 5 min, 30 min, 2 h, and 16–20 h (*see* **Note 7**).
3. After incubation, QD-labeled hMSCs are washed several times with PBS to remove unbound bioconjugated QDs (*see* **Note 5**) and then suspended in 2 ml of DMEM.
4. Brightfield and fluorescence microscopy (*see* **Note 8**) are performed to determine the optimal QD concentration and time for labeling hMSCs (pictures not shown).

3.4. Test the Effects of QD Labeling on Cell Proliferation

1. The presence of cadmium and selenium in the core of QDs makes QDs susceptible to toxicity (33, 34). To determine whether QD bioconjugates are cytotoxic, hMSCs (5,000 cell/well) are incubated with the bioconjugated QDs with an optimized 30 nM concentration (*see* **Note 8**) and optimized incubation time of 16–20 h.
2. After incubation, QD-labeled hMSCs are washed several times with PBS to remove unbound bioconjugated QDs (*see* **Note 5**) and then suspended in 2 ml of DMEM for up to an additional 22 days, with DMEM change every 3–4 days.
3. Brightfield and fluorescence microscopy (*see* **Note 8**) are performed at various time points (days 0, 4, 7, and 22) to determine whether QD labeling negatively affects cell proliferation and QD labeling is retained in replicated hMSCs (**Fig. 4.1**).
4. Cell viability is assessed using trypan blue solution (**Fig. 4.2**) (22, 34). QD labeled and unlabeled hMSCs are trypsinized and centrifuged at 500 rcf for 5 min to produce a pellet. Cells are then suspended in 2 ml of DMEM. A total of 10 μl of this cell suspension is mixed with 10 μl of trypan blue dye in a sterile glass tube. Cell viability for various time points (Day 0, 7, 14 and 22) is determined by using a hemacytometer and counting the number of live cells vs. dead cells.

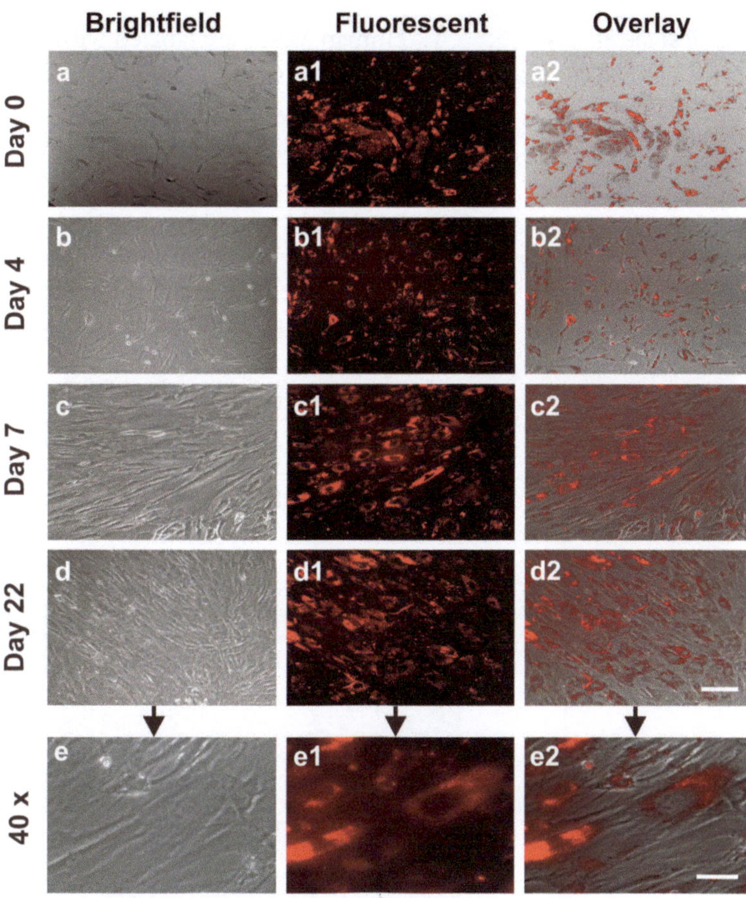

Fig. 4.1. Human mesenchymal stem cells (hMSCs) labeled with bioconjugated quantum dots (QDs) undergo proliferation up to the tested 22 days. hMSCs after 16-h incubation with bioconjugated QDs (30 nM) (**a–a2**). Following the removal of extracellular QDs, QD-labeled hMSCs and unlabeled hMSCs of the same subpopulation were continuously cultured for 4, 7, and 22 days (**b–b2, c–c2, d–d2**, respectively). Scale bar: 30 μm. QDs were internalized in the cytoplasm, even after 22 days of culture-expansion (**e–e2**), clearly observed in fluorescent (**e1**) and overlay (**e2**) images, apparently endocytosed as aggregates. Scale bar: 5 μm.

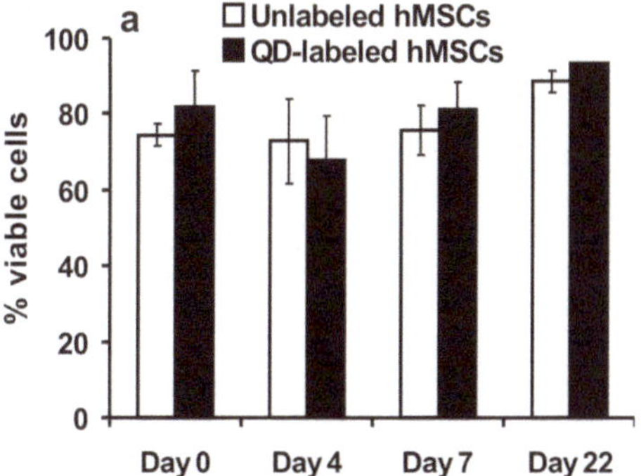

Fig. 4.2. Cell viability. Cell viability lacked statistically significant difference between QD-labeled hMSCs and unlabeled hMSCs. With or without QD labeling, substantial number of hMSCs remained viable (range: 67–93%).

3.5. Test the Effects of QD Labeling on Osteogenic Differentiation of hMSCs

1. Human MSCs are labeled with QD bioconjugates overnight (*see* **Notes 6** and 7) and unlabeled hMSCs served as control.
2. QD labeled and unlabeled hMSCs are treated with osteogenic medium for up to 28 days (22–24) with osteogenic medium changes every 3–4 days.
3. Brightfield and fluorescence microscopy (*see* **Note 8**) are performed to determine whether QD labeling negatively affects osteogenic cell differentiation as compared to unlabeled cells and QD labeling is retained in differentiated cells (**Fig. 4.3**).
4. Differentiation of labeled and unlabeled hMSCs into osteogenic cells is determined qualitatively by alkaline phosphatase reactivity for 14 days and calcium content for 28 days (25–28).

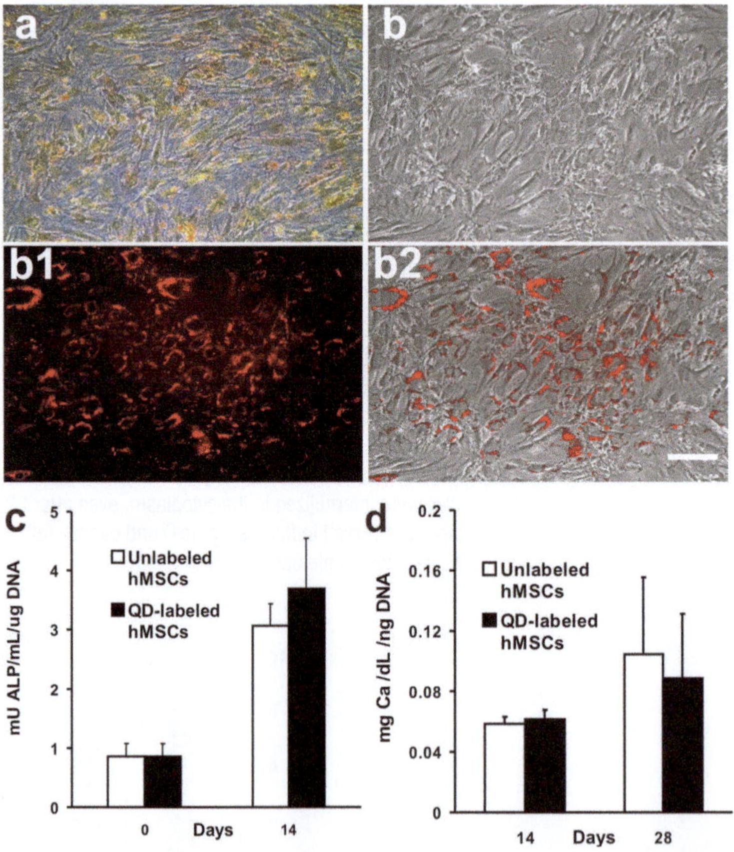

Fig. 4.3. Quantum dot (QD) labeling of human mesenchymal stem cells (hMSCs) during osteogenic differentiation. **a** Expression of alkaline phosphatase (ALP) during osteogenic differentiation of QD-labeled hMSCs. **b–b2** QDs remained in hMSCs during osteogenic differentiation (**b**) brightfield image of hMSCs labeled with QDs; **b1** fluorescent image of **b1** showing QD labeling; **b2** overlay of (**b**) and (**b1**) (**c** and **d**) No significant differences in ALP content and calcium production between QD-labeled and unlabeled hMSC-derived osteoblasts, respectively. Scale: 30 μm.

3.6. Test the Effects of QD Labeling on Chondrogenic Differentiation of hMSCs

1. Human MSCs are labeled with QD bioconjugates overnight (*see* **Notes 6** and 7) and unlabeled hMSCs served as control.
2. Chondrogenic differentiation of QD labeled and unlabeled hMSCs is performed in pellet culture since 2D culture of hMSCs and/or chondrocytes may lead to induce de-differentiation (22, 32). Upon 80–90% confluence, QD-labeled or unlabeled hMSCs are trypsinized, centrifuged for 8 min at 500 rcf, and then suspended with a final density of 5 M cells/ml. Drops of 50 μl cell suspension (approx. 250,000 cells) are slowly placed into each of 24-well untreated culture dishes, followed by 3-h incubation at 37°C to allow for cell attachment.
3. After incubation, QD-labeled and unlabeled hMSCs are incubated in chondrogenic medium for up to 28 days with chondrogenic medium changes every 3–4 days.
4. Brightfield and fluorescence microscopy (*see* **Note 8**) was performed to determine whether QD labeling negatively affects chondrogenic cell differentiation as compared to unlabeled cells and QD labeling is retained in differentiated cells (**Fig. 4.4**).
5. Alcian blue labels glycosaminoglycans and is a conventional marker for chondrogenesis. Differentiation of labeled and unlabeled hMSCs into chondrogenic cells is determined by measuring Glycosaminoglycan (GAG) content, an indication of biosynthesis of cartilage matrix (23, 26, 27, 29).

3.7. Test the Effects of QD Labeling on Adipogenic Cell Differentiation of hMSCs

1. Human MSCs are labeled with QD bioconjugates overnight (*see* **Notes 6** and 7) and unlabeled hMSCs served as control (*see* **Note 9**).
2. QD labeled and unlabeled hMSCs are treated with adipogenic medium for up to 28 days with adipogenic medium changes every 3–4 days (26, 31–33).
3. Brightfield and fluorescence microscopy (*see* **Note 8**) are performed to determine whether QD labeling negatively affects adipogenic cell differentiation as compared to unlabeled cells and QD labeling is retained in differentiated cells (**Fig. 4.5**).
4. Oil-Red O staining is used to detect lipid vacuole formation in QD labeled and unlabeled hMSCs (26, 31–33).
5. Differentiation of QD labeled and unlabeled hMSCs into adipogenic cells is also determined by measuring Glycerol content (26, 33).

3.8. Data Analysis and Statistics

Quantitative analyses are applied to all numerical data including cell viability, alkaline phosphatase (ALP) and calcium content for osteogenic differentiation, glycosaminoglycan (GAG) content for

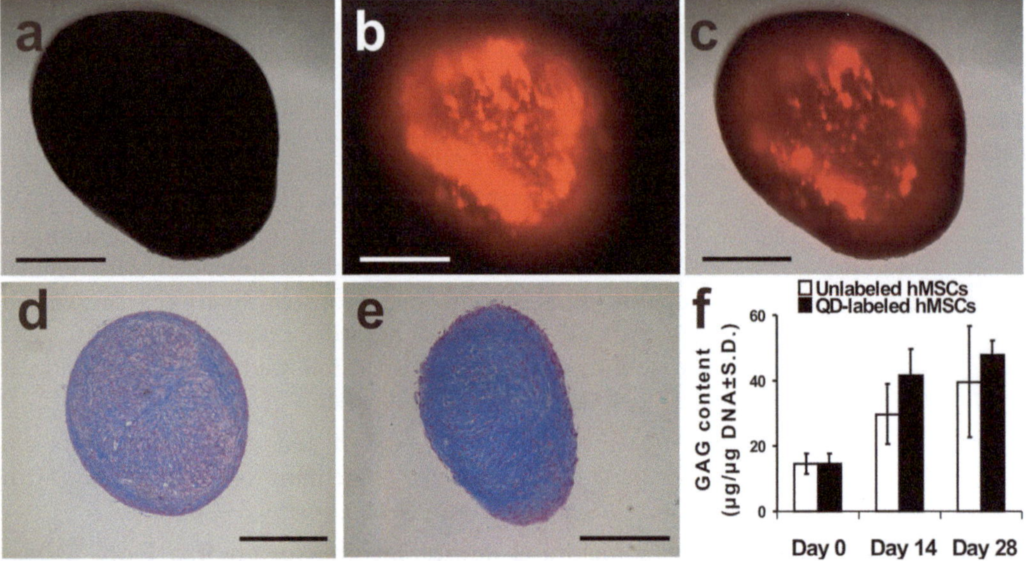

Fig. 4.4. Quantum dot (QD) labeling of human mesenchymal stem cells (hMSCs) during chondrogenic differentiation (**a–c**) QD labeling of hMSCs during chondrogenic differentiation in pellet culture (**a**: Brightfield; **b**: Fluorescent; **c**: Overlay). **d** and **e** Positive alcian blue staining of QD labeled or unlabeled hMSCs during chondrogenic differentiation. **f** No statistically significant difference in glycosaminoglycan (GAG) content between QD labeled and unlabeled hMSC-derived chondrocytes. Scale bar: 250 μm.

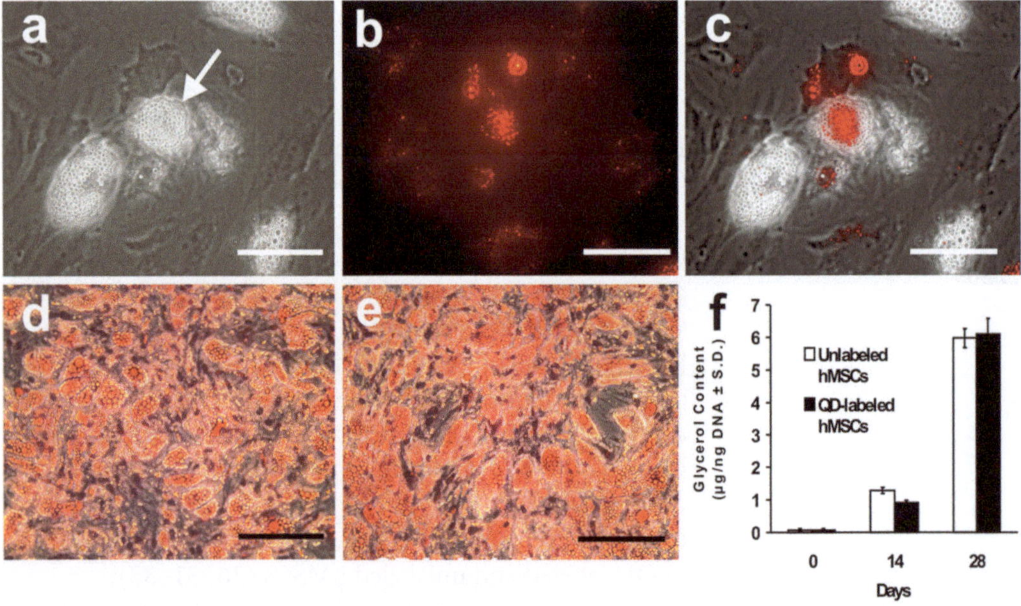

Fig. 4.5. Quantum dot (QD) labeling of human mesenchymal stem cells (hMSCs) during adipogenic differentiation. **a–c** Formation of intracellular lipid vacuoles in QD-labeled hMSCs during adipogenic differentiation. *Arrow points* to intracellular lipid vacuole. Scale bar: 50 μm. **d** and **e** *Oil-red* O staining showing adipogenesis formation without (**d**) or with (**e**) QD labeling. Scale bar: 100 μm. **f** No statistically significant difference in glycerol content between QD labeled and unlabeled hMSC-derived adipocytes.

chondrogenic differentiation, and glycerol content for adipogenic differentiation at various time points. ANOVA with bonferroni tests are applied at an alpha level of 0.05.

4. Notes

1. This protocol can be adapted probably for all adherent cells such as hMSCs, osteoblasts, fibroblasts, etc. (35, 36).
2. Multiplexing QDs (multiple color QDs) from different companies come in a different concentration, which should be taken into account before conjugation.
3. QD bioconjugation protocol should be strictly followed under sterile conditions after sterilizing various solutions. Use syringe and 0.22-μm filter to sterilize solutions.
4. We have tested both Evident Technology's Fort Orange QDs and Invitrogen's Green Dots for labeling hMSCs. This presently described protocol should work with QDs of different colors from both Evident and Invitrogen.
5. Upon overnight labeling of hMSCs with QD bioconjugates, it is difficult to remove unbound QDs as they remain stuck to the plate. Despite washing several (5, 6) times, some unboumd QDs are likely to remain in culture.
6. Since QD bioconjugates are endocytosed by hMSCs, overnight labeling likely provides sufficient time for QD internalization.
7. While incubating 5,000 cells/well overnight with QD bioconjugates, mix 30 nM QDs in 0.5 ml of DMEM prior to addition to cell culture.
8. Visualize QD-labeled cells in a dark room under fluorescent filter.
9. For adipogenic differentiation, ensure that the cells are confluent before adding adipogenic differentiating medium.

Acknowledgments

The following individuals are gratefully acknowledged for discussion and technical assistance: Dr. Paul Clark, Dr. Eduardo Moioli, Mr. Hai Do, and Mr. Neehar Bhatnagar. This research was supported by NIH grants DE15391 and EB02332 to J.J.M.

References

1. Dubertret, B., Skourides, P., Norris, D. J., Noireaux, V., Brivanlou, A. H., and Libchaber, A. (2002) In vivo imaging of quantum dots encapsulated in phospholipid micelles. *Science* **298**, 1759–62.
2. Orlic, D., Hill, J. M., and Arai, A. E. (2002) Stem cells for myocardial regeneration. *Circ. Res.* **91**, 1092–102.
3. Rahaman, M. N. and Mao, J. J. (2005) Stem cell based composite tissue constructs for regenerative medicine. *Biotechnol. Bioeng.* **91**, 261–84.
4. Terasaki, M. (1989) Fluorescent labeling of endoplasmic recticulum. *Methods Cell Biol.* **29**, 125–35.
5. Srivastava, S. C., Straub, R. F., and Meinken, G. E. (1990) Recent developments in blood cell labeling research. *Acta Radiol. Suppl.* **374**, 103–08.
6. Sugaya, A., Chudler, E. H., and Byers, M. R. (1994) Uptake of exogenous fluorescent Di-I by intact junctional epithelium of adult rats allows retrograde labeling of trigeminal sensory neurons. *Brain Res.* **653**, 330–34.
7. Marks, K. M. and Nolan, G. P. (2006) Chemical labeling strategies for cell biology. *Nat. Methods* **3**, 591–96.
8. Lippincott-Schwartz, J. and Smith, C. L. (1997) Insights into secretory and endocytic membrane traffic using green fluorescent protein chimeras. *Curr. Opin. Neurobiol.* **7**, 631–39.
9. Daly, C. J. and McGrath, J. C. (2003) Fluorescent ligands, antibodies, and proteins for the study of receptors. *Pharmacol. Ther.* **100**, 101–18.
10. Stahl, A., Wu, X., Wenger, A., Klagsbrun, M., and Kurschat, P. (2005) Endothelial progenitor cell sprouting in spheroidcultures is resistant to inhibition by osteoblasts: a model for bone replacement grafts. *FEBS Lett.* **579**, 5338–842.
11. Frangioni, J. V. (2003) In vivo near-infrared fluorescence imaging. *Curr. Opin. Chem. Biol.* **7**, 626–34.
12. Frangioni, J. V. (2006) Self-illuminating quantum dots light the way. *Nat. Biotechnol.* **24**, 326–28.
13. Bruchez, M. P. (2005) Turning all the lights on: quantum dots in cellular assays. *Curr. Opin. Chem. Biol.* **9**, 533–37.
14. Chan, W. C. (2006) Bionanotechnology progress and advances. *Biol. Blood Marrow Transplant.* **12**, 87–91.
15. Bruchez, M., Jr., Moronne, M., Gin, P., Weiss, S., and Alivisatos, A. P. (1998) Semiconductor nanocrystals as fluorescent biological labels. *Science* **281**, 2013–6.
16. Chan, W. C., Maxwell, D. J., Gao, X., Bailey, R. E., Han, M., and Nie, S. (2002) Luminescent quantum dots for multiplexed biological detection and imaging. *Curr. Opin. Biotechnol.* **13**, 40–6.
17. Peng, Z. A. and Peng, X. (2001) Formation of high-quality CdTe, CdSe, and CdS nanocrystals using CdO as precursor. *J. Am. Chem. Soc.* **123**, 183–4.
18. Alivisatos, P. (2004) The use of nanocrystals in biological detection. *Nat. Biotechnol.* **22**, 47–52.
19. Jaiswal, J. K. and Simon, S. M. (2004) Potentials and pitfalls of fluorescent quantum dots for biological imaging. *Trends Cell Biol.* **14**, 497–504.
20. Jaiswal, J. K., Mattoussi, H., Mauro, J. M., and Simon, S. M. (2003) Long-term multiple color imaging of live cells using quantum dot bioconjugates. *Nat. Biotechnol.* **21**, 47–51.
21. Estrada, C. R., Salanga, M., Bielenberg, D. R., Harrell, W. B., Zurakowski, D., Zhu, X., et al. (2006) Behavioral profiling of human transitional cell carcinoma ex vivo. *Cancer Res.* **66**, 3078–86.
22. Alhadlaq, A. and Mao, J. J. (2004) Mesenchymal stem cells: isolation and therapeutics. *Stem Cells Dev.* **13**, 436–48.
23. Alhadlaq, A. and Mao, J. J. (2005) Tissue-engineered osteochondral constructs in the shape of an articular condyle. *J. Bone Joint Surg. Am.* **87**, 936–44.
24. Moioli, E. K., Hong, L., Guardado, J., Clark, P. A., and Mao, J. J. (2006) Sustained release of TGFbeta3 from PLGA microspheres and its effect on early osteogenic differentiation of human mesenchymal stem cells. *Tissue Eng.* **12**, 537–46.
25. Alhadlaq, A., Elisseeff, J. H., Hong, L., Williams, C. G., Caplan, A. I., Sharma, B., et al. (2004) Adult stem cell driven genesis of human-shaped articular condyle. *Ann. Biomed. Eng.* **32**, 911–23.
26. Alhadlaq, A. and Mao, J. J. (2005) Tissue-engineered osteochondral constructs in the shape of an articular condyle. *J. Bone Joint Surg. Am.* **87**, 936–44.
27. Marion, N. W., Liang, W., Reilly, G. C., Day, D. E., Rahaman, M. N., and Mao, J. J. (2005) Borate glass supports the in vitro osteogenic differentiation of human mesenchymal stem cells. *Mech. Adv. Mat. Struct.* **12**, 1–8.

28. Yourek, G. A., Patel, R., McCormick, S., Reilly, G. C., and Mao, J. J. (2004) Nanophysical properties of living cells: the Cytoskeleton. *Biol. Nanostruct. Appl. Nanostruct. Biol.* **2**, 69–97.
29. Stosich, M. S. and Mao, J. J. (2007) Adipose tissue engineering from human adult stem cells: clinical implications in plastic and reconstructive surgery. *Plast. Reconstr. Surg.* **119**, 71–83.
30. Stosich, M. S. and Mao, J. J. (2005) Stem cell based soft tissue grafts for plastic and reconstructive surgeries. *Sem. Plast. Surg.* **19**, 251–60.
31. Peptan, I. A., Hong, L., and Mao, J. J. (2006) Comparison of osteogenic potentials of visceral and subcutaneous adipose-derived cells of rabbits. *Plast. Reconstr. Surg.* **117**, 1462–70.
32. Jaiswal, J. K. and Simon, S. M. (2004) Potentials and pitfalls of fluorescent quantum dots for biological imaging. *Trends Cell Biol.* **14**, 497–504.
33. Derfus, A. M., Chan, W. C. W., and Bhatia, S. N. (2004) Probing the cytotoxicity of semiconductor quantum dots. *Nano Lett.* **4**, 11–18.
34. Alhadlaq, A. and Mao, J. J. (2003) Tissue-engineered neogenesis of human-shaped mandibular condyle from rat mesenchymal stem cells. *J. Dent. Res.* **82**, 950–55.
35. Friedenstein, A. J., Deriglasova, U. F., Kulagina, N. N., Panasuk, A. F., Rudakowa, S. F., Luria, E. A., and Ruadkow, I. A. (1974) Precursors for fibroblasts in different populations of hematopoietic cells as detected by the in vitro colony assay method. *Exp Hematol* **2**, 83–92.
36. Friedenstein, A. J., Gorskaja, J. F., and Kulagina, N. N. (1976) Fibroblast precursors in normal and irradiated mouse hematopoietic organs. *Exp Hematol* **4**, 267–74.

Chapter 5

Quantification of miRNA Abundance in Single Cells Using Locked Nucleic Acid-FISH and Enzyme-Labeled Fluorescence

Jing Lu and Andrew Tsourkas

Abstract

The ability to quantify miRNA abundance at the single-cell level and image its spatial distribution could lead to unique insight into the biological roles of miRNAs and miRNA-associated gene regulatory networks. This protocol describes a method for quantitatively imaging miRNAs in single cells using fluorescence in situ hybridization (FISH). The method combines the unique miRNA recognition properties of locked nucleic acid (LNA) with the signal amplification technology known as enzyme-labeled fluorescence (ELF). Although both approaches have previously been shown to increase detection specificity and/or sensitivity in FISH, combining these techniques into one protocol allows for single molecule detection. Specifically, individual miRNAs are identified as bright, photostable fluorescent spots. The dynamic range was found to span over three orders of magnitude and the average miRNA copy number per cell was within 17.5% of measurements acquired by quantitative RT-PCR.

Key words: miRNA, fluorescence in situ hybridization (FISH), locked nucleic acid (LNA), enzyme-labeled fluorescence (ELF), single molecule detection.

1. Introduction

In recent years, it has become well established that small RNAs are key regulators of gene expression and translation. In fact, one class of short noncoding RNAs (18–25 nt in length), termed microRNAs (MiRNAs), have been predicted to influence the regulation of over one third of all human genes (1). They have also been implicated in most major cellular processes

K. Shah (ed.), *Molecular Imaging*, Methods in Molecular Biology 680,
DOI 10.1007/978-1-60761-901-7_5,

including proliferation, apoptosis, developmental timing, hematopoiesis, and organogenesis (2). To date, there have over 600 miRNAs identified in humans (http://www.sanger.ac.uk/Software/Rfam/mirna/) (3).

Despite recent progress in miRNA discovery and our understanding of miRNA biogenesis and mechanism, the influence of miRNA on central signaling pathways and cell cycle control is still largely unknown (4). Elucidating these physiological roles of miRNA will likely require miRNA expression to be correlated with mRNA and protein abundance at the single-cell level, especially considering the complex stochastic nature of gene expression in mammalian cells and the impact of these fluctuations on phenotypic diversity and cell fate (5–8).

Although numerous techniques are available for studying miRNA expression, including Northern blot, microarrays, RNA-primed array-based Klenow enzyme assay (RAKE), and mirVana miRNA labeling and detection kits (Ambion), these techniques all require the lysis of a population of cells and thus do not allow miRNA abundance to be quantified at single-cell level. Single-cell PCR could provide one option for the quantification of RNA transcripts within single cells, but this technique can only be used to examine a small number of cells. Moreover, single-cell RT-PCR is laborious and can often result in poor sample quality, which can lead to ambiguous findings and erroneous conclusions. Therefore, a more suitable option for the single-cell analysis of miRNA may be fluorescence in situ hybridization (FISH). It has already been well established that locked nucleic acid (LNA) oligonucleotides can be used as effective hybridization probes, allowing miRNA to be visualized at the tissue, cellular, and even subcellular level (9–13). Further, LNA probes exhibit a remarkable affinity and specificity against RNA targets, allowing for the discrimination of even single-base mismatches (14–17). Unfortunately, traditional miRNA-FISH does not possess the sensitivity for the detection of single miRNAs, and thus cannot be used provide a quantitative measure of miRNA abundance within single cells.

To overcome the limited sensitivity of LNA-FISH, we have recently combined LNA-FISH with enzyme-labeled fluorescence (ELF) (18). ELF is a process whereby cleavage of a pro-luminescent substrate by phosphatase yields a brilliant, yellow-green fluorescent product at the site of enzymatic activity. The ELF precipitate is not only photostable compared to commonly used fluorophores but also results in labeling that is up to 40 times brighter than signals achieved with probes directly labeled with fluorophores (19). Consequently, individual miRNAs are identified as bright, photostable fluorescent spots and can be simply counted on a fluorescence microscopy image.

2. Materials

2.1. Cell Culture

1. Dulbecco's Modified Eagle's Medium (DMEM) supplemented with 10% fetal bovine serum (FBS) for HeLa and MCF-7 cell culture.
2. L-15 medium supplied with 2 mM glutamine and 15% FBS for MDA-MB-231 cell culture.
3. Solution of trypsin (0.25%) and ethylenediamine tetraacetic acid (EDTA) (1 mM).
4. Multi-chambered coverglass slides and 10-cm cell culture dishes (Lab-Tek, Nalge Nunc, Rochester, New York, United States).

2.2. Locked Nucleic Acid (LNA) Probes

LNA probes, e.g., 5′-CACAAACCATTATGTGCTGCTA-3′ for miR-15a and 5′-CCCCTATCACGATTAGCATTAA-3′ for miR-155, with digoxigenin (DIG) on the 3′ end. LNA probes can be purchased from Exiqon (*see* **Note 1**). 2.5 pmol of probe will be used for each hybridization. Probes purchased from Exiqon usually have a concentration of 25 μM. Dilute probes in a total volume of 250 μl nuclease-free water for a concentration of 100 nM as stock. Aliquot the stocks of LNA probe and store at –20°C or below (*see* **Note 2**). When in use, the probe will be further diluted in Hybridization buffer at a 1:10 ratio.

2.3. Fluorescence In Situ Hybridization (FISH)

1. 4% (wt/vol) paraformadelhyde in PBS, pH7.4. Dissolve EM-grade formaldehyde powder in 1× DEPC-PBS with stirring and heating. Cover the flask with aluminum foil to limit evaporation. Do not heat the solution to a boil. Once the powder is dissolved, let the solution cool to room temperature and subsequently filter it through a 0.2-μM filter (*see* **Note 3**).
2. Diethylpyrocarbonate (DEPC) (*see* **Note 4**).
3. Deionized formamide. Add 100 ml of ultra pure formamide to 5 g resin (AG501-XB, BioRad) and stir for 1 h at room temperature. Remove resin using Whatman No. 1 filter paper or a 0.2-μm filter (*see* **Note 5**).
4. 20× SSC.
5. 50× Denhardt's solution.
6. 20× (200 mM) Ribonucleoside Vanadyl Complex, RVC.
7. 50% dextran sulfate. Add 25 g of dextran sulfate to 50 ml DEPC-treated water and stir overnight.
8. *Escherichia coli* tRNA.

9. Hybridization buffer: 25% formamide, 0.05 M EDTA, 4× SSC, 10% dextran sulfate, 1× Denhardt's solution, 0.5 mg/ml *E. coli* tRNA and 20 mM RVC. To 14 ml DEPC-treated water, add 12.5 ml of deionized formamide, 10 ml of 20× SSC, 10 ml 50% dextran sulfate, 1 ml of 50× Denhardt's solution, and 2.5 ml 20× RVC for a total volume of 50 ml. Add 50 mg *E. coli* tRNA directly to the solution. Divide the hybridization buffer into 5-ml aliquots and store at –80°C. The hybridization buffer has a pH of approximately 6–6.5 (*see* **Note 6**).
10. Goat anti-DIG-alkaline phosphatase antibody (*see* **Note 7**).
11. ELF 97 mRNA in situ hybridization kit (Molecular Probes, Inc, Eugene, OR, USA).
12. Post-fixation solution: 2% formaldehyde, 20 mg/ml BSA in 1× PBS.

2.4. Hybridizer

Slide Moat (Model 240000, Boekel Scientific) (*see* **Note 8**).

2.5. Microscope

Olympus IX81 motorized inverted fluorescence microscope equipped with a back-illuminated EMCCD camera (Andor), an X-cite 120 excitation source (EXFO), and Sutter excitation and filter wheels. A UPLN 60× oil immersion objective, N.A. 0.9.

2.6. Filter Sets

All filter sets were purchased from Chroma Technology.

ELF (e460spuv, HQ535/50, Q505lp)

Hoescht (D350/50, D460/50, 400dclp)

2.7. Software

IPLab acquisition software with AutoQuant plug-in

ImageJ software (available from NIH website http://rsbweb.nih.gov/ij/).

3. Methods

We have previously demonstrated the utility of LNA-FISH and ELF signal amplification for the absolute quantification of miRNA in single cells (18). In brief, the cells cultured in multiple chambered slides were fixed using fresh 4% (wt/vol) paraformaldehyde (PFA) and prehybridized. This was followed by a 1-h hybridization step using a DIG-labeled LNA oligonucleotide probe complementary to the mature miRNA. The LNA probes were then labeled with alkaline phosphatase-conjugated anti-DIG antibodies. A highly fluorescent signal at the site of LNA hybridization was generated using ELF 97. Fluorescent images were acquired using an Olympus IX81 motorized inverted fluorescence microscope equipped with a back-illuminated EMCCD camera (Andor), an X-cite 120 excitation source (EXFO), and Sutter excitation and filter wheels. A UPLN 60× oil-immersion objective, N.A. 0.9, was used for all imaging experiments. For image analysis and signal quantification, the software IPlabs and ImageJ were used.

We described this method as highly sensitive and specific for miRNA detection. Specifically, by combining LNA hybridization probes with ELF signal amplification, single miRNAs could be visualized and counted to yield quantitative measures of miRNA expression. The dynamic range of this approach spanned more than three orders of magnitude (i.e., 1 to ~1,000 miRNAs per cell) directly and through the construction of standardization curves could also yield quantitative measurements on cells with higher miRNA copy numbers. Overall, LNA-ELF-FISH is extremely simple and yields reproducible data. Further, in contrast to RT-PCR, no cell lysis, miRNA purification, or sample enrichment steps are required and spatial information is retained.

Additional advantages of LNA-ELF-FISH include the long stokes shift and high photostability of the fluorescent precipitate formed with ELF. The long stokes shift results in low autofluorescence and the high photostability allows for repeated imaging. Moreover, the fluorescent precipitate is extremely bright and thus only short exposure times are needed (i.e., ~10 ms).

One potential shortcoming of LNA-ELF-FISH that is important to recognize is its reliance on the hybridization of a single LNA probe. Any nonspecific binding will result in a false-positive signal that can be mistaken for miRNA. Conversely, inefficient hybridization will result in an underestimate of target mRNA. Therefore, it becomes extremely important to use both positive and negative control probes to optimize the experimental conditions. Comparisons between the average copy number per cell determined by LNA-ELF-FISH and measurements obtained by quantitative RT-PCR is also recommended as an additional control.

3.1. LNA-ELF-FISH

1. Seed cells into multi-chambered coverglass slides and incubate under normal growth conditions overnight, reaching 50–70% confluency.
2. Wash cells in 500 μl 1× PBS three times, 5 min per wash (*see* **Note 9**).
3. Fix the cells with 500 μl 4% formaldehyde for 30 min at room temperature.
4. Wash slides three times with 500 μl 1× DEPC-treated PBS, 5 min per wash.

5. Permeabilize at 4°C in 500 μl 70% ethanol at least overnight. To prevent evaporation, cover the chamber slide with parafilm. The parafilm should be placed under the plastic cover.
6. Remove 70% ethanol and wash slides in 500 μl 1× DEPC-treated PBS once for 5 min.
7. Prehybridize cells in 250 μl Hybridization buffer, cover with parafilm and incubate in a humid chamber at 60°C for 2–4 h (*see* **Note 10**).
8. Perform FISH using 250 μl of LNA probes at a concentration of 10 nM at ~55°C for 1~3 h after prehybridization (*see* **Notes 11** and **12**).
9. Perform four stringent washes in 4× SSC (briefly), 2× SSC (30 min), 1× SSC (30 min), and 0.1× SSC (20 min) at 37°C (*see* **Note 13**).
10. Generate bright fluorescent precipitate at sites of miRNA hybridization according to the manual of ELF 97 mRNA In Situ Hybridization Kit.
11. Wash the cells in 500 μl 1× wash buffer (make 50 ml of 1× wash buffer from the 10× stock provided with the ELF kit) three times, 5 min each at room temperature (*see* **Note 14**).
12. Incubate cells in 200 μl blocking buffer (component B of ELF kit) in a humid chamber at room temperature for 1 h.
13. Add 2 μg/ml of goat anti-DIG-AP antibody in blocking buffer (diluted 1–250) to the cells and incubate at room temperature for 1 h. Use 250 μl per well (*see* **Note 15**).
14. After three washes in 1× wash buffer (5 min per wash), incubate cells in 200 μl ELF 97 phosphatase substrate working solution for 10–15 min. To make ELF 97 phosphatase substrate working solution, dilute ELF 97 phosphatase substrate (component D) tenfold into the developing buffer (component C). Filter the resulting solution into a sterile vial using a 0.2-μM pore-size filter. After filtration, dilute the substrate additive 1 (component E) and substrate additive 2 (component F) each 1:500 into the substrate working solution, vortex the solution well, and use it immediately or store it at 4°C in a sterile container for up to 48 h (*see* **Note 16**).
15. For long-term in situ signal preservation, quickly wash the sample with 1× wash buffer, two times. Postfix the samples by incubating the slides in post-fixation solution for 30 min at room temperature (*see* **Note 17**).

16. Counterstain the cells in 1 μg/ml Hoechst 33342 and mount in mounting solution (*see* **Note 18**).
17. Fluorescence imaging. The slides can be checked quickly for hybridization efficiency and background levels 1 h after mounting. However, fluorescence needs to be retrieved overnight to give the best results for visualization. Slides can be stored for months without losing their signals if kept at 4°C.

3.2. Image Acquisition and Analysis

1. Following in situ hybridization, acquire fluorescent images of cells. IPLab acquisition software can be used to acquire 3D images.
2. After randomly selecting cells in a field, take a 3D stack viewed image of single cells with 0.3-μm increments in the *z*-direction and a total of 35 sections.
3. Deconvolve the 3D images in IPLab using AutoQuant plug-in software.
4. Create a 2D image in IPLab using a maximum intensity merged image.
5. Process images in ImageJ using the following commands:(I) Process -> Sharpen, (II) Image -> type -> 8-bit and (III) Process -> binary -> make binary. Fluorescent images of individual miRNAs in single mammalian cells that have been processed are shown in **Fig. 5.1**.
6. Count the total number of isolated signals within single cells in ImageJ using the particle analysis counter program (Analyze -> analyze particles).
7. In cells where the number of miRNAs exceeds ~1,000 copies, it will become increasingly difficult to discern individual fluorescent spots. At very high miRNA copy numbers (>2,000), the entire cell will likely exhibit a nearly uniform fluorescent signal. For these cells, it is necessary to construct a standard curve to acquire a measure of miRNA copy number. This approach is described in Steps 8–12.
8. First, identify as many ‘countable’ cells as possible from the slide, i.e., cells that possess low enough miRNA copies to be accurately counted.
9. In ImageJ, count the miRNA copy numbers of these selected cells following Steps 1–6.
10. Measure the total integrated fluorescence of the ‘countable’ cells. Specifically, draw a region of interest (ROI) around individual cells and use the following command in ImageJ: Analyze->measure. Record the value listed under ‘IntDen’. Move the ROI to another location within the image that is devoid of cells to acquire a background

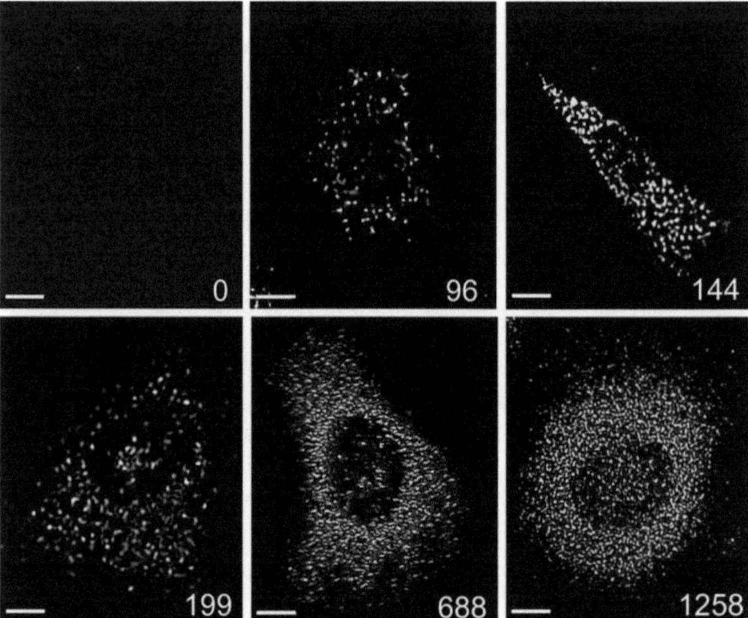

Fig. 5.1. Fluorescent images of individual miRNAs in HeLa cells. HeLa cells were stained with an LNA probe for miR-15a followed by ELF signal amplification. Each bright fluorescent spot represents a single miRNA. The total number of miRNAs identified in each cell is shown in the lower right corner of each panel. Scale bars, 5 μm.

measure of 'IntDen'. Determine the difference between these two measurements. This value is the total integrated fluorescence of the cell.

11. Draw a linear correlation between the total integrated fluorescence and the miRNA copy number for all of the 'countable' cells. Fit the data with a trend line.
12. Measure the total integrated fluorescence of 'uncountable' cells, i.e., cells in which individual miRNA cannot be discerned, using the same method as described in Step 10.
13. Plug the total integrated fluorescence measurement acquired from each uncountable cell into the trend line equation from Step 11. Solve for the unknown, i.e., miRNA copy number. Quantitative analysis of miRNA in three cancer cell lines is provided in **Fig. 5.2**.

4. Notes

1. Each probe was designed to hybridize to the mature miRNA sequences. On average, 30% of the oligonucleotides within the sequence are modified to an LNA.

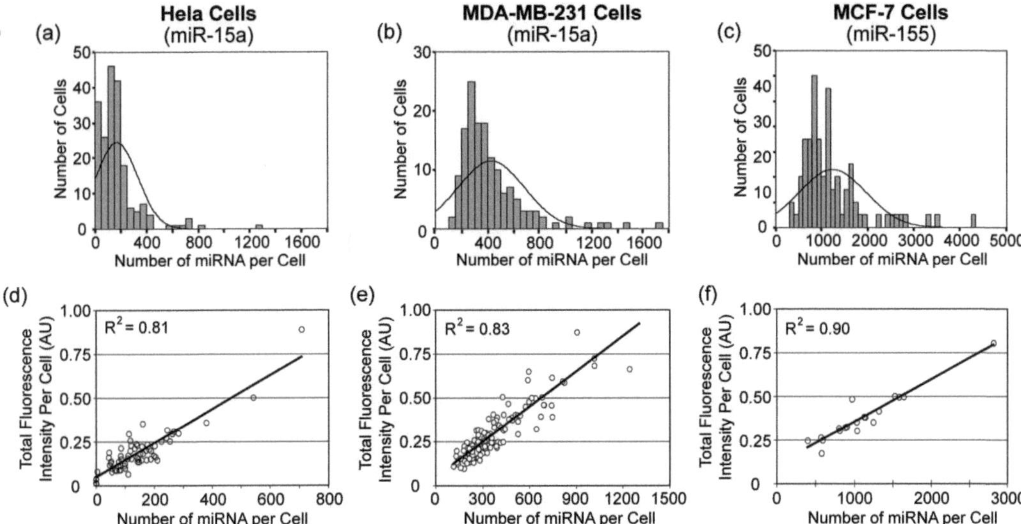

Fig. 5.2. Quantitative analysis of miRNA copy number in HeLa, MDA-MB231, and MCF-7 cells. The total number of miR-15a molecules in (**a**) Hela cells ($n = 198$) and (**b**) MDA-MB-231 cells ($n = 148$) was determined following LNA-ELF-FISH. Similarly, the total number of miR-155 in (**c**) MCF-7 cells ($n = 84$) was also quantified. Since individual miRNA could not be discerned in some cells with high miRNA copy number, an estimate was obtained by first drawing a linear correlation between miRNA copy number and total cellular fluorescence. The correlations for (**d**) Hela, (**e**) MDA-MB-231, and (**f**) MCF-7 cells are shown. The equation describing each correlation was used to calculate the miRNA copy numbers in cells with high expression, based on their fluorescence intensity (from Lu and Tsourkas (18)).

Probes in this study were prelabeled with DIG on the 3′ end, but they can also be unlabeled or labeled with FITC or biotin etc on 5′ and/or 3′ ends. It is very important to use control probes to check the reliance of the method, including a positive probe, for example, U6; and a scrambled sequence as negative probe.

2. Labeled LNA probes should be aliquoted when received since their efficiency decreases with multiple freeze and thaw cycles. Labeled probes can be stored for up to 2 years at –20°C until use.
3. PFA is a possible carcinogen and harmful by inhalation, ingestion or skin absorption. Use gloves and work in a fume hood. Aliquot and store at –20°C; thaw on the same day, before the fixation step.
4. DEPC is an eye skin and respiratory tract irritant and toxic by ingestion. Use gloves and work in fume hood.
5. Formamide is a teratogen and a mutagen. Can cause harm to lungs and liver by high doses of inhalation. Contact with eyes and skin should be prevented. Work in a fume hood to avoid inhaling fumes. Formamide waste should be collected and disposed according to local rules and regulations. It should be kept in the dark at 4°C.

6. If the hybridization temperature exceeds 55°C, add citric acid to 9.2 mM final concentration, as the pH of formamide increases at high temperatures leading to loss of hybridization efficiency.
7. If a biotin labeled LNA probe is used, streptavidin-AP should be used. However, if LNA-ELF-FISH is extended to tissue sections such as the liver, where a large amount of biotin may be present, endogenous biotin has to be blocked before applying streptavidin-AP.
8. It is very important to put slides in a humid chamber during hybridization. This is accomplished by placing wet (western blot) filter paper or a wet paper towel in the incubator. The liquid used to humidify the chamber should ideally possess the same concentration of formamide and SSC as in the hybridization buffer; however, in most cases DEPC-treated water is sufficient.
9. Some cells types such as NIH3T3 cells are sensitive to temperature; use warm PBS or even warm fixative.
10. We prehybridize at temperatures of 17–22°C below the predicted Tm value of the LNA oligonucleotide probe used.
11. The optimal level of formamide can be determined to gain maximal signal-to-background ratio. Here the optimal level of formamide used during hybridization and washing was empiricaly determined to be 25%.
12. The optimal hybridazation temperature is 20–22°C below the Tm of the LNA probes. Due to enhanced hybridization properties of LNA, hybridizing for longer than 3 h does not improve the signal intensity. Most of the probe will hybridize within the first hour.
13. Use prewarmed SSC solution (37°C). Stringency washes can be adjusted to achieve the best signal-to-noise ratio.
14. It is very important that do not let the slide dry out at any stage of the ELF detection protocol.
15. If the sample is expected to contain significant endogenous phosphastase activity, we recommend incubating samples for 1 h in 1 mM levamisole diluted with the blocking reagent, just prior to adding the phosphatase conjugate.
16. Do not allow the fluorescent signal to develop for more than 2 h because a high background consisting of large fluorescent crystals and nonspecific labeling may result.
17. It is very important to postfix the cells, or else the localized punctuate fluorescence may suffer from diffusion.

18. In general, Hoescht was preferred over DAPI because DAPI would often exhibit a bright fluorescent signal even with the ELF filter set, making it difficult to count the individual bright spots corresponding to single miRNA.

Acknowledgments

The authors thank Dr. Steven Bartush from Exiqon for LNA probe design. This work was supported by the National Institutes of Health (NCI) R21-CA125088 and R21-CA116102; the National Science Foundation BES-0616031; and the American Cancer Society RSG-07-005-01.

References

1. Lewis, B. P., Burge, C. B., and Bartel, D. P. (2005) Conserved seed pairing, often flanked by adenosines, indicates that thousands of human genes are microRNA targets. *Cell* **120**, 15–20.
2. Kim, V. N. (2005) MicroRNA biogenesis: coordinated cropping and dicing. *Nat. Rev. Mol. Cell Biol.* **6**, 376–85.
3. Griffiths-Jones, S. (2004) The microRNA Registry. *Nucleic Acids Res.* **32**, D109–11.
4. Chang, T. C. and Mendell, J. T. (2007) MicroRNAs in vertebrate physiology and human disease. *Annu. Rev. Genomics Hum. Genet.* **8**, 215–39.
5. Hume, D. A. (2000) Probability in transcriptional regulation and its implications for leukocyte differentiation and inducible gene expression. *Blood* **96**, 2323–8.
6. Kepler, T. B. and Elston, T. C. (2001) Stochasticity in transcriptional regulation: origins, consequences, and mathematical representations. *Biophys. J.* **81**, 3116–36.
7. Ross, I. L., Browne, C. M., and Hume, D. A. (1994) Transcription of individual genes in eukaryotic cells occurs randomly and infrequently. *Immunol. Cell Biol.* **72**, 177–85.
8. Swain, P. S., Elowitz, M. B., and Siggia, E. D. (2002) Intrinsic and extrinsic contributions to stochasticity in gene expression. *Proc. Natl. Acad. Sci. USA* **99**, 12795–800.
9. Kloosterman, W. P., Wienholds, E., de Bruijn, E., Kauppinen, S., and Plasterk, R. H. (2006) In situ detection of miRNAs in animal embryos using LNA-modified oligonucleotide probes. *Nat. Methods* **3**, 27–29.
10. Nelson, P. T., Baldwin, D. A., Kloosterman, W. P., Kauppinen, S., Plasterk, R. H., and Mourelatos, Z. (2005) RAKE and LNA-ISH reveal microRNA expression and localization in archival human brain. *RNA.* **12**, 187–91.
11. Politz, J. C., Zhang, F., and Pederson, T. (2006) MicroRNA-206 colocalizes with ribosome-rich regions in both the nucleolus and cytoplasm of rat myogenic cells. *Proc. Natl. Acad. Sci. USA* **103**, 18957–62.
12. Silahtaroglu, A. N., Nolting, D., Dyrskjot, L., Berezikov, E., Moller, M., Tommerup, N., and Kauppinen, S. (2007) Detection of microRNAs in frozen tissue sections by fluorescence in situ hybridization using locked nucleic acid probes and tyramide signal amplification. *Nat. Protoc.* **2**, 2520–8.
13. Wienholds, E., Kloosterman, W. P., Miska, E., Alvarez-Saavedra, E., Berezikov, E., de Bruijn, E., Horvitz, H. R., Kauppinen, S., and Plasterk, R. H. (2005) MicroRNA expression in zebrafish embryonic development. *Science* **309**, 310–1.
14. Chou, L. S., Meadows, C., Wittwer, C. T., and Lyon, E. (2005) Unlabeled oligonucleotide probes modified with locked nucleic acids for improved mismatch discrimination in genotyping by melting analysis. *Biotechniques* **39**, 644, 646, 648 passim.
15. Johnson, M. P., Haupt, L. M., and Griffiths, L. R. (2004) Locked nucleic acid (LNA)

single nucleotide polymorphism (SNP) genotype analysis and validation using real-time PCR. *Nucleic Acids Res.* **32**, e55.

16. Valoczi, A., Hornyik, C., Varga, N., Burgyan, J., Kauppinen, S., and Havelda, Z. (2004) Sensitive and specific detection of microRNAs by northern blot analysis using LNA-modified oligonucleotide probes. *Nucleic Acids Res.* **32**, e175.
17. You, Y., Moreira, B. G., Behlke, M. A., and Owczarzy, R. (2006) Design of LNA probes that improve mismatch discrimination. *Nucleic Acids Res.* **34**, e60.
18. Lu, J. and Tsourkas, A. (2009) Imaging individual microRNAs in single mammalian cells in situ. *Nucleic Acids Res.* **37**, e100.
19. Paragas, V. B., Zhang, Y. Z., Haugland, R. P., and Singer, V. L. (1997) The ELF-97 alkaline phosphatase substrate provides a bright, photostable, fluorescent signal amplification method for FISH. *J. Histochem. Cytochem.* **45**, 345–57.

Section II

Imaging in Pre-clinical Settings

Chapter 6

Imaging Fate of Stem Cells at a Cellular Resolution in the Brains of Mice

Khalid Shah

Abstract

Transplantation of genetically engineered cells into the central nervous system (CNS) offers immense potential for the treatment of several neurological disorders. Monitoring expression levels of transgenes and following changes in cell function and distribution over time is critical in assessing therapeutic efficacy of such cells in vivo. We detail a unique method to visualize the fate of human neural stem cells (NSC) and tumor cells at a cellular resolution in glioma bearing brains in vivo by using intravital-scanning microscopy in real-time. The ability to monitor fate of stem cells in disease models enables studies aimed at evaluating the efficacy of their treatment for CNS disorders.

Key words: Stem cells, glioma, in vivo intravital microscopy.

1. Introduction

Neural stem cells (NSC) are defined by their ability to self-renew and give rise to mature progenitors of neural lineages. The ability of NSC to migrate to diseased areas of the brain (1–3) and their capacity to differentiate into all neural and glial phenotypes (4) provides a powerful tool for targeting the treatment of both diffuse and localized neurologic disorders. Several studies have demonstrated the effectiveness of NSC transplantation in the treatment of neurodegenerative diseases, including spinal cord injury and brain tumors (1, 5–8). While these studies demonstrate the feasibility of NSC-based therapy, cellular delivery of therapeutic proteins via NSC grafts will likely require long-term transgene expression. In vivo assays that permit rapid assessment of the fate

K. Shah (ed.), *Molecular Imaging*, Methods in Molecular Biology 680,
DOI 10.1007/978-1-60761-901-7_6,

of transplanted NSC, transgene expression, and differentiation are urgently needed to objectively compare therapeutic efficacies of different paradigms. Several imaging modalities, including magnetic resonance imaging (MRI) and fluorescence imaging provide means of tracking transplanted cells in vivo (9–11) but these techniques are often constrained by limited sensitivity and/or retention of the label (12, 13). Laser scanning microscopic methods, e.g., intravital and multiphoton microscopy are becoming more widely used to image cellular details in vivo as they permit in vivo detection of fluorescent reporter proteins within intact tissue (14). To view stem cell fate in mouse model of glioma in real time, we have designed a surgical protocol and used fluorescently labeled stem cell and brain tumor cells. This chapter will detail anesthesia, surgical preparation, craniotomy, animal recovery, and imaging procedures in mouse glioma models using glioma cells and stem cells expressing different fluorescent proteins.

2. Materials

2.1. Cell Culture

1. Neural stem cells (NSC) expressing DsRed2 (NSC-DsRed2) (15)
2. Glioma cells (Gli36) expressing GFP (Gli36-GFP) (15)
3. Glioma cell medium: Dulbecco's Modified Eagle's Medium (DMEM) (Gibco/BRL, Bethesda, MD) supplemented with 10% fetal bovine serum (FBS, HyClone, Ogden, UT)
4. NSC medium: (DMEM/F-12 Gibco, 0.6% D-glucose (Sigma-Aldrich), 0.5% albumax (Gibco), 0.5% glutamine (Gibco), recombinant human FGF (20 ng/ml) (R & D Systems), recombinant human EGF (20 ng/ml) (R & D Systems), N2 supplements (Gibco), and 1% non-essential amino acids (Cellgro), 1 mM sodium pyruvate (Cellgro), 26 mM sodium bicarbonate)
5. Solution of trypsin (0.25%) and ethylenediamine tetraacetic acid (EDTA) (1 mM) from Gibco/BRL
6. 1× penicillin/streptomycin (from 200× stock, Invitrogen)

2.2. Cell Transplantation and Imaging In Vivo

1. SCID mice (6–8 weeks old; Charles River Laboratories, Wilmington, MA)
2. Anesthesia: ketamine, 120 mg/kg; xylazine 16.0 mg/kg
3. Stereotaxic frame (Harvard Apparatus, Cambridge, MA)
4. Hand-held micro-drill (Fine Science tools, Foster city, CA)
5. 0.45-mm Round drill burr (VWR, Willard, OH).

6. Fine scissors (Fine Science tools, Foster city, CA)
7. 1-ml syringes with 27-gauge needle (Becton and Dickinson, Franklin Lakes, NJ)
8. Cotton-tipped applicators (Scientifics)
9. Forceps, angled and straight and ultrafine angled (Fine Science tools, Foster city, CA)
10. Stereo dissecting microscope – variable magnification (1× to 4.5×) (Nikon, Melville, NY)
11. 10-μl 26-gauge Hamilton Gastight 1701 syringe (Hamilton, Reno, NV)
12. 70% Isopropyl alcohol (Fisher Scientific, Pittsburgh, PA)
13. Betadyne solution (Bruce Medical, Waltham, MA)
14. Bone wax (Ethicon, Somerville, NJ)

2.3. Intravital Laser Scanning Microscope

To acquire optical sections in the cranial window in the brain, we use a prototype multichannel upright laser scanning fluorescent microscope IV100 (Olympus, Japan). The microscope has a custom-designed stage, which is equipped with a heating plate regulated by a thermostat (37°C). Lasers used for excitation include a 488-nm argon laser, a 561-nm solid-state yellow laser, and a 633-nm HeNe-R laser. Emission signal is filtered using 505–525, 586–615, and 660–730 nm band-pass filters, respectively. Images are acquired with Fluoview imaging software (Olympus) and quantification is performed using Image J analysis software (version 1.40, freeware, NIH, http://rsbweb.nih.gov/ij/download.html).

3. Methods

3.1. Cell Culture

1. Culture human neural stem cells (NSC) and glioma cells (Gli36) in culturing medium as described below. For our studies, we used:
   (a) Human fetal neural stem cell line expressing DsRed2 (NSC-DsRed2) derived from the human diencephalic and telencephalic regions of 10–10.5 weeks gestational age from an aborted human Caucasian embryo (*see* **Note 1**).
   (b) Gli36-GFP, a human glioma cell line expressing GFP whose in vitro and in vivo characteristics have been described elsewhere (1, 16) (*see* **Note 1**).
2. Culture NSC-DsRed2 and glioma cells in their respective culturing medium at 37°C in a humidified atmosphere with

5% CO_2 and $1\times$ penicillin/streptomycin (Invitrogen, Grand Island, NY). When cells reach 70–80% confluency, subculture cells in a 1:4 (NSC-DsRed2) or 1:5 (glioma cell) ratio.

3.2. Cell Transplantation and Imaging

This protocol is used for transplantation of glioma cells expressing different fluorescent markers in mice and describes the dual imaging of NSC fate and glioma progression in mice glioma model.

3.2.1. Anesthetizing and Handling the Animal

1. Grasp the animal firmly with one hand and anesthetize by injecting ketamine and xylazine intraperitoneally (120 mg/kg ketamine and 16 mg/kg xylazine) (*see* **Note 2**).

3.2.2. Surgery

1. Secure animal on a stereotactic head frame and trim dorsal surface of the animal's head (*see* **Note 3**) (**Fig. 6.1**).

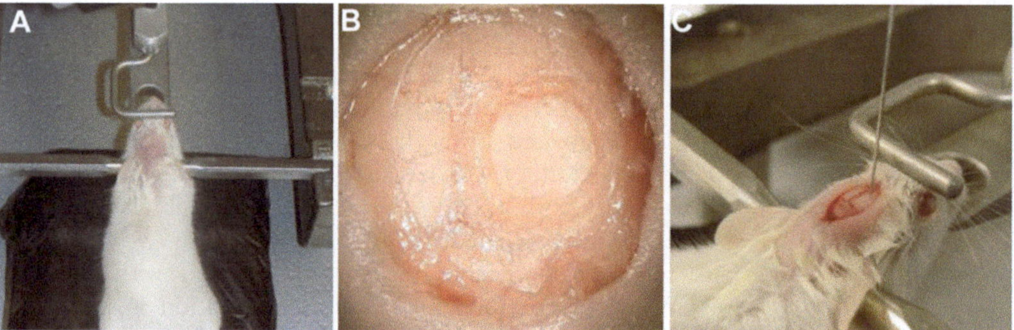

Fig. 6.1. Creation of a cranial window and implantation of cells: **a** Anesthetized mouse in a stereotax being implanted with glioma cells. **b** Cranial window created after drilling through the bone and exposing the cortical surface. **c** Implantation of cells in a cranial window using a Hamilton syringe.

2. Disinfect the shaved area by applying alternating two coats of Betadyne and isopropyl alcohol.
3. Using scissors and forceps, remove the skin from the disinfected region and use a dry cotton swab to completely remove the periosteum membrane from the exposed skull surface (*see* **Note 4**)
4. Gently create a square approximately 4 × 4 mm diameter into the right hemisphere of the skull surface with the drill. Position the drill with the prospective window site and begin drilling through the bone, exposing the cortical surface. Place several pieces of saturated gel foam over the crevice (*see* **Note 5**).
5. Using an absorbent wedge, soak-up excess PBS and blood while being careful to prevent over-drying. Using a syringe, apply additional PBS to the gel foam as needed to maintain a moist environment. Depending on the extent of

bleeding, multiple washes and re-application of gel foam may be necessary.

3.2.3. Tumor Cell Implantation

1. Place 4-μl of Gli36-GFP glioma cells (100,000 cells) in a 10-μl 26-gauge Hamilton Gastight 1701 syringe needle and insert the needle to a specified depth into the left frontal lobe. In our experiments we use the following stereotactic co-ordinates (2.5 mm lateral and 0.5 mm caudal to bregma; depth 1.0 mm from dura).
2. Implant cells over a period of 4 min with 30 s intervals (*see* **Note 6**).
3. After implantation is complete, wait for 5 min and remove needle over a period of 10 min with an interval of 1 min.
4. Seal the burrow hole with Matrigel and close the wound with 4.0 vicryl or surgical staples.

3.3. Animal Recovery

For the most part, the animal should survive the procedure despite the absence of an external heat source. Make certain the animal is restrained and that it cannot cause harm to itself relative to the probe. When the animal is maintaining its own normal body temperature and has a reflexive response to toe-pinch stimulation, it is ready to be returned to a clean and un-occupied cage. The usual recovery time for this procedure can range from 2 to 12 h. If the animal has not resumed normal grooming and eating behavior beyond this time frame, it may require additional medical attention or euthanasia.

3.3.1. Preparation of Mouse for Intravital Fluorescence Microscopy

1. One week after glioma cell implantation, prepare mice for intravital microscopy.
2. Anesthetize the mouse by injecting ketamine and xylazine intraperitoneally (120 mg/kg ketamine and 16 mg/kg xylazine).
3. Secure animal on a stereotactic head frame and open the surgical staples to expose the cortical surface.
4. Transfer surgically exposed animal to the intravital imaging system.

3.3.2. Intravital Fluorescence Microscopy of Glioma Cells

1. Choose 4× objective for imaging and rapidly scan glioma cells with desired excitation at moderate speed with medium laser power and high PMT gain. For Gli36-GFP cells, we typically use 488-nm channel. Gradually increase power if unable to localize glioma cells within the field (*see* **Notes 7** and **8**).
2. To obtain a z-series of an average-sized tumor (20–40 μm in diameter) use 1-to 5-μm z-steps. For kinetic studies, a four-dimensional movie (z-series overtime) can be created

by acquiring multichannel image stack as well as varying power settings

3.3.3. Image Analysis

1. Transfer image stacks from the IV100 system which are stored as multi-layer tiff files.
2. Analyze images with Image J analysis software programme.

3.4. Stem Cell Implantation

1. Anesthetize and secure the same animals implanted with glioma cells on a stereotactic head frame as described in **Section 3.2**.
2. Drill the hole in the contralateral, right frontal lobe at the following coordinates: 2.5 mm lateral and 0.5 mm caudal to bregma; depth 1.0 mm from dura.
3. Place 4–5 μl of NSC-DsRed2 (500,000 cells) in a 10-μl 26-gauge Hamilton Gastight 1701 syringe needle and implant cells as described in **Section 3.2**.
4. Seal the burrow hole with Matrigel and close the wound with 4.0 vicryl or surgical staples and let the animal recover as described in **Section 3.3**.

3.5. In Vivo Intravital Microscopy of NSC and Glioma Cells

1. Three days post stem cell implantation, prepare mice for intravital microscopy by anesthetizing mouse by injecting ketamine and xylazine intraperitoneally.
2. Choose 4× objective for imaging and rapidly scan stem cells with desired excitation at moderate speed with medium laser power and high PMT gain as described in **Section 3.4.3**. For NSC-DsRed2 cells, we typically use 580-mn excitation channels.
3. Scan the animals again on day 7 and day 10 post-NSC implantation. In our case we look for migration of NSC toward gliomas (*see* **Note 9**) (**Fig. 6.2**).
4. Analyze image stacks from the IV100 system which are stored as multi-layer tiff files. There will be 200 images in a 2 -channel experiment and if 100 slices are acquired for each channel, the first 100 would be from channel 1 (488 nm channel), the next 100 would be from channel 2 (580 nm channel).

3.6. Tissue Processing

1. Immediately following the last imaging session, sacrifice mice and immerse brains in Tissue-Tek (Sakura Finetek, Torrence, California) on dry ice.
2. Using cryostat, cut 7 μm of coronal brain and mount them on slides.

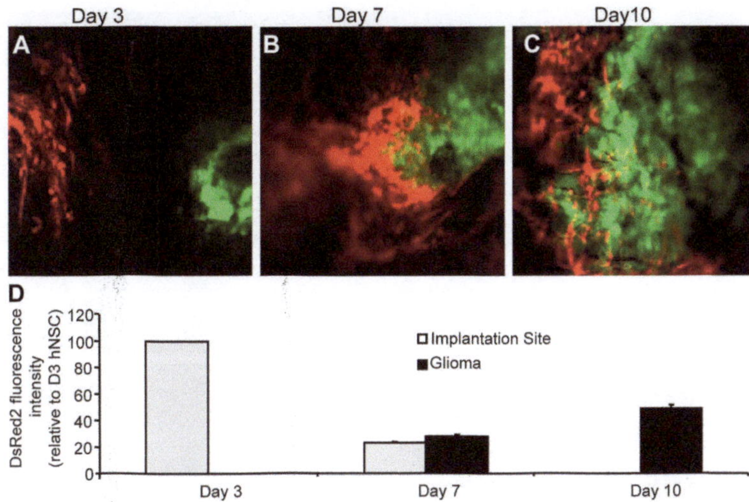

Fig. 6.2. NSC migrate into gliomas in vivo. Intravital microscopy of NSC-DsRed2 implanted in mice with established GFP-GFP gliomas on days 3 (**a**), 7 (**b**), and 10 (**c**) after NSC implantation. **d** Summary data of NSC cell density at the site of NSC implantation and co-localized with established glioma at 3, 7, and 10 days post-implantation (* $p < 0.05$ vs. NSC at implantation site). Magnification ×10. Adapted from Shah et al. (15) with permission from Society for Neuroscience.

3. Visualize slides on microscopy GFP and DsRed2 fluorescence on a confocal microscope (LSM Pascal, Zeiss).
4. View slides under phase contrast microscopy (to locate the cells and identify the focal plane) and finally under confocal microscopy (LSM Pascal, Zeiss). Excitation at 488 nm induces the green fluorescence for EGFR-GFP expression, while excitation at 510 nm induces red fluorescence for DsRed2 expression. Examples of the signals for Gli36-GFP and NSC-DsRed2 expression are shown in **Fig. 6.3**.
5. Sections can also be stained with different antibodies. In our studies, we stain for Nestin, GFAP, MAP-2, and Ki67 for 1 h in a blocking solution (0.3% BSA, 8% goat serum, and 0.3% Triton-X100) at room temperature (RT), followed by incubation at 4°C overnight with following primary antibodies diluted in blocking solution: (1) anti-human nestin (clone 10C2; Chemicon), (2) anti-human GFAP (Chemicon), and (3) anti-Ki67 (clone MIB-1; DAKO) and anti-MAP-2 (Chemicon).
6. Sections are washed three times with PBS, incubated in appropriate secondary antibody, and visualized using confocal microscope (LSM Pascal, Zeiss) (**Fig. 6.3**).

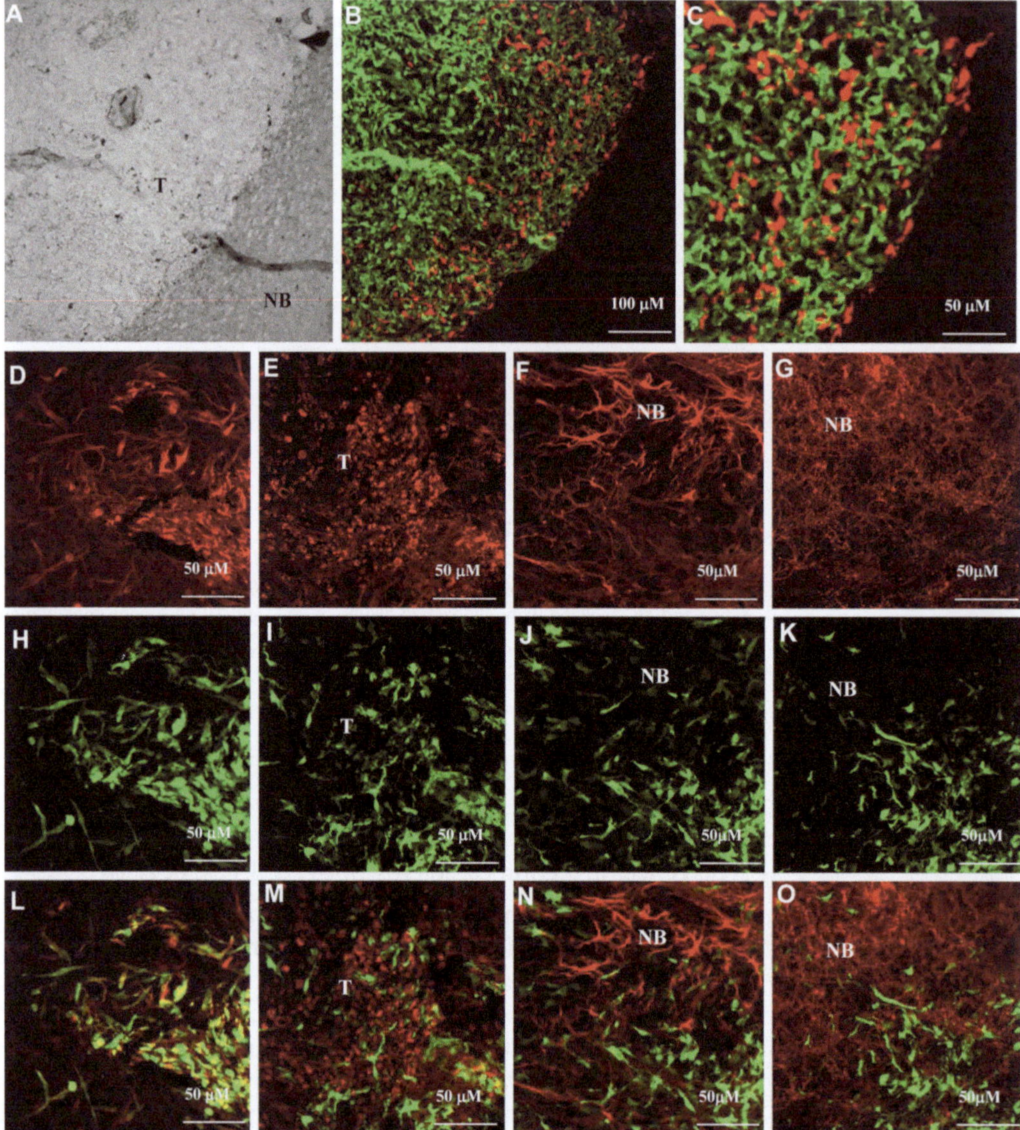

Fig. 6.3. NSC are present specifically in the gliomas in an undifferentiated state. Mice implanted with Gli36-GFP-Rluc glioma cells stereotactically into the right frontal lobe were implanted with Fluc-DsRed2 NSC 2 days later. Mice were imaged by intravital microscopy and sacrificed on day 10 after NSC implantation. Mice brains were sectioned and confocal microscopy was performed. **a** Light image showing the normal brain (NB) and the tumor (T); **b** Fluorescent image of **panel a** showing NSC (*red*) infiltrating the tumor (*green*); 10× magnification. **c** Higher magnification (40×) image of **panel b**. **d–o** Immunohistochemistry on brain sections from Gli36-glioma bearing mice implanted with NSC expressing GFP-Fluc, 10 days post-implantation. Representative images of brain sections immunostained for nestin (**d**, **h**, **l**), Ki67 (**e**, **i**, **m**), GFAP (**f**, **j**, **n**), and MAP-2 (**g**, **k**, **o**). (Green-GFP expression; Red-Ki67, GFAP, or MAP-2 expression; Yellow-co-expression of GFP and nestin.) Adapted from Shah et al. (15) with permission from Society for Neuroscience.

4. Notes

1. The in vitro and in vivo properties of human neural stem cells used in this study (including the absence of transformation, clonality, multipotency, stability, and survival) have been described in detail elsewhere (17–19). An efficient and robust way to follow cells both in culture and in vivo is to transduce them with lentiviral vectors expressing fluorescent marker genes. These vectors have the ability to integrate transgenes into the genome of dividing and non-dividing cells (20) and provide means of efficient long-term expression in cells and their progeny without using any antibiotic selection marker.
2. The ideal dosage of anesthesia for each animal will vary primarily based upon the animal's body mass.
3. We use custom-built circular-based stereotaxic assemblies that fit directly into our microscope stage (**Fig. 6.1**). Any design that can be secured to a microscope stage and incorporates pointed earbars and a noseclamp should suffice. To effectively immobilize the animal's head, the ear bars must be clamped firmly just anterior to the ears. Once the mouse appears to be secured, confirm by observing absence of head movement.
4. The skull should be kept moist by frequent application of sterile PBS following the removal of the periosteum.
5. When marking the skull, it is best to err on the side of caution, drilling only deep enough to produce a visible outline. It is important to keep the skull cool and moist with sterile PBS. Selectively dry only the area that will be immediately drilled, and reapply PBS when moving on to another area. The skull thickness varies considerably; the skull will be thickest toward the posterior portion and can be quite thin in the anterior region, especially near the midline. It can be challenging to judge whether or not the drill has completely penetrated the skull especially because it is quite transparent once it becomes very thin.
6. Care should be taken to consistently implant tumors at the same location and depth to facilitate imaging interpretation from within this relative point source.
7. Although multiphoton excitation is relatively benign at low power, long-term repetitive scans can yield tissue damage and photo-bleaching. It is best to calculate an estimated total scan-exposure time, keeping the time between z-series intervals to a maximum; essentially establishing a balance between

temporal resolution and photo-damage. The goal is to maximize dynamic range without saturating the data. It is ideal to have two power settings: a low power and high power setting for each mice. Using the same power settings thought study facilitates comparison between subjects.

8. Higher magnification objectives (10× and above) often reduce image quality because of pulsation motion artifact sensitivity. Of note is that the IV100 system allows a twofold zoom feature without changing objectives, so that the user can acquire 8× magnification images with the 4× objective.
9. Animals can be imaged by intravital microscopy every day. However, imaging the animal requires exposing the cortical surface and could influence the survival of mice. It is recommended to image mice with cranial windows every 3–5 days.

References

1. Shah, K., Bureau, E., Kim, D. E., Yang, K., Tang, Y., Weissleder, R., and Breakefield, X. O. (2005) Glioma therapy and real-time imaging of neural precursor cell migration and tumor regression. *Ann. Neurol.* **57**, 34–41.
2. Snyder, E. Y. and Macklis, J. D. (1995) Multipotent neural progenitor or stem-like cells may be uniquely suited for therapy for some neurodegenerative conditions. *Clin. Neurosci.* **3**, 310–6.
3. Tang, Y., Shah, K., Messerli, S. M., Snyder, E., Breakefield, X., and Weissleder, R. (2003) In vivo tracking of neural progenitor cell migration to glioblastomas. *Hum. Gene Ther.* **14**, 1247–54.
4. Gage, F. H. (2000) Mammalian neural stem cells. *Science* **287**, 1433–8.
5. Ehtesham, M., Kabos, P., Gutierrez, M. A., Chung, N. H., Griffith, T. S., Black, K. L., and Yu, J. S. (2002) Induction of glioblastoma apoptosis using neural stem cell-mediated delivery of tumor necrosis factor-related apoptosis-inducing ligand. *Cancer Res.* **62**, 7170–4.
6. Hofstetter, C. P., Holmstrom, N. A., Lilja, J. A., Schweinhardt, P., Hao, J., Spenger, C., Wiesenfeld-Hallin, Z., Kurpad, S. N., Frisen, J., and Olson, L. (2005) Allodynia limits the usefulness of intraspinal neural stem cell grafts; directed differentiation improves outcome. *Nat. Neurosci.* **8**, 346–53.
7. Iwanami, A., Kaneko, S., Nakamura, M., Kanemura, Y., Mori, H., Kobayashi, S., Yamasaki, M., Momoshima, S., Ishii, H., Ando, K., Tanioka, Y., Tamaoki, N., Nomura, T., Toyama, Y., and Okano, H. (2005) Transplantation of human neural stem cells for spinal cord injury in primates. *J. Neurosci. Res.* **80**, 182–90.
8. Lindvall, O., Kokaia, Z., and Martinez-Serrano, A. (2004) Stem cell therapy for human neurodegenerative disorders-how to make it work. *Nat. Med.* **10**(Suppl), S42–S50.
9. Bulte, J. W., Duncan, I. D., and Frank, J. A. (2002) In vivo magnetic resonance tracking of magnetically labeled cells after transplantation. *J. Cereb. Blood Flow Metab.* **22**, 899–907.
10. Graves, E. E., Weissleder, R., and Ntziachristos, V. (2004) Fluorescence molecular imaging of small animal tumor models. *Curr. Mol. Med.* **4**, 419–30.
11. Lewin, M., Carlesso, N., Tung, C. H., Tang, X. W., Cory, D., Scadden, D. T., and Weissleder, R. (2000) Tat peptide-derivatized magnetic nanoparticles allow in vivo tracking and recovery of progenitor cells. *Nat. Biotechnol.* **18**, 410–4.
12. Jendelova, P., Herynek, V., Urdzikova, L., Glogarova, K., Kroupova, J., Andersson, B., Bryja, V., Burian, M., Hajek, M., and Sykova, E. (2004) Magnetic resonance tracking of transplanted bone marrow and embryonic stem cells labeled by iron oxide nanoparticles in rat brain and spinal cord. *J. Neurosci. Res.* **76**, 232–43.
13. Lee, I. H., Bulte, J. W., Schweinhardt, P., Douglas, T., Trifunovski, A., Hofstetter, C.,

Olson, L., and Spenger, C. (2004) In vivo magnetic resonance tracking of olfactory ensheathing glia grafted into the rat spinal cord. *Exp. Neurol.* **187**, 509–16.
14. Mempel, T. R., Scimone, M. L., Mora, J. R., and von Andrian, U. H. (2004) In vivo imaging of leukocyte trafficking in blood vessels and tissues. *Curr. Opin. Immunol.* **16**, 406–17.
15. Shah, K., Hingtgen, S., Kasmieh, R., Figueiredo, J. L., Garcia-Garcia, E., Martinez-Serrano, A., Breakefield, X., and Weissleder, R. (2008) Bimodal viral vectors and in vivo imaging reveal the fate of human neural stem cells in experimental glioma model. *J. Neurosci.* **28**, 4406–13.
16. Shah, K., Tung, C. H., Yang, K., Weissleder, R., and Breakefield, X. O. (2004) Inducible release of TRAIL fusion proteins from a proapoptotic form for tumor therapy. *Cancer Res.* **64**, 3236–42.
17. Villa, A., Navarro-Galve, B., Bueno, C., Franco, S., Blasco, M. A., and Martinez-Serrano, A. (2004) Long-term molecular and cellular stability of human neural stem cell lines. *Exp. Cell Res.* **294**, 559–70.
18. Rubio, F. J., Bueno, C., Villa, A., Navarro, B., and Martinez-Serrano, A. (2000) Genetically perpetuated human neural stem cells engraft and differentiate into the adult mammalian brain. *Mol. Cell Neurosci.* **16**, 1–13.
19. Navarro-Galve, B., Villa, A., Bueno, C., Thompson, L., Johansen, J., and Martinez-Serrano, A. (2005) Gene marking of human neural stem/precursor cells using green fluorescent proteins. *J. Gene Med.* 7, 18–29.
20. Naldini, L., Blomer, U., Gallay, P., Ory, D., Mulligan, R., Gage, F. H., Verma, I. M., and Trono, D. (1996) In vivo gene delivery and stable transduction of nondividing cells by a lentiviral vector. *Science* **272**, 263–7.

Chapter 7

Magnetic Resonance Imaging of Brain Inflammation Using Microparticles of Iron Oxide

Martina A. McAteer, Constantin von Zur Muhlen, Daniel C. Anthony, Nicola R. Sibson, and Robin P. Choudhury

Abstract

For molecular magnetic resonance imaging (mMRI), microparticles of iron oxide (MPIO) create potent hypointense contrast effects that extend a distance far exceeding their physical size. The potency of the contrast effects derive from their high iron content and are significantly greater than that of ultra-small particles of iron oxide (USPIO), commonly used for MRI. Due to their size and incompressible nature, MPIO are less susceptible to nonspecific vascular egress or uptake by endothelial cells. Therefore, MPIO may be useful contrast agents for detection of endovascular molecular targets by MRI. This Chapter describes the methodology of a novel, functional MPIO probe targeting vascular cell adhesion molecule-1 (VCAM-1), for detection of acute brain inflammation in vivo, at a time when pathology is undetectable by conventional MRI. Protocols are included for conjugation of MPIO to mouse monoclonal antibodies against VCAM-1 (VCAM-MPIO), the validation of VCAM-MPIO binding specificity to activated endothelial cells in vitro, and the application of VCAM-MPIO for in vivo targeted MRI of acute brain inflammation in mice. This functional molecular imaging tool may potentially accelerate accurate diagnosis of early cerebral vascular inflammation by MRI, and guide specific therapy.

Key words: Microparticles of iron oxide, MPIO, MRI, inflammation, brain, molecular imaging, vascular cell adhesion molecule 1, VCAM-1.

1. Introduction

Multiple sclerosis is a disease of the central nervous system (CNS) characterized by multifocal inflammatory white matter lesions, demyelination, and axonal loss (1). Endothelial vascular cell adhesion molecule-1 (VCAM-1; CD106) and its ligand, $\alpha_4\beta_1$ integrin (also known as very late antigen-4, VLA-4), are key mediators of

K. Shah (ed.), *Molecular Imaging*, Methods in Molecular Biology 680,
DOI 10.1007/978-1-60761-901-7_7,

leukocyte recruitment and plaque development (2). VCAM-1 is not expressed constitutively on cerebral vascular endothelium but is upregulated upon endothelial activation (3). Selective inhibitors that bind to the α_4 subunit of $\alpha_4\beta_1$, blocking association with VCAM-1, substantially reduce new or enlarging lesions on MRI and clinical relapse in MS (4). VCAM-1 is therefore an attractive molecular imaging target of early cerebral vascular inflammation. Molecular imaging techniques that can accurately identify markers of early inflammation in the brain are needed to accelerate accurate diagnosis and guide specific therapy.

Microparticles of iron oxide (MPIO) are super-paramagnetic particles consisting of a magnetite (Fe_3O_4) and/or maghemite (Fe_2O_3) core surrounded by a polymer coat. MPIO possess several characteristics that are potentially useful for imaging endovascular molecular targets. First, MPIO have a high iron content, orders of magnitude greater than that contained in ultrasmall particles of iron oxide (USPIO) commonly used for MRI contrast. Due to the high iron content, MPIO create potent negative contrast effects on T2*-weighted images that extend to a distance roughly 50 times the physical diameter of the MPIO. Second, the potency of MPIO contrast has recently enabled in vivo cell tracking (5) and in vivo detection of single MPIO-labelled cells by MRI (6). Third, due to their size, MPIO are less susceptible than USPIO to non-specific uptake by endothelial cells and therefore they retain specificity for endovascular molecular targets (7). Finally, MPIO are commercially available with a range of reactive surface groups, providing the opportunity for covalent conjugation of protein, antibodies or small peptides. Commercial sources of MPIO include Invitrogen (Paisley, UK), Bangs Laboratories (Fishers, IN, USA), and Miltenyi Biotec Ltd (Surrey, UK).

We have recently developed a novel VCAM-1 targeted MPIO probe that identifies VCAM-1 expression in vivo in mouse acute brain inflammation with exceptional conspicuity and at a time when pathology is undetectable by conventional MRI techniques (8). MPIO (1 μm diameter), with reactive tosyl groups, are used for covalent conjugation of mouse monoclonal VCAM-1 antibodies (VCAM-MPIO). Activated mouse endothelial cells, stimulated with tumor necrosis factor α (TNF-α), are used to test the capacity of VCAM-MPIO constructs for specific and quantitative binding in vitro. For in vivo studies, acute brain inflammation is induced by stereotactic injection of interleukin 1β (IL-1β) into the left corpus striatum of mice. VCAM-MPIO are administered intravenously and in vivo MRI of the brain is performed at 7 Tesla using a T_2*-weighted 3D gradient-echo sequence, with a final isotropic resolution of 88 μm^3. VCAM-MPIO generate highly specific, potent hypointense contrast effects that delineate the architecture of activated cerebral blood vessels, with minimal background contrast.

The commercial availability of MPIO and VCAM-1 antibodies supports a straightforward protocol for producing targeted MPIO probes for early detection of brain inflammation in vivo. An additional advantage of this protocol is that MPIO are readily adaptable for diagnostic imaging of other endothelial-specific targets, simply by modifying the protein ligand. We have recently used similar MPIO-based constructs to image adhesion molecules in atherosclerosis (9) and activated platelets in mouse models of cerebral malaria (10) and atherothrombosis (11, 12). This targeted MPIO-based approach may provide a useful tool for early identification of vascular inflammation by MRI, which may accelerate accurate diagnosis and guide delivery of specific therapy.

2. Materials

2.1. Conjugation of VCAM-1 Antibody to MyOne™ Tosylactivated MPIO

1. MyOne™ Tosylactivated superparamagnetic polystyrene Dynabeads® (1.08 μm diameter) (Invitrogen, Paisley, UK). Store at 4°C (*see* **Note 1**).
2. Dynal MPC® -S magnetic particle concentrator (magnet) (Invitrogen).
3. Pre-washing and Coating buffer: 0.1 M sodium borate, pH 9.5. Store at 4°C (*see* **Note 2**).
4. 3 M Ammonium sulphate.
5. Antibody ligand (*see* **Notes 3** and **4**): Purified monoclonal rat anti-mouse CD106/VCAM-1 antibody (clone M/K2) (Cambridge Bioscience, Cambridge, UK). Store at 4°C (*see* **Note 5**). Purified isotype negative control IgG-1 antibody (clone Lo-DNP-1) (Serotec, Oxford, UK). Store at 4°C.
6. Blocking buffer: phosphate buffered saline (PBS), pH 7.4, 0.5% bovine serum albumin (BSA), and 0.05% Tween 20. Store at 4°C.
7. Washing and Storage buffer: PBS, pH 7.4, 0.1% BSA, and 0.05% Tween 20. Store at 4°C.

2.2. In Vitro VCAM-MPIO Binding to TNF-α Stimulated sEND-1 Cells

1. Dulbecco's Modified Eagle's Medium (DMEM) supplemented with 10% fetal bovine serum, 2 mM L-glutamine, 100 U penicillin, and 0.1 mg/ml streptomycin. Store at 4°C.
2. Trypsin/EDTA solution. Store at 4°C.
3. Round microscope cover slips (19 mm).
4. Murine recombinant tumor necrosis factor alpha (TNF-α, R&D systems, Abingdon, UK). Reconstitute with sterile

PBS and store aliquots at –20°C. Reconstituted TNF-α is stable at –20°C for 3 months.

5. Recombinant mouse VCAM-1 Fc chimera (Fc-VCAM-1) and recombinant mouse ICAM-1 Fc chimera (Fc-ICAM-1) (R&D systems). Reconstitute with sterile water (50 μg/ml) and store aliquots at –20°C. Once reconstituted, Fc-VCAM-1 and Fc-ICAM-1 are stable at –20°C for 4 weeks.
6. Paraformaldehyde. Prepare a 1% (w/v) solution fresh for each experiment.
7. Purified monoclonal rat anti-mouse CD106/VCAM-1 antibody (clone M/K2) (Cambridge Bioscience). Store at 4°C.
8. Alexa Fluor 488 conjugated rabbit secondary antibody to rat IgG (Vector Laboratories, Peterborough, UK). Store at 4°C.
9. Vectashield mounting media containing 4′,6-Diamidino-2-Phenylindole (DAPI) nuclear stain (Vector Laboratories). Store at 4°C.

2.3. In Vivo Mouse Protocol

1. Adult male NMRI mice (mean body weight 35 g).
2. 2.0–2.5% isofluorane anaesthesia (in 70% N_2O: 30% O_2).
3. 1 mg/ml mouse recombinant IL-1β (R&D systems). Reconstitute with sterile PBS and store in aliquots at –20°C. Once reconstituted, IL-1β is stable for 3 months at –20°C.
4. Low endotoxin saline containing 0.1% BSA.

2.4. MRI

1. Quadrature birdcage coil with an in-built stereotaxic frame.
2. 7 Tesla horizontal bore magnet with a Varian Inova spectrometer (Varian, Inc., Palo Alto, CA, USA).
3. Physiological monitoring and regulation: subcutaneous ECG electrodes (in-house); circulating warm-water system and rectal probe (Harvard Apparatus).

2.5. MR Image Analysis

1. ImagePro Plus Image analysis software (Media Cybernetics, Marlow, UK).
2. 3D Constructor plug-in for ImagePro Plus (Media Cybernetics).

3. Methods

MyOne™ Tosylactivated MPIO (1 μm diameter) are used for direct covalent conjugation of mouse monoclonal VCAM-1 antibodies (VCAM-MPIO). Tosylactivated MPIO do not require surface activation, unlike, for example, iron oxide particles with reactive carboxylic acid surface groups, which require activation prior to conjugation, using either carbodiimide, most commonly 1-ethyl-3-(3-dimethylaminopropyl) (EDC), or a combination of EDC and *N*-hydroxyl succinimide ester (NHS). Furthermore, the hydrophobic properties of tosylactivated MPIO facilitate optimal antibody orientation since Fc regions of the antibody, which are generally more hydrophobic than the Fab portion, will adsorb to the hydrophobic surface of MPIO followed by rapid covalent bond formation This exposes the Fab-regions of the antibody, thus maximizing the binding potential of antibody-conjugated MPIO to the target protein. The antibody-conjugated MPIO are stable at 4°C for several months without loss of antigen binding.

It is important to test and validate the capacity of VCAM-MPIO constructs for specific and quantitative binding in vitro prior to in vivo studies. This can be accomplished by incubating VCAM-MPIO or negative control IgG-MPIO with activated mouse endothelial cells, stimulated with graded doses of tumor necrosis factor alpha (TNF-α). After extensive washing to remove unbound MPIO, specific MPIO binding to cells can be visualized and quantified using differential interference confocal microscopy. To further validate binding specificity, VCAM-MPIO can be pre-blocked with soluble chimeric protein containing the extracellular domain of VCAM-1 (Fc-VCAM-1) or with negative control soluble extracellular ICAM-1 (Fc-ICAM-1). Fc-blocked VCAM-MPIO can be incubated with activated endothelial cells as above and subsequently VCAM-1 demonstrated using immunofluorescence. Cells can be assessed by confocal microscopy for VCAM-MPIO binding and VCAM-1 immunofluorescence on the cell surface.

For in vivo MRI studies, acute brain inflammation in mice is induced by unilateral stereotactic injection of IL-1β into the left corpus striatum. After 3 h, VCAM-MPIO or negative control IgG-MPIO is intravenously injected into a tail vein and allowed to circulate for 1.5–2 h prior to MRI. This allows time for specific MPIO binding in the brain and clearance of unbound MPIO from the blood. Control groups of mice may undergo identical treatments with substitution of IgG-MPIO or injected with VCAM-1 antibody (0.2 mg/kg body weight) 30 min prior to VCAM-MPIO administration to block VCAM-1 binding sites in vivo. MR images are acquired using a T_2*-weighted 3D gradient-echo sequence, with a final isotropic resolution of 88 μm^3. For MR image analysis, hypotense signal areas are segmented using an automated histogram-based tool using Image-Pro Plus and rendered to create a three-dimensional volumetric map of MPIO binding in the brain (*see* Fig. **7.2**).

3.1. Conjugation of VCAM-1 Antibody to MyOne™ Tosylactivated MPIO

1. MyOne™ Tosylactivated MPIO (5 mg, 5×10^9 MPIO) are transferred into a 1.5-ml microcentrifuge tube (*see* **Note 6**). The tube is placed in a Dynal MPC-S magnet (*see* **Note 7**) until MPIO have formed a pellet at the side of the tube and the liquid is clear. The supernatant is discarded.
2. The tube is removed from the magnet and MPIO resuspended in 1 ml of pre-washing and coating buffer (0.1 M sodium borate buffer, pH 9.5). The tube is placed in the magnet to pellet MPIO. The supernatant is removed and this step is repeated once more.
3. The MPIO pellet is resuspended in 200 μg antibody (*see* **Notes 8** and **9**).
4. Ammonium sulphate (3 M) is immediately added to give a concentration of 1 M in the final coating solution.
5. The tube is placed in a rotating wheel and incubated, with constant head-over-head rotation, at 37°C for 20 h.
6. MPIO are pelleted and the supernatant discarded to remove unbound antibody.
7. Blocking buffer is added at the same volume used for coating the MPIO, i.e., in this example 600 μl.
8. The tube is placed in a rotating wheel and incubated, with constant head-over-head rotation, at 37°C overnight to block any remaining unbound active tosyl sites.
9. MPIO are pelleted using the magnet and the supernatant discarded.
10. The tube is removed from the magnet and MPIO resuspended in Washing and Storage buffer (1 ml). The tube is placed in a rotating wheel and incubated, with constant head-over-head rotation, at 4°C for 5 min. MPIO are pelleted using the magnet and the supernatant discarded. This step is repeated three times.
11. Antibody-conjugated MPIO are stored in Washing and Storage buffer at concentration of 2.5×10^{10} MPIO/ml. The solution is stable at 4°C for several months without loss of antigen binding (*see* **Note 10**).

3.2. In Vitro VCAM-MPIO Binding to TNF-α Stimulated sEND-1 Cells

1. Cells of a mouse endothelial cell line, sEND-1 are passaged when approaching confluency with trypsin/EDTA. Cells are plated at a density of 8×10^5 per 35 mm well in a 6-well plate, each well containing a sterile 19-mm round cover slip.
2. Cells are stimulated for 20 h at 37°C with graded doses of mouse recombinant TNF-α (0–10 ng/ml DMEM).

3. The TNF-α media is then removed by aspiration.
4. Stimulated cells are incubated with VCAM-MPIO or IgG-MPIO (2.5×10^7 MPIO in 2 ml DMEM) in duplicate. The cell plate is immediately placed onto a sample rocker to avoid sedimentation of MPIO, and incubated for 30 min at room temperature with continual mixing.
5. The media is removed by aspiration and unbound MPIO removed by extensive washing with PBS.
6. 1% paraformaldehyde (2 ml) is added for 30 min at room temperature to fix cells.
7. The cell coverslip is mounted onto a glass slide by slowly inverting the coverslip onto mounting medium (13 μl) on a microscope slide. Nail varnish is used to seal the sample (*see* **Note 11**).
8. MPIO binding to cells are viewed using differential interference contrast microscopy. Four fields of view are acquired per sample. The number of bound MPIO per field are quantified using ImagePro plus.
9. For blocking experiments, VCAM-MPIO are pre-blocked with 5 μg Fc-VCAM-1 or Fc-ICAM-1 per μg MPIO for 1 h at room temperature (13).
10. Fc-blocked MPIO (2.5×10^7 MPIO in 2 ml DMEM) are incubated with cells stimulated with 50 ng/ml TNF-α or unstimulated cells, extensively washed with PBS and fixed as described above (*see* Steps 4–6). Experiments are performed in triplicate.
11. Fc-blocked MPIO binding to cells are viewed using an inverted microscope (20× objective). Four fields of view are acquired per sample. The number of bound MPIO per field are quantified using ImagePro plus.
12. For immunofluorescent VCAM-1 staining, MPIO-bound cells are incubated with rat anti-mouse VCAM-1 (5 μg per ml PBS) for 1 h at room temperature.
13. Primary antibody is removed and the cells washed three times for 5 min each with PBS.
14. Cells are incubated with secondary Alexa Fluor 488 conjugated rabbit antibody to rat IgG (1:100) for 1 h at room temperature (*see* **Note 12**).
15. The secondary antibody is removed and the cells washed three times for 5 min each with PBS.
16. The cell coverslip is carefully mounted onto a glass slide as described above (*see* Step 7) using mounting media containing DAPI nuclear stain. Cells are kept in the dark at 4°C

until imaged using confocal microscopy. Slides are viewed on the same day of preparation.

17. Cells are assessed for VCAM-MPIO binding (*see* **Note 13**) and VCAM-1 immunofluorescent staining using confocal microscopy (*see* **Note 14**). An example is shown in **Fig. 7.1**.

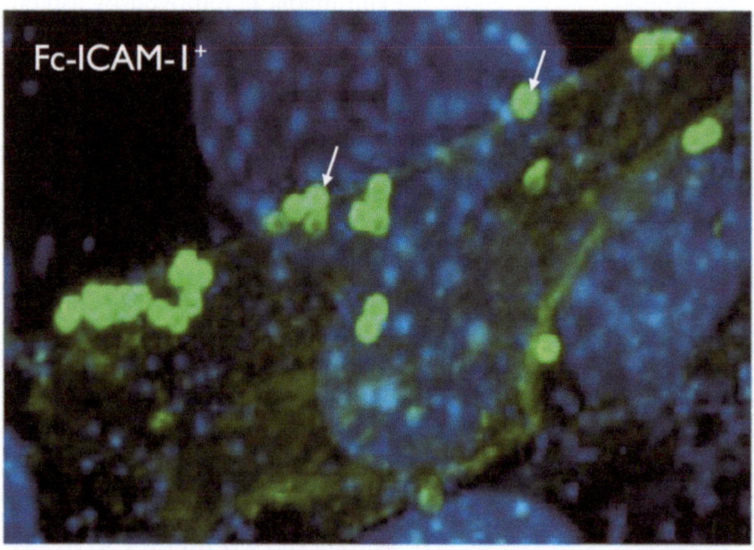

Fig. 7.1. VCAM-MPIO binding co-localises with VCAM-1 immunofluorescence on the surface of sEND-1 cells, stimulated with TNF-α (50 ng/ml). VCAM-MPIO were pre-incubated with soluble extracelluar VCAM-1 (Fc-VCAM-1) or ICAM-1 (Fc-ICAM-1) (5 μg/μg MPIO) for 1 h at room temperature. Fc-blocked MPIO were incubated with stimulated cells, extensively washed using PBS and immunostained for VCAM-1. Confocal images were obtained on a Zeiss LSM150 using ×60 oil-immersion lens. Pre-incubation of VCAM-MPIO with FcICAM-1 did not inhibit VCAM-MPIO binding. VCAM-MPIO were visualized as autofluorescent spheres (*see arrows*) on the cell surface that co-localised with VCAM-1 immunofluorescence. Pre-incubation of VCAM-MPIO with Fc-VCAM-1 abolished VCAM-MPIO binding, despite cell surface expression of VCAM-1, as confirmed by immunofluorescence.

3.3. In Vivo Mouse Protocol

1. Mice are deeply anaesthetised using 2.0–2.5% isofluorane (in 70% N_2O:30% O_2).
2. Mice are positioned in a stereotaxic frame under a Wild M650 operating microscope (Leica Microsystems, Milton Keynes, UK).
3. Using a glass pipette with a tip <50 μm, mouse recombinant IL-1β (1 ng in 1 μl of low endotoxin saline containing 0.1% BSA) is stereotactically injected into the left striatum, 0.5 mm anterior and 2 mm lateral to the bregma, at a depth of 2.5 mm, over a 10-min period.
4. After 3 h, a cannula is inserted into the tail vein for administration of MPIO (4 × 10^8 MPIO in 200 μl low

endotoxin saline containing 0.1% BSA) (*see* **Note 15**). VCAM-MPIO (4×10^8) is also administered to control mice that receive intracerebral injections of saline or no intracerebral injections.

5. To block VCAM binding sites in vivo, a further group of mice are injected with VCAM-1 antibody (0.2 mg/kg body weight) 3 h after IL-1β injection and VCAM-MPIO administered 15 min later.

6. Following MPIO injection, mice are positioned in a quadrature birdcage coil with an in-built stereotaxic frame. All mice are closely monitored for any signs of ill-health or toxicity (*see* **Note 16**).

3.4. MRI

1. MRI is performed using a 7 Tesla horizontal bore magnet with a Varian Inova spectrometer. During MRI, anesthesia is maintained with 1.0–1.5% isofluorane in 70% N_2O:30% O_2, ECG is monitored via subcutaneous electrodes, and body temperature maintained at 37°C by a circulating warm-water system.

2. MR images of the brain are acquired using a T_2*-weighted 3D gradient-echo sequence with the following parameters; flip angle 35°, repetition time (TR) = 50 ms, echo time (TE) = 5 ms, field of view (FOV) $22.5 \times 22.5 \times 31.6$ mm, matrix size $192 \times 192 \times 360$, two averages. The total acquisition time is approximately 1 h (*see* **Note 17**). The data is zero-filled to $256 \times 256 \times 360$ and reconstructed off-line, to give a final isotropic resolution of 88 μm^3.

3.5. MR Image Analysis

1. Extra-cerebral structures in each MR image are manually masked using ImagePro Plus.

2. Low signal areas are segmented in ten evenly spaced slices per brain using the automated signal intensity histogram-based tool in ImagePro Plus to obtain the median low signal intensity value (*see* **Note 18**).

3. Low signal areas are segmented in 41 contiguous slices of the brain, spanning a depth of 3.6 mm from the dorsal hippocampus ventrally. To ensure true laterality, the left and right hemispheres are segmented simultaneously, 1 mm from the midline outwards.

4. The median signal intensity value is applied to the 41 slice sequence to correct for minor variations in absolute signal intensity between individual scans.

5. Masks of the segmented low signal areas in 41 contiguous slices are merged and reconstructed using the 3-D Constructor plug-in for ImagePro Plus to visualize MPIO binding patterns in the inflamed (left) and non-inflamed

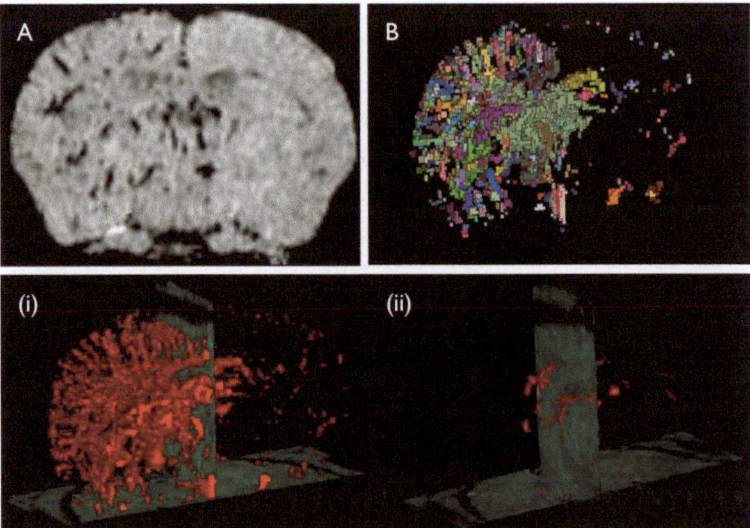

Fig. 7.2. 3-dimensional (3-D) volumetric maps of VCAM-MPIO binding pattern in the brain. **a** T_2*-weighted 3-D gradient echo MR image of mouse brain, 1–2 h post-MPIO injection, from a 7-Tesla magnet, approximately 90 μm isotropic resolution. Mouse was given a stereotactic injection of IL-1β into the left corpus striatum (1 ng in 1 μl saline), 3 h prior to intravenous injection of VCAM-MPIO (4×10^8 MPIO). Intense low signal areas on the left hemisphere reflect specific VCAM-MPIO retention on acutely activated vascular endothelium with virtually absent contrast effect in the contra-lateral control hemisphere. **b** Low signal contrast effects were segmented in 41 contiguous MR slices using an automated signal intensity histogram tool using ImagePro Plus. Masks of low signal areas were merged and 3-D reconstructed to create a 3-D volumetric map of low signal voxels. **c** Surface rendered 3-D volumetric map of VCAM-MPIO binding patterns. (i) VCAM-MPIO contrast effects delineated the architecture of inflamed cerebral vasculature in the IL-1β-stimulated hemisphere (*image left*) with almost total absence of binding on the contra-lateral, non-activated side. The *midlines* are indicated by vertical sections. (ii) Absence of MPIO contrast effects in mouse intravenously injected with VCAM-1 antibody (0.2 mg per kg), prior to VCAM-MPIO intravenous injection, which effectively blocked VCAM-MPIO binding.

(right) cerebral hemispheres. Examples of three-dimensional (3-D) volumetric maps of VCAM-MPIO binding patterns are shown in **Fig. 7.2**.

4. Notes

1. MPIO should be kept in liquid suspension during storage at 4°C as drying will reduce the performance of MPIO. We found it useful to store the MPIO vial on a sample roller at 4°C in order to prevent sedimentation of MPIO. MPIO should never be frozen as this will cause irreversible aggregation.

2. The pre-washing and coating sodium borate buffer must not contain any protein or amino groups (e.g., glycine, Tris) as these will bind to MPIO surface, inhibiting specific antibody binding. A higher pH favours optimal antibody binding.
3. MyOne^{TM} Tosylactivated MPIO can be conjugated to any ligand containing amino or sulphydryl groups (i.e., antibody, protein, peptide, or glycoprotein). However the antibody or protein must be purified since all proteins or amino groups will bind to the MPIO surface.
4. Preservatives such as sodium azide may disturb antibody conjugation to MPIO. In addition, sodium azide is cytotoxic and therefore not suitable for in vivo application. Therefore, antibodies free from stabilisers should be used or else remove stabilisers from the antibody/protein solution prior to conjugation.
5. The VCAM-1 antibody is commercially supplied in sodium borate buffer, pH 8.0, free from stabilisers. We found this antibody to be excellent for immunofluorescence imaging.
6. MPIO should be thoroughly resuspended prior to use by vortexing.
7. The Dynal MPC-S magnet can be used to prepare up to 6 microcentrifuge tubes of antibody-conjugated MPIO simultaneously.
8. For antibody conjugation, a concentration of 40 μg antibody per mg of MPIO is optimal. Conjugating less than recommended amounts of antibody may cause aggregation of MPIO. We found it best to use a stock purified antibody concentration of 0.5–1 mg/ml in order to achieve a sufficient antibody coating concentration. More dilute antibodies may require methods to concentrate the antibody prior to conjugation with MPIO.
9. MPIO should be suspended in the antibody solution with very efficient mixing using a vortex and transferred immediately to the sample rotating wheel for incubation. MPIO should not be allowed to come out of suspension at any stage.
10. We store our antibody-conjugated MPIO, continually mixing on a sample roller at 4°C to avoid sedimentation and drying of MPIO, which would reduce their binding capacity.
11. Air bubbles are undesirable in the mounting medium. Therefore, the coverslip should be inverted slowly onto the mounting media using fine forceps.

12. We found Alexa Fluor 488 conjugated rabbit secondary antibody to be excellent for visualizing VCAM-1 immunofluorescent staining by confocal microscopy as it is not prone to bleaching. This is particularly important when constructing z-stacks.

13. MPIO autofluoresce under confocal microscopy due to their high iron content and can be viewed using either red or green emission.

14. Due to the diameter of the MPIO, it may be difficult to find a focal plane that is suitable for simultaneously visualizing bound MPIO and immunofluorescent staining using confocal microscopy. We found it useful to create a z-stack of images throughout the depth of the MPIO and use the merged image to view co-localisation of immunfluorescence and MPIO.

15. For in vivo administration, we found it best to perform intravenous MPIO injections away from the MR magnet. We previously tried injecting MPIO into mice positioned inside the magnet. However, MPIO rapidly came out of solution when they were within the magnetic field and sedimented prior to administration.

16. We have found antibody-conjugated MPIO to be well tolerated in all mice, with no animals showing any signs of ill effect during close observation for up to 5 h post-injection.

17. We have serially imaged the same mouse and found maximal contrast at 1–2 h with diminution by 4 h.

18. Image analysis should be performed by an operator blinded to the origin of data.

References

1. Compston, A. and Coles, A. (2002) Multiple sclerosis. *Lancet* **359**, 1221–31.
2. Elices, M. J., Osborn, L., Takada, Y., Crouse, C., Luhowskyj, S., Hemler, M. E., and Lobb, R. R. (1990) VCAM-1 on activated endothelium interacts with the leukocyte integrin VLA-4 at a site distinct from the VLA-4/fibronectin binding site. *Cell* **60**, 577–84.
3. Carlos, T. M., Schwartz, B. R., Kovach, N. L., Yee, E., Rosa, M., Osborn, L., Chi-Rosso, G., Newman, B., Lobb, R., et al. (1990) Vascular cell adhesion molecule-1 mediates lymphocyte adherence to cytokine-activated cultured human endothelial cells. *Blood* **76**, 965–70.
4. Polman, C. H., O'Connor, P. W., Havrdova, E., Hutchinson, M., Kappos, L., Miller, D. H., Phillips, J. T., Lublin, F. D., Giovannoni, G., Wajgt, A., Toal, M., Lynn, F., Panzara, M. A., and Sandrock, A. W. (2006) A randomized, placebo-controlled trial of natalizumab for relapsing multiple sclerosis. *N. Engl. J. Med.* **354**, 899–910.
5. Shapiro, E. M., Skrtic, S., and Koretsky, A. P. (2005) Sizing it up: cellular MRI using micron-sized iron oxide particles. *Magn. Reson. Med.* **53**, 329–38.
6. Shapiro, E. M., Sharer, K., Skrtic, S., and Koretsky, A. P. (2006) In vivo detection of single cells by MRI. *Magn. Reson. Med.* **55**, 242–9.
7. Briley-Saebo, K. C., Johansson, L. O., Hustvedt, S. O., Haldorsen, A. G., Bjornerud, A., Fayad, Z. A., and Ahlstrom, H. K. (2006) Clearance of iron oxide

particles in rat liver: effect of hydrated particle size and coating material on liver metabolism. *Invest. Radiol.* **41**, 560–71.

8. McAteer, M. A., Sibson, N. R., von Zur Muhlen, C., Schneider, J. E., Lowe, A. S., Warrick, N., Channon, K. M., Anthony, D. C., and Choudhury, R. P. (2007) In vivo magnetic resonance imaging of acute brain inflammation using microparticles of iron oxide. *Nat. Med.* **13**, 1253–8.
9. McAteer, M. A., Schneider, J. E., Ali, Z. A., Warrick, N., Bursill, C. A., von zur Muhlen, C., Greaves, D. R., Neubauer, S., Channon, K. M., and Choudhury, R. P. (2008) Magnetic resonance imaging of endothelial adhesion molecules in mouse atherosclerosis using dual-targeted microparticles of iron oxide. *Arterioscler. Thromb. Vasc. Biol.* **28**, 77–83.
10. von Zur Muhlen, C., Sibson, N. R., Peter, K., Campbell, S. J., Wilainam, P., Grau, G. E., Bode, C., Choudhury, R. P., and Anthony, D. C. (2008) A contrast agent recognizing activated platelets reveals murine cerebral malaria pathology undetectable by conventional MRI. *J. Clin. Invest.* **118**, 1198–207.
11. von Zur Muhlen, C., Peter, K., Ali, Z. A., Schneider, J. E., McAteer, M. A., Neubauer, S., Channon, K. M., Bode, C., and Choudhury, R. P. (2008) Visualization of activated platelets by targeted magnetic resonance imaging utilizing conformation-specific antibodies against glycoprotein IIb/IIIa. *J. Vasc. Res.* **46**, 6–14.
12. von Zur Muhlen, C., von Elverfeldt, D., Moeller, J. A., Choudhury, R. P., Paul, D., Hagemeyer, C. E., Olschewski, M., Becker, A., Neudorfer, I., Bassler, N., Schwarz, M., Bode, C., and Peter, K. (2008) Magnetic resonance imaging contrast agent targeted toward activated platelets allows in vivo detection of thrombosis and monitoring of thrombolysis. *Circulation* **118**(3), 258–67.
13. Kelly, K. A., Allport, J. R., Tsourkas, A., Shinde-Patil, V. R., Josephson, L., and Weissleder, R. (2005) Detection of vascular adhesion molecule-1 expression using a novel multimodal nanoparticle. *Circ. Res.* **96**, 327–36.

Chapter 8

Optical Characterization of Arterial Apoptosis

Maarten F. Corsten and Abdelkader Bennaghmouch

Abstract

Apoptosis is a biological hallmark of both acute and chronic vascular pathology. It contributes to erosion and rupturing of atherosclerotic plaques, causing stroke and myocardial infarction, and plays an important role in post-angioplastic remodeling. Therefore, apoptosis is intensively studied in both explanatory and interventional vascular studies. Real-time molecular imaging of vascular processes, such as apoptosis, promises to improve our understanding and control over vascular micropathology, and could accelerate the development of novel therapies. Annexin A5 binds to apoptotic cells and is a well-established molecular imaging tool for detecting cell death in vivo. Here we describe a relatively straightforward approach to visualizing cell death in a murine carotid artery injury model using fluorescently tagged annexin A5. Our methods allow investigators to monitor gross apoptotic burden in real-time, as well as to assess in detail the apoptotic cell population and localization.

Key words: Molecular imaging, apoptosis, vascular injury, carotid artery, atherosclerosis, vulnerable plaque, annexin A5, annexin V, optical imaging, vital imaging, multiphoton imaging.

1. Introduction

The concept of programmed cell death (apoptosis) has revolutionized our understanding of physiology and disease. In vascular biology, apoptosis has been shown to play an important role in pathological processes such as plaque erosion, rupture, restenosis, and vascular remodelling (1–4). These processes underlie clinical conditions including myocardial infarction and stroke, rendering vascular apoptosis an intensively studied research topic.

Non-invasive detection of apoptosis has become feasible since the introduction of annexin A5. Because of its high binding affinity to phosphatidyl serine (PS), a cell membrane marker of

K. Shah (ed.), *Molecular Imaging*, Methods in Molecular Biology 680,
DOI 10.1007/978-1-60761-901-7_8,

apoptotic cells (5), labeled annexin A5 has been used to non-invasively image cell death in cancer, myocardial infarction, and atherosclerosis in both pre-clinical and clinical studies (6–10). Although nuclear imaging of annexin A5 is a powerful technique that can reveal crude presence of vascular apoptosis (11), and perhaps predict risk of plaque rupturing (10), it cannot provide the temporal and spatial detail required to study the elementary biology and evolution of vascular damage. Fluorescence imaging does meet these specific requirements to a large extent.

Compared to other molecular imaging modalities, optical imaging is a fast and relatively low-cost technique that offers high resolution and multiplexing capability. Additionally, short acquisition times usually permit sequential imaging to capture molecular processes throughout time. Here we describe a straightforward protocol for detecting vascular apoptosis using fluorescently tagged annexin A5. Progression of annexin A5 uptake following acute vascular injury can be visualized in vivo using a vital fluorescence reflectance imaging setup, and subsequently, localization and identity of the annexin A5 positive cells can be better defined by two-photon laser scanning microscopy and immunohistochemistry. Imaging techniques such as described here offer considerable opportunities for studying vascular pathologies, such as atherosclerosis and post-angioplasty remodeling, and for accelerated screening of novel anti-apoptotic drugs.

2. Materials

2.1. Labeled Annexin A5

1. Biotinylated or fluorescently labeled 2nd generation annexin A5 (*see* **Note 1**) can be purchased from MosaMedix (second generation annexin-A5, Maastricht, the Netherlands) or Invitrogen (Annexin V, Invitrogen, Carlsbad, CA) (*see* **Note 2**) and should be stored at 2–6°C, away from light. Avoid freezing (*see* **Note 3**). To exclude non-specific attachment to injured vessels, a labeled mutant annexin A5 that does not bind to phosphatidylserine (annexin A5-M1234, Mosamedix) is ideally incorporated in the study setup.
2. Dilute and aliquot annexin A5 – wild-type or M1234 mutant control – labeled with either Alexa568, Oregon Green (OG, for multispectral experiments) or biotin at 1 mg/ml and store at 2–6°C away from light.

2.2. Murine Model of Carotid Artery Endothelial Injury

1. Standard small animal surgical equipment including stereomicroscope, electrocardiogram (ECG) monitoring system, and heating pad.

2. Six- to eight-week-old specified pathogen free Swiss mice (Charles River/Jackson Laboratories) (*see* **Note 4**).
3. A cannula, consisting of a blunted 30G$^{1}/_{2}$ needle inserted into a polyethylene tube (PE-10, Portex Limited, England), attached to a saline-filled syringe.
4. Flexible wire with a 0.35 μm diameter (Guidant Europe NV, Belgium).
5. Pentobarbital (Nembutal) dissolved in PBS at 20 mg/ml (*see* **Note 5**).
6. Unfractioned heparin (5,000 IE/ml) (LEO Pharma, the Netherlands), stored at room temperature.

2.3. Vital Epifluorescence Imaging of Arterial Injury Temporal Dynamics

1. A stereomicroscope (Leica MZ FL III, Leica, Switzerland) equipped with a fluorescent module.
2. A peltier-cooled 12-bit B/W charge-coupled-device (CCD) camera (Hamamatsu C4742-95, Hamamatsu Photonics Systems, Japan) interfaced to a computer and operated by AquaCosmos 1.2 or HiPic 5.1 software, provided by the camera manufacturer.
3. Image processing software (Hipic/Aquacosmos, Hamamatsu).
4. Appropriate band-pass filters (Omega Optical, Brattleboro, Vermont) for selective fluorophore detection: for Oregon Green (OG), a 470/5 nm and a 525/5 nm band-pass filter (for excitation and collection, respectively) can be used. For Alexa568, 560/5 nm (excitation) and 620/5 nm (collection) band-pass filters are appropriate.
5. Premade concentrations of labeled annexin as described above.

2.4. Multiphoton Characterization of Apoptotic Cell Population

1. Arterial perfusion chamber (IDEE, Maastricht, the Netherlands).
2. Hanks' balanced salt solution (HBSS, Invitrogen, the Netherlands) having a pH of 7.4.
3. Syto13 (Molecular Probes, Leiden, the Netherlands) can be purchased as a 5-mM stock solution in dimethylsulfoxide and should be stored at 2–6°C away from light. Shortly before usage, dilute Syto13 in PBS to a 4-μM labeling solution, which can be kept at room temperature.
4. Biorad 2100 MP Laser Scanning System (Biorad, Hemel Hempstead, GB).
5. A 140-fs-pulsed Spectra Physics Tsunami Ti-sapphire laser (Mountain View, CA, USA) is used for excitation, tuned and locked at 800 nm.

6. Microscope objective of 60×, water dipping, numerical aperture 1.0, working distance 2 mm.
7. To detect emitted fluorescence, multiple photo multiplier tubes (PMT) are required.
8. A Nikon E600FN microscope (Nikon, Germany).
9. Image-Pro Plus 6.0 software (Media Cybernetics, Silver Spring, MD, USA) for image processing. For three-dimensional reconstructions one can use 3D Constructor 5.1 software (Media Cybernetics).

2.5. Ex Vivo Localization of Annexin A5 Binding

1. For tissue fixation, use freshly prepared 2% paraformaldehyde (PFA) (*see* **Note 6**) buffered in HEPES 10 mM, NaCl 140 mM, $CaCl_2$ 2.5 mM, and pH 8.0.
2. For deparaffinization: xylol, ethanol (100, 96, and 70%), 1% H_2O_2 in methanol, phosphate buffered saline (PBS).
3. Vectastain ABC-kit (PK-6100, Vector Laboratories, Burlingame, CA, USA) is used for biotin detection and should be stored at 2–6°C. Use 1% bovine serum albumin (BSA) in PBS to buffer ABC-kit reagents.
4. Diaminobenzidine tetrahydrochloride (DAB) (Sigma-Aldrich, Zwijndrecht, the Netherlands) is stored at –20°C.
5. Imidazole (Sigma-Aldrich, Zwijndrecht, the Netherlands) is stored at 2–6°C.
6. 30% H_2O_2 for activation of DAB/imidazole substrate mix, kept at 2–6°C.
7. Haematoxylin, kept at room temperature.
8. Mounting solution (Enthalan, Merck, Germany), kept at room temperature, and regular cover slips.
9. For imaging and storing of stained sections, use a regular light microscope with camera and interfaced to a computer equipped with a dedicated software package for image processing and analysis (QWin V3, Leica, Switzerland).

3. Methods

The murine carotid artery wall is sufficiently thin to be penetrated by a readily detectable portion of intraluminally emitted fluorescent photons. Therefore, a programmed cell death ligand such as annexin A5 can be optically labeled to visualize in vivo and throughout time the evolution of apoptosis in the arterial wall following experimental de-endothelialization. Since vital, planar imaging is limited by resolution in high magnification fields, primarily due to inability to reject out-of-focus signal, it can provide valuable information about the onset, extent, and propagation of apoptosis, but reveals little information about the vascular layer and cellular subset of annexin A5 positivity. Multiphoton imaging does allow gathering such additional information and thus represents a helpful extension of vital imaging.

3.1. Fluorescently Labeled Annexin A5

1. Fluorescently labeled annexin A5 should be kept at 2–6°C away from light until shortly before experiments. Prior to administration, the compound to be administered is allowed to settle at room temperature for approximately 30 min to minimize physiological disturbances due to temperature gradients.

3.2. Murine Model of Mechanical Carotid Artery Endothelial Injury

1. The heating pad should be preheated and material for surgery prepared, including sutures, cannula, and flexible wire.
2. Anesthetize the mouse with an intraperitoneal injection of pentobarbital 70 mg/kg.
3. The animal is placed in supine position on the heating pad and the cannula is carefully inserted into the right jugular vein. Take great care in avoiding air bubbles in the cannula as they might cause lethal emboli in the murine circulation.
4. After cannulation, animals are administered Heparin 20 μl (5,000 IE/ml) per cannula to prevent vessel occlusion by thrombus (*see* **Note 7**).
5. The animal is kept in supine position and a 15- to 20-mm incision is made in the ventral neck area. The bifurcation of right communal carotid artery is now carefully exposed. Also expose the left communal carotid artery, which will serve as a control artery for imaging, and should thus experience the same amount of environmental exposure. Throughout the procedure, keep both vessels moist as much as possible by superfusion with saline (*see* **Note 8**).
6. For temporary blood flow control, three sutures are placed: one suture proximal of the bifurcation around the commune artery, the other two distal of bifurcation, around the internal and external carotid artery, respectively. The sutures should be tightened around the vessel to abrogate blood flow, but should not be knotted (**Fig. 8.1**).
7. An iris scissor is used to create a small incision in the external carotid artery to provide an entrance for the 0.35-μm flexible guide wire. The wire is carefully introduced in the artery and advanced to the common carotid. Then, the wire is pushed and pulled back three times over a 10-mm distance

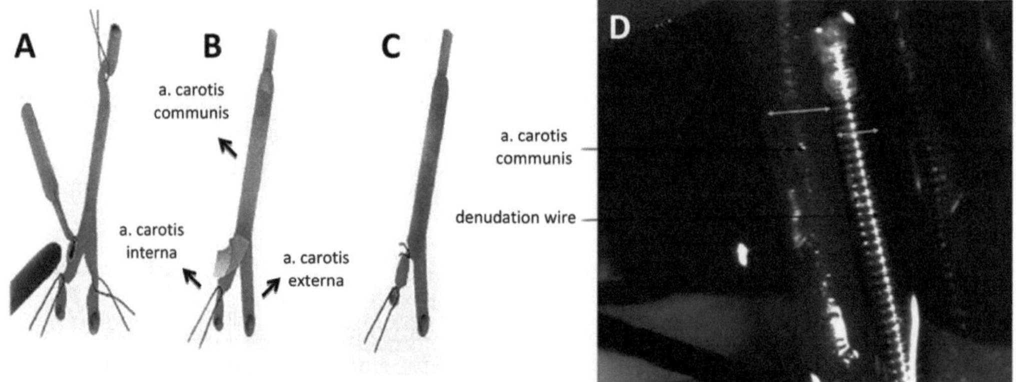

Fig. 8.1. Schematic representation of carotid artery endothelial denudation procedure. **a** Sutures are placed around the commune, internal and external carotid artery for blood flow abrogation. Only the suture around the external artery is knotted. Through a small incision in the external artery, distal of the knotted suture, the wire is introduced into the carotid artery. **b** Proceed the wire past the bifurcation and advance into the common carotid artery. Push and pull the wire three times over a 10-mm distance to ensure complete endothelial denudation. **c** After removing the wire, sacrifice the external carotid artery by placing and knotting a suture distal of the incision point. Then restore blood flow through the internal and commune carotid arteries by releasing their respective sutures. **Panel d** demonstrates the relative sizes of wire and commune carotid artery. Reproduced from Sata et al., with permission from Elsevier (copyright 2000) (15).

for complete removal of the endothelium. The wire is then removed.

8. After removing the wire, the external carotid artery is sacrificed proximally of the incision by knotting the suture. Remaining blood flow is then restored by releasing and removing the sutures around commune and internal carotid arteries.

3.3. Vital Epifluorescence Imaging of Arterial Injury Temporal Dynamics

1. During surgery and imaging mouse temperature is kept constant at 36.5° and ECG is monitored.
2. Timing of injection of labeled annexin(s) depends on study goal. For regular visualization and quantification of annexin uptake following endothelial injury inject annexin A5-Alexa568 (4 mg/kg) (*see* **Notes 9** and **10**) before endothelial injury. For multispectral imaging of early and late vascular apoptosis following arterial injury, inject annexin A5-Alexa568 (4 mg/kg) before endothelial injury and inject annexin-OG (4 mg/kg) at 120 min after injury, or at any alternative time-point relevant to the studied hypothesis.
3. For immunohistochemical purposes, inject annexin A5-biotin (12 mg/kg) before injury and sacrifice at any time point relevant to studied hypothesis (*see* **Note 11**).
4. When injecting labeled annexin A5, strictly avoid introducing air bubbles into the circulation.

5. To prevent bleaching as much as possible, aim to work in a dark or dimmed environment as much as possible following fluorophore administration.
6. For optimal contrast and to decrease background signal, a piece of black plastic (*see* **Note 12**) is placed behind the arterial region of interest.
7. Select the preferred magnification for imaging the entire region of interest and select the appropriate filter set. When imaging, be sure to acquire a parallel set of images of the contralateral control carotid artery. For an example of hence obtained images, *see* **Fig. 8.2**.
8. The exposed segments (around 1 cm) of the injured and non-injured vessels are imaged sequentially using an acquisition time of 2,000 ms (*see* **Note 13**) at appropriate time intervals, e.g., every 10 min until the end of the experiment (90 min) in a longitudinal study setup (*see* **Note 14**).

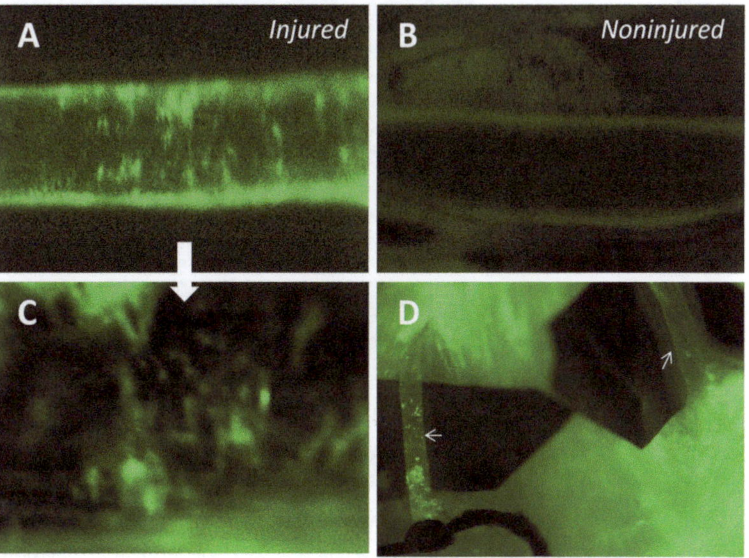

Fig. 8.2. In vivo planar imaging of annexin A5 accumulation in the damaged carotid artery wall. **a** and **b**: Annexin A5-Oregon Green (*green*) uptake after endothelial denudation in injured and contralateral control artery, respectively. **c** High magnification (160×) of **panel a**. **d** Low magnification overview of the mouse neck area during surgery and imaging, showing the ventral neck area with exposed *right* (damaged) and *left* (control) carotid arteries.

3.4. Multiphoton Characterization of Apoptotic Cell Population

1. For two-photon light scanning microscopy (TPLSM), animals were sacrificed by flushing saline through the left ventricle for 4 min. Arteries were immediately explanted, freed from adipose tissue, and stored in HBSS at 4°C for a maximum of 20 min.

2. Subsequently, arteries were mounted on two glass micropipettes (tip diameter 80–100 μm) in a homebuilt perfusion chamber filled with 37°C HBSS, and carefully flushed with HBSS (12).

3. Syto13 was added to the HBSS solution in the perfusion chamber to a final concentration of 4 μm and applied both intra- and extraluminally for fluorescent nuclear counterstaining (green).

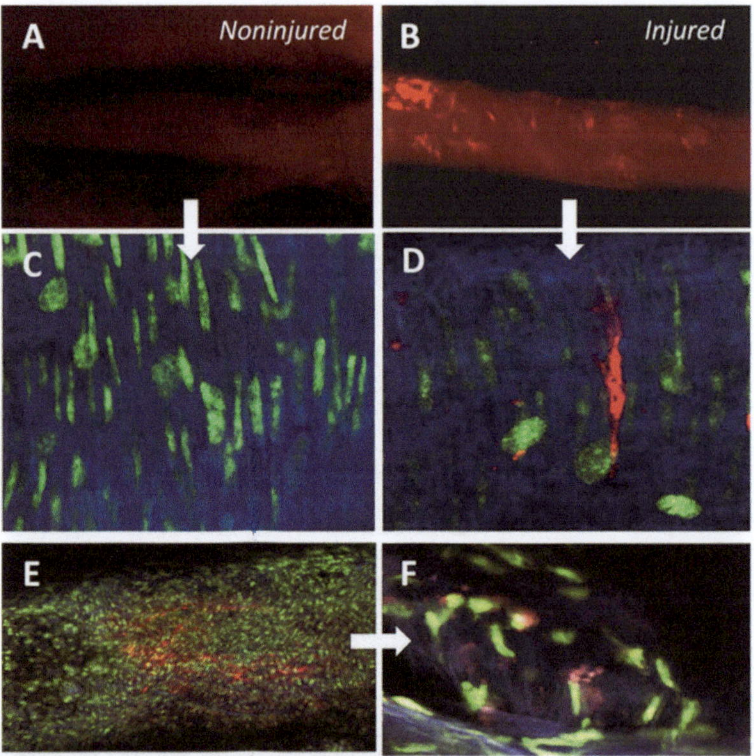

Fig. 8.3. Two-photon imaging allows for characterizing the fluorescent vascular cell population. **a** and **b** In vivo vital imaging of annexin-Alexa568 (*red*) localization 5 min after endothelial denudation shows marked localized uptake in the damaged carotid artery (**b**) and no uptake in the contra-lateral control vessel (**a**). **c** and **d** Corresponding ex vivo two-photon image reconstructions after treatment with Syto-13 green nuclear dye. Two-photon images reveal an absence of annexin A5-positive cells in the control vessel (**c**), whereas the damaged vessel harbors a population of annexin A5-positive, stretched, spindle-shaped cells, with a long axis perpendicular to the direction of blood flow. These characteristics are highly indicative for smooth muscle cells residing in the medial vascular layer. To emphasize the discriminatory ability of two-photon imaging for cellular identity, **e** and **f** show low-magnification and high-magnification two-photon images, respectively, of annexin A5 uptake (*red*) in undamaged carotid arteries of a 50-week old ApoE-knockout mouse. The annexin A5-positive cells do not display an organized arrangement or orientation and are not spindle-shaped. This corroborates with atherosclerotic plaque biology, where annexin A5 uptake is known to occur predominantly in inflammatory cells.

4. Flushing is adjusted to reach a physiological transluminal pressure of 80 mmHg, using a modified Big Ben sphygmomanometer (Riester, Germany) (12).
5. All imaging is performed on the central part of the artery, at 37°C, and in absence of luminal flow.
6. The perfusion chamber is positioned on the Nikon microscope.
7. For TPLSM imaging (13), pinholes are fully opened and two photomultipliers are used, accepting wavelengths of either 500–540 nm (for Syto13) or above 570 nm (Alexa568) (*see* **Note 15**).
8. Imaging speed is set at 0.1 Hz with a pixel dwelling time of 39 μs, or at 0.3 Hz with a dwelling time of 12 μs combined with Kalman filtering ($n = 3$ cycles). Laser power is minimized to prevent thermal damage to the arteries, e.g., at 8 mW (12).
9. Separate images are stored per PMT and then merged to a single two-dimensional image. For an example of thus produced images, *see* **Fig. 8.3**. Series of two-dimensional images can additionally be merged into a z-stack using Image-Pro and 3D Constructor software to create a three-dimensional model of the studied artery.

3.5. Ex Vivo Localization of Annexin A5 Binding

1. Ex vivo annexin A5 staining is ideally performed on vessels of animals that were injected with biotinylated annexin A5 (*see* **Note 16**) or biotinylated M1234 (serving as a non-binding control) 30 min before sacrifice.
2. The anesthetized animal is sacrificed by perfusion with 0.9% Saline via the left ventricle with for 3 min, followed by perfusion fixation with 20 ml of 2% PFA. The injured right and uninjured left common (internal control) carotid arteries are subsequently excised, post-fixed in 2% PFA, incubated in 70% ethanol, embedded in paraffin, and cut into longitudinal sections (4 μm).
3. The sections are de-waxed in xylol and rehydrated by proceeding through a series of decreasing ethanol concentrations (100, 96, and 70%, respectively).
4. To block endogenous peroxidase activity, sections are incubated with 1% H_2O_2 in methanol for 15 min, and subsequently washed in PBS.
5. Vectastain ABC-kit (PK-6100, Vector Laboratories, Burlingame, CA) is prepared 30 min before usage, by mixing the supplied components. For each section, 1 μl of reagent A and 1 μl of reagent B are added to 98 μl of PBS/BSA (1%).

6. Sections are incubated in buffered ABC-kit for 30 min and subsequently washed in PBS.
7. The peroxidase detection solution is freshly prepared directly before usage by adding 8 ml of Tris-HCl, 1 ml of imidazole, and 1 ml of DAB. Activate by adding 2.5 μl of 30% H_2O_2 (*see* **Note 17**).
8. The DAB/imidazole mixture is applied to the sections and staining is monitored under a light microscope. When sufficiently stained, the reaction is stopped by washing in PBS.
9. Sections are counterstained by 30 s incubation in haematoxylin and subsequently washed in tap water.
10. Dehydrate sections by proceeding through ethanol (70, 96, and 100%, respectively) and xylol and cover sections with enthalan and glass cover slips.
11. Stained sections are microscopically photographed with a magnification of 400× and quantified using a convenient Leica software package (QWin, Leica, Switzerland).
12. For quantitative study purposes, the apoptotic index (defined as the percentage annexin A5 positive cells in the total wall area) can be calculated in the (neo)intima, media and adventitia. Evaluating multiple representative sections from different heights of the mouse vessel and comparing to non-injured control arteries provides a referenced readout.

4. Notes

1. Second generation annexin A5 differs from wild-type annexin A5 in conjugation chemistry. A cysteine modification at the biologically non-functional side of the molecule allows routine thiol conjugation and ensures 1:1 stoichiometrical binding without perturbing the biological affinity for phosphatidyl serine (PS). In contrast, fluorophore coupling to wild-type annexin A5 is non-site specific and may interfere with PS binding sites. Throughout this chapter, 'annexin A5' refers to 2nd generation, not wild-type annexin A5.
2. Alternatively, 2nd generation annexin A5 can be generated from cDNA using a bacterial expression vector such as pET-5a (Novagen), and expressed in *Escherichia coli*. After performing fluorophore conjugation, confirm PS binding affinity of the labeled annexin by ellipsometry (14).

3. When stored at 2–6°C and away from light, annexin A5-fluorescent conjugates should be stable for at least 6 months (manufacturer's protocol), but we have obtained good results with conjugates stored over 12 months.
4. For these purposes, the authors do not have any animal gender preferences. Males are usually preferred to exclude fluctuating hormonal influences on wound healing, but this is not relevant in acute, terminal experiments. Younger animals, however, are preferred over older ones, as older mice tend to have more adipose and connective tissue, which complicates both surgery and imaging.
5. The authors have good experiences with the use of pentobarbital in terminal experiments; however, replacement of the anesthetic with ketamine/xylazine or isoflurane might be well-suited alternatives.
6. PFA 4% is regularly used for tissue fixation. However, for fragile tissues, such as carotid arteries, less concentrated (and aggressive) PFA is recommended. To reduce the burden of making fresh PFA every week, prepare an excess amount at once and freeze aliquots in glass at −20°C. After thawing an aliquot, discard what has not been used at the end of the week.
7. We recommend using high dose heparin since the experiment in question is terminal and prevention of thrombotic vessel occlusion is a key factor to imaging success.
8. Do aim to keep the arteries permanently moist to avoid dehydration damage, as this may lead to false positive results with imaging.
9. The fluorophore quantity required for imaging depends on the fluororescent molecule's brightness. When using alternative fluorophores, dose optimization may prevent low sensitivity or wasting of valuable imaging probe.
10. Administering 4 mg/kg of a 1 mg/ml solution to a 6-week-old Swiss mouse (typically weighing 35–50 g) implies injecting up to 200 μl. When performing multispectral experiments, keep in mind that 400 μl is a rather large volume to inject into a Swiss mouse. Consider to reduce dosing, or use higher concentrations of labeled annexin A5 for this application if necessary.
11. Both fluorescent and immunohistochemical (biotin) detection of annexin A5 uptake should be adequately controlled with non-injured carotids and, preferably, non-binding mutant M1234 annexin A5.
12. The type of plastic material used is of modest interest (garbage bags have served these investigators well), as long

as it is flexible and is put in place with minimal manipulation and stretching of the carotid artery.

13. As carotid arteries are typically subject to minimal movement, longer acquisition times such as recommended here can be used to improve optical imaging resolution.
14. When performing a sequential imaging study, take care to avoid too long cumulative exposure time to prevent bleaching. Limit excitation exposure to instants required for imaging and minimize frequency of imaging to the necessary.
15. For any given set of fluorescent emission spectra, PMT filter settings should be adjusted to optimize photon detection of 1 fluorophore per PMT, while minimizing bleed-through from the other markers used.
16. When annexin A5-biotin is not available or undesired, a direct immunohistochemical stain for annexin A5 can be performed using anti-annexin A5 antibodies (Hyphen Biomed, France).
17. The total volume prepared can be scaled up or down while keeping the constituents' relative proportions equal.

References

1. Kolodgie, F. D., Narula, J., Burke, A. P., Haider, N., Farb, A., Hui-Liang, Y., Smialek, J., and Virmani, R. (2000) Localization of apoptotic macrophages at the site of plaque rupture in sudden coronary death. *Am. J. Pathol.* **157**, 1259–68.
2. Clarke, M. C., Figg, N., Maguire, J. J., Davenport, A. P., Goddard, M., Littlewood, T. D., and Bennett, M. R. (2006) Apoptosis of vascular smooth muscle cells induces features of plaque vulnerability in atherosclerosis. *Nat. Med.* **12**, 1075–80.
3. Korshunov, V. A. and Berk, B. C. (2008) Smooth muscle apoptosis and vascular remodeling. *Curr. Opin. Hematol.* **15**, 250–4.
4. Mnjoyan, Z. H., Doan, D., Brandon, J. L., Felix, K., Sitter, C. L., Rege, A. A., Brock, T. A., and Fujise, K. (2008) The critical role of the intrinsic VSMC proliferation and death programs in injury-induced neointimal hyperplasia. *Am. J. Physiol. Heart Circ. Physiol.* **294**, H2276–84.
5. Martin, S. J., Reutelingsperger, C. P., McGahon, A. J., Rader, J. A., van Schie, R. C., LaFace, D. M., and Green, D. R. (1995) Early redistribution of plasma membrane phosphatidylserine is a general feature of apoptosis regardless of the initiating stimulus: inhibition by overexpression of Bcl-2 and Abl. *J. Exp. Med.* **182**, 1545–56.
6. Haas, R. L., de Jong, D., Valdes Olmos, R. A., Hoefnagel, C. A., van den Heuvel, I., Zerp, S. F., Bartelink, H., and Verheij, M. (2004) In vivo imaging of radiation-induced apoptosis in follicular lymphoma patients. *Int. J. Radiat. Oncol. Biol. Phys.* **59**, 782–7.
7. Hofstra, L., Dumont, E. A., Thimister, P. W., Heidendal, G. A., DeBruine, A. P., Elenbaas, T. W., Boersma, H. H., van Heerde, W. L., and Reutelingsperger, C. P. (2001) In vivo detection of apoptosis in an intracardiac tumor. *JAMA* **285**, 1841–2.
8. Dumont, E. A., Reutelingsperger, C. P., Smits, J. F., Daemen, M. J., Doevendans, P. A., Wellens, H. J., and Hofstra, L. (2001) Real-time imaging of apoptotic cell-membrane changes at the single-cell level in the beating murine heart. *Nat. Med.* **7**, 1352–5.
9. Hofstra, L., Liem, I. H., Dumont, E. A., Boersma, H. H., van Heerde, W. L., Doevendans, P. A., De Muinck, E., Wellens, H. J., Kemerink, G. J., Reutelingsperger, C. P., and Heidendal, G. A. (2000) Visualisation of cell death in vivo in patients with acute myocardial infarction. *Lancet* **356**, 209–12.

10. Kietselaer, B. L., Reutelingsperger, C. P., Heidendal, G. A., Daemen, M. J., Mess, W. H., Hofstra, L., and Narula, J. (2004) Non-invasive detection of plaque instability with use of radiolabeled annexin A5 in patients with carotid-artery atherosclerosis. *N. Engl. J. Med.* **350**, 1472–3.
11. Kolodgie, F. D., Petrov, A., Virmani, R., Narula, N., Verjans, J. W., Weber, D. K., Hartung, D., Steinmetz, N., Vanderheyden, J. L., Vannan, M. A., Gold, H. K., Reutelingsperger, C. P., Hofstra, L., and Narula, J. (2003) Targeting of apoptotic macrophages and experimental atheroma with radiolabeled annexin V: a technique with potential for noninvasive imaging of vulnerable plaque. *Circulation* **108**, 3134–9.
12. Megens, R. T., Reitsma, S., Schiffers, P. H., Hilgers, R. H., De Mey, J. G., Slaaf, D. W., oude Egbrink, M. G., and van Zandvoort, M. A. (2007) Two-photon microscopy of vital murine elastic and muscular arteries. *J. Vasc. Res.* **44**, 87–98.
13. van Zandvoort, M., Engels, W., Douma, K., Beckers, L., Oude Egbrink, M., Daemen, M., and Slaaf, D. W. (2004) Two-photon microscopy for imaging of the (atherosclerotic) vascular wall: a proof of concept study. *J. Vasc. Res.* **41**, 54–63.
14. Andree, H. A., Reutelingsperger, C. P., Hauptmann, R., Hemker, H. C., Hermens, W. T., and Willems, G. M. (1990) Binding of vascular anticoagulant alpha (VAC alpha) to planar phospholipid bilayers. *J. Biol. Chem.* **265**, 4923–8.
15. Sata, M., Maejima, Y., Adachi, F., Fukino, K., Saiura, A., Sugiura, S., Aoyagi, T., Imai, Y., Kurihara, H., Kimura, K., Omata, M., Makuuchi, M., Hirata, Y., and Nagai, R. (2000) A mouse model of vascular injury that induces rapid onset of medial cell apoptosis followed by reproducible neointimal hyperplasia. *J. Mol. Cell. Cardiol.* **32**, 2097–104.

Chapter 9

Intravital Fluorescence Microscopic Molecular Imaging of Atherosclerosis

Farouc A. Jaffer

Abstract

Atherosclerosis is a lipid deposition and inflammatory disease that results in considerable morbidity and mortality worldwide. Advances in molecular imaging, particularly near-infrared fluorescence imaging, are now enabling the in vivo study of fundamental biological processes that govern atherogenesis and its complications. Here we describe applications of near-infrared fluorescence reporter technology and intravital fluorescence microscopy to elucidate important biological processes in atherosclerosis in vivo.

Key words: Atherosclerosis, near-infrared fluorescence, molecular imaging, intravital microscopy, inflammation.

1. Introduction

Progression and complication of atherosclerotic plaques may produce unheralded sudden cardiac death, myocardial infarction, stroke, and ischemic limbs. Unraveling of the underlying biology of atherosclerosis has provided new opportunities to limit these devastating complications; however, improved understanding and treatment of atherosclerosis remains urgently needed.

Molecular imaging, specifically optical molecular imaging, is well positioned to provide novel insight into atheroma initiation, progression, and complications in vivo (1–3). The development of multichannel intravital fluorescence imaging systems in concert with versatile fluorescence reporter agents is permitting a

NIH R01 HL108229, American Heart Association Scientist Development Grant #0830352N, and Howard Hughes Medical Institute Career Development Award.

K. Shah (ed.), *Molecular Imaging*, Methods in Molecular Biology 680,
DOI 10.1007/978-1-60761-901-7_9, © Springer Science+Business Media, LLC 2011

high-resolution window into atherosclerosis biology in vivo. In particular, a multitude of new near-infrared fluorescence (NIRF) imaging agents has significantly expanded the capabilities of intravital microscopy. Imaging in the NIR window offers several advantages compared to visible light fluorochromes, including increased penetration depth of NIR photons due to markedly reduced blood photon absorption, as well as reduced tissue background autofluorescence (4, 5). Recent studies employing NIRF reporters have shed light in vivo insight on macrophage phagocytic activity, cysteine protease activity, and osteogenesis in atherosclerosis (6–8). Substantial growth in intravital fluorescence imaging studies is anticipated in the next several years as NIRF imaging agents and intravital systems become routine components of vascular biology research centers.

2. Materials

2.1. Intravital Laser Scanning Microscope

1. For acquisition of optical sections through atheromata in vivo, a commercially available system is the IV100 (Olympus, Japan). The system is capable of rapid, interleaved detection of three fluorochromes for multicolor fluorescence detection. The system has laser excitations at 488, 561, 633, and 748 nm (the latter two channels allowing detection of NIRF agents) (9). Objectives (standard and "stick") allow imaging from 1× to 50× optical zoom. Optical sections (similar to confocal microscopy) are obtained using a motorized platform. Anesthesia for small animals may be delivered via a gas regulator with isoflurane.
2. Digital camera – the Olympus IV 100 does not have white light reflectance based imaging capability. Digital photography of the imaged atheroma, particularly in serial studies, is helpful.
3. ImageJ Software Analysis Program (version 1.40, freeware, NIH, http://rsbweb.nih.gov/ij/download.html).

2.2. Near-Infrared Fluorescence Imaging Agents

1. Selection depends on the specific molecular/cellular target(s) to be investigated.
2. Phosphate buffered saline (1× PBS) or 0.9% (normal) saline for dilution of imaging agents.
3. Mouse tail vein injection setup (narrow diameter plastic intravenous tubing that can snugly house a 30-gauge needle; 0.5- to 1.0-ml syringe).

2.3. Angiographic Fluorescence Imaging Agents

1. Fluorescein isothiocyanate (FITC)-dextran (MW 2,000,000, Sigma catalog FD2000 s). Excitation/emission 490/520 nm. Stable for 2–3 years at 4°C.
2. Alternatively, if a near-infrared channel is available, a long half-life NIRF intravascular agent may be used (Angiosense680 (10) or Angiosense750, Visen Medical) or shorter half-life agent indocyanine green (ICG, 5 mg/kg, excitation 780 nm).

2.4. Murine Atherosclerosis Model

1. Apolipoprotein E deficient ($ApoE^{-/-}$, females, B6.129P2-Apoe<tm1Unc>/J Jackson Labs, 8–9 weeks on arrival, *see* **Note 1**).
2. High-cholesterol diet (0.2% commonly used).
3. Optional: cholesterol measurement kit (cholesterol kit; colorimetric assay, spectrophotometer for absorption measurement).

2.5. Surgical Setup for Carotid Arterial Dissection

1. Stereomicroscope, standard rodent animal surgical equipment for vascular dissection (surgical instruments; ketamine/xylazine for anesthesia (*see* **Note 2**)).
2. Place intrvaneous tubing (0.3 mm diameter) to be placed underneath the vessel, to aid localization of atheromata (will absorb light).
3. Tail vein catheter (intravenous tubing with 30 G needle on the front end).

2.6. NIRF-Enabled Fluorescence Microscope for Fluorescence Microscopy

1. A commercially available NIRF-capable system is the Eclipse 80i epifluorescence microscope (Nikon, Japan, *see* **Note 3**).
2. Standard histopathological setup for obtaining frozen sections: optical cutting temperature (OCT) compound (Sakura Finetek), cryotome, and glass slides.
3. Microscopy image acquisition and analysis software.

3. Methods

Carotid atheromata of $ApoE^{-/-}$ mice are surgically exposed for intravital microscopy (6–8). Multichannel intravital fluorescence microscopy is next performed using near-infrared and visible light fluorochromes. Compared to visible light fluorochromes, near-infrared fluorescence (NIRF) reporters offer greater depth penetration and signal-to-noise detection due to reduced photon absorption and less tissue autofluorescence, respectively. Multichannel high-resolution optical sections ($10 \times 10 \times 10$ μm resolution) are next obtained allowing multiplexing of various biological targets/processes in vivo. The following step-by-step method plan details the experimental procedure.

3.1. Development of Atherosclerosis

1. Obtain institutional animal committee approval for planned experiments.
2. Initiate ApoE$^{-/-}$ mice on high-cholesterol diet from age 10–24 weeks (*see* **Note 4**).
3. Confirm the effect of high-cholesterol diet by cholesterol measurement (*see* **Note 5**).

3.2. Injection of Imaging Agents

1. Inject (via i.v. tail vein) long-circulating atherosclerosis-targeted agents 24 h prior to imaging: magnetic nanoparticles (e.g., iron oxide)-based agents typically at a dose of 5–10 mg Fe/kg; protease-activatable agents typically at a dose of 80–200 nmol/kg.
2. Inject vascular angiographic agents immediately prior to imaging: FITC-dextran 0.5 mg per mouse (excitation 488 nm) or Angiosense 2 nmol/mouse (excitation 680 nm or 750 nm), or indocyanine green 5 mg/kg (excitation 780 nm).

3.3. Preparation of Mouse for IVFM

1. Induce anesthesia with ketamine (IP 100 mg/kg) and xylazine (IP 5 mg/kg); give maintenance doses every 30–45 min (*see* **Note 2**).
2. Place tail vein catheter (*see* **Note 6**).
3. Make a vertical surgical neck incision just off the midline on the side of the carotid of interest; typically the right carotid artery is selected.
4. Bluntly dissect and expose the distal common carotid artery (*see* **Note 7**). Plaques are typically at the distal vessel (towards the head) and usually extend into the bifurcation/trifurcation of this vessel.
5. Place a small piece of plastic tubing gently underneath the artery to facilitate vessel localization on IVFM.
6. Obtain high-magnification digital photograph of exposed surgical field/carotid plaque – particularly helpful for serial imaging studies where precise registration of the initial imaging field is necessary.
7. Transfer surgically exposed animal to the intravital imaging system.

3.4. IVFM Data Acquisition

1. Choose 4× objective for imaging (*see* **Note 8**) (**Figs. 9.1 and 9.2**).
2. Rapidly localize carotid atheromata on fluorescence images by an absorbing or fluorescent phantom under the vessel (*see* **Note 9**).

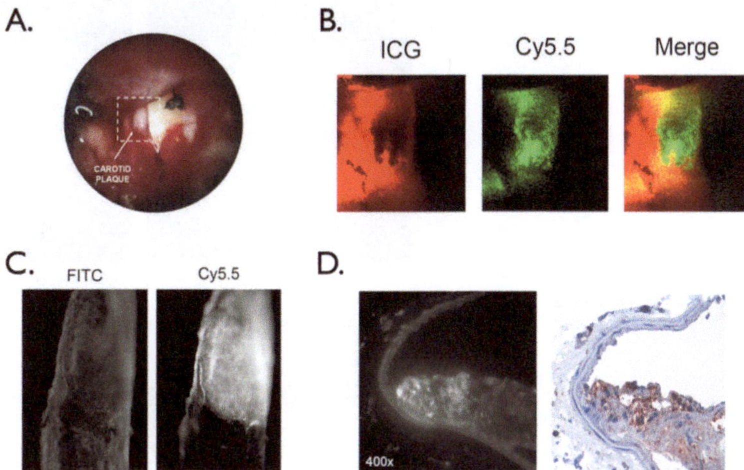

Fig. 9.1. In vivo detection of macrophage phagocytic activity in atherosclerosis using a macrophage-targeted near-infrared fluorescent nanoparticle (CLIO-Cy5.5). **a** Following CLIO-Cy5.5 (ex/em 673/694 nm, dose 10 mg iron/kg) injection 24 h beforehand, the right carotid artery of an $ApoE^{-/-}$ mouse is surgically exposed in preparation for intravital laser scanning fluorescence microscopy. A typical yellowish-white atherosclerotic plaque is present at the distal common carotid artery bifurcation. A fluorescent phantom is used as reference during imaging (placed adjacent to the plaque). The *dashed box* represents the region displayed in laser scanning fluorescence microscopy imaged in (**b**). **b** Following indocyanine green (ICG) injection, a vascular angiogram becomes evident, along with an intravascular filling defect due to the plaque. In the Cy5.5 NIR channel, strong focal plaque signal is evident. Merged image of the ICG and Cy5.5 signal confirms colocalization of the macrophage Cy5.5 signal to the filling defect seen on the angiogram. **c** Fluorescence reflectance imaging of an excised carotid atheroma from an $ApoE^{-/-}$ CLIO-Cy5.5-injected animal shows bright enhancement in the Cy5.5 channel, consistent with NIR nanoparticle uptake by plaque macrophages, and distinct from FITC-channel autofluorescence. **d** Correlative immunohistochemistry confirms that the NIRF signal colocalizes with immunoreactive plaque macrophages (*right*). Modified by permission from Pande et al. (6).

3. Set laser power and gains for target channels. This takes some individualization based on the anticipated signal-to-noise in vivo. The goal is to maximize dynamic range without saturating ("clipping") the data. A helpful strategy is to have two power settings, a low power and a high power setting for each subject/each study. Using the same power settings thought the study facilitates comparison between subjects (*see* **Note 10**).
4. Set imaging boundaries in the z-direction – this defines the IVFM stack. In practice NIR fluorochromes can be detected up to 300 μm below the external surface (adventitia) of the plaque. Typical parameters thus utilize 30 slices with a slice thickness of 10 μm.
5. Inject vascular angiographic agent (e.g., FITC-dextran, Angiosense, ICG) via tail vein. Begin live imaging (choose a

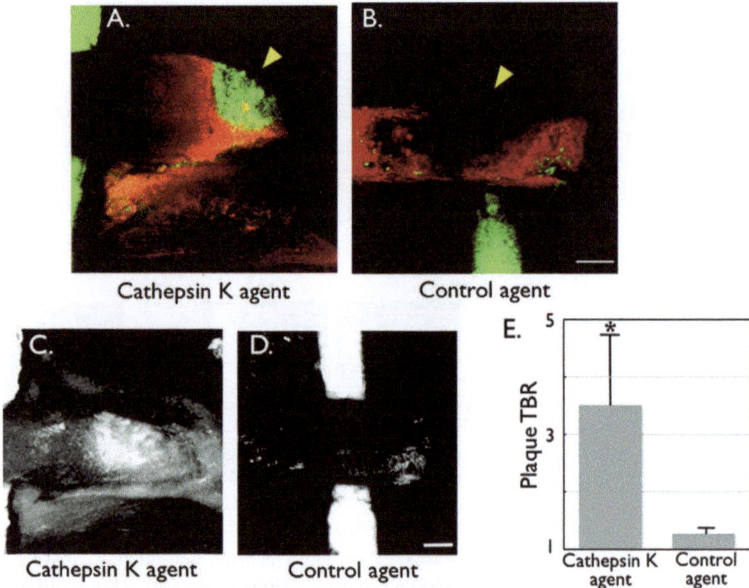

Fig. 9.2. Two-channel intravital fluorescence microscopy (IVFM) of cathepsin K protease activity in carotid plaques of ApoE$^{-/-}$ mice. At 24 h prior to imaging, a cathepsin K NIRF agent (ex/em 670/690 nm, dose 200 nmol/kg) was injected intravenously. During IVFM, a second spectrally distinct NIRF agent (Angiosense750, ex/em 750/770 nm, dose 2 nmol) was co-injected to provide a vascular angiogram. **a** Fusion images of cathepsin K protease activity (*green*) and Angiosense750 signal (*red angiogram*) reveal focal NIRF signal (*arrowhead*) indicating abundant cathepsin K activity. **b** A control NIRF agent (the amino acid analog of the cathepsin K agent) shows relatively scant NIRF signal, indicating that cathepsin K cleavage of the peptide substrate is required to generate substantial NIRF signal. **c** and **d** Summation projection images (obtained by ImageJ analysis) demonstrate greater plaque signal with the cathepsin K agent compared to the control, uncleavable D-analog agent. **e** Quantification of plaque target-to-background ratio distinguishes the cathepsin K NIRF agent from the control NIRF agent. Reproduced by permission from Jaffer et al. (7).

slice in the middle of the imaging stack containing the vessel) until a vascular angiogram is apparent.

6. Acquire multichannel image stack, and repeat as indicated if temporal data is required, as well as varying power settings and zooms. In the usual multichannel acquisition, one channel will be for the angiogram, and the other one or two channels will be used for molecular/cellular targets of interest.

7. For survival experiments, remove phantom and surgically close the incision, and provide analgesia per animal committee-approved protocol.

3.5. Image Analysis

1. Obtain and analyze image stacks from the IV100 system. Images are typically stored as multi-layer tiff files. In a three-channel experiment, if 50 slices were acquired, there will be

50*3 = 150 images. The first 50 would be from channel 1 (typically the 488-nm channel), the next 50 would be from channel 2 (typically the 633-nm channel), and last 50 would be from channel 3 (typically the 748-nm channel).

2. Analyze images with NIH ImageJ: Choose "Z-Project" from the menu. Input the start slice (e.g., 51) and the end slice (e.g., 100). Next choose projection type: Sum slices (not maximal intensity or other choices). An example summation projection image is provided in **Fig. 9.2** (*see* **Note 11**).
3. Use the manual ROI tool (either freehand or polygon tool) to circle the fluorescent region of interest. It is imperative to recognize that the fluorescent signals may define only part of the atheroma. It is therefore very helpful to review the digital photographic images and angiograms obtained to looking for plaque, vascular filling defects, and side branches. This information increases the accuracy/confidence of these measurements.
4. After drawing the ROI of the target area, select Measure from the menu. Record the area (check header for units, typically in cm^2) and mean (average signal intensity = total signal in ROI/# pixels in ROI).
5. Repeat ROI measurement for a background fluorescence signal in the vessel (non-plaque region as confirmed by digital photography and angiogram image). The target-to-background ratio is calculated as average signal intensity(plaque)/average signal intensity(background). This can be repeated for each channel of interest. An example is provided in **Fig. 9.2**.

3.6. Fluorescence Microscopy

1. Fluorescence microscopy of plaque sections provides critical corroborative data for intravital imaging results (i.e., **Fig. 9.1**).
2. At the end of the study, sacrifice and perfuse the animal with saline to clear residual fluorochromes from the vasculature (*see* **Note 12**).
3. Resect carotid artery and embed fresh in OCT compound and freeze at –80°C.
4. Perform fluorescence microscopy of cryocut 5-μm fresh-frozen sections. The typical exposure times on the Nikon 80i 680 channel: 1–5 s; 750 channel 5–30 s (*see* **Note 13**).
5. Obtain 488 channel fluorescence (exposure time 0.5–1 s) to obtain tissue autofluorescence and confirm unique fluorescence distribution of targeted NIR fluorochromes (*see* **Note 14**).

6. Perform microscopy image data analysis – one can obtain merged/blended fluorescence images and perform ROI threshold analysis for quantification of the fluorescence signal distribution in plaque sections.
7. Perform correlative immunohistochemistry/histopathology to confirm specificity of NIRF signal obtained on fluorescence microscopy.

4. Notes

1. In addition to ApoE$^{-/-}$ mice, LDL-receptor-deficient mice are also commonly used but develop atherosclerosis more slowly.
2. Isoflurane gas anesthesia may be used, but compared to ketamine/xylazine, we have observed that isoflurane increases carotid arterial pulsation artifacts presumably due to its vasodilatory properties.
3. Fluorescence microscopy is an excellent molecular research tool that naturally supports intravital fluorescence imaging studies. Of note is that most commercial fluorescence microscopes do not have the routine filters to detect NIR channels; this requires customized NIR filters. The Nikon 80i epifluorescence microscope can resolve two NIR channels (e.g., 680 and 750 nm) using appropriate bandpass excitation and emission filters as well as dichroic mirrors. As an alternative, the IV100 system itself, while not optimized for confocal microscopy of slides, could also be investigated for this purpose (n.b. routine confocal microscopes are not able to detect far red fluorochromes (>700 nm)).
4. This high cholesterol diet protocol produces animals with visible carotid atheromata approximately 85–90% of the time; dermatitis and stopped posture may occur in cholesterol-fed animals > 30 weeks of age.
5. Cholesterol values for 20–50 week ApoE$^{-/-}$ mice on chow diet is 275 mg/dl and increases to >450 mg/dl on the above 0.2% cholesterol supplemented diet (11).
6. It may be easier to place tail vein under isoflurane, which is vasodilatory, then switch over to ketamine/xylazine for the remainder of the experiment.
7. Avoid excessive trauma to vagus nerve running along side the carotid artery or the mouse may suffer a respiratory arrest.

8. Higher magnification objectives (10× and above) often reduce image quality because of pulsation motion artifact sensitivity. Of note is that the IV100 system allows a twofold zoom feature without changing objectives, so that the user can acquire 8× magnification images with the 4× objective.
9. As PE-10 tubing is absorptive in many fluorescent channels, the associated signal void can be used to localize the carotid artery, obviating the need to fill the PE-10 phantom with a fluorochrome.
10. Fluorescence image artifact, particularly in the 750 channel, may occasionally be seen. Adding saline to the field may help to reduce this artifact.
11. While time consuming, it may be helpful to analyze each slice within the image stack, as the individual images are higher resolution than projection image.
12. Perfusion with harsh fixatives such as formaldehyde may damage bound fluorochromes. Fresh frozen tissue is the safest way to ensure the integrity of tissue fluorochromes.
13. Typical broadband halogen light sources have relatively fewer excitatory photons in the NIR window, thus requiring relatively longer exposure times compared to visible light fluorochromes.
14. In the 488-nm channel, atheroma sections usually show substantial signal in the media of the vessel due to elastin fiber autofluorescence, as well as plaque autofluorescence from collagen and macrophages (hence the rationale for using NIR fluorochromes for targeted imaging).

References

1. Jaffer, F. A., Libby, P., and Weissleder, R. (2007) Molecular imaging of cardiovascular disease. *Circulation* **116**, 1052–61.
2. Chang, K. and Jaffer, F. (2008) Advances in fluorescence imaging of the cardiovascular system. *J. Nucl. Cardiol.* **15**, 417–28.
3. Jaffer, F. A., Libby, P., and Weissleder, R. (2009) Optical and multimodality molecular imaging: insights into atherosclerosis: *Arterioscler Thromb Vasc Biol.* **29**, 1017–24.
4. Weissleder, R. and Ntziachristos, V. (2003) Shedding light onto live molecular targets. *Nat. Med.* **9**, 123–8.
5. Ntziachristos, V., Ripoll, J., Wang, L. V., and Weissleder, R. (2005) Looking and listening to light: the evolution of whole-body photonic imaging. *Nat. Biotechnol.* **23**, 313–20.
6. Pande, A. N., Kohler, R. H., Aikawa, E., Weissleder, R., and Jaffer, F. A. (2006) Detection of macrophage activity in atherosclerosis in vivo using multichannel, high-resolution laser scanning fluorescence microscopy. *J. Biomed. Opt.* 11, 021009.
7. Jaffer, F. A., Kim, D. E., Quinti, L., Tung, C. H., Aikawa, E., Pande, A. N., et al. (2007) Optical visualization of cathepsin K activity in atherosclerosis with a novel, protease-activatable fluorescence sensor. *Circulation* **115**, 2292–8.
8. Aikawa, E., Nahrendorf, M., Sosnovik, D., Lok, V. M., Jaffer, F. A., Aikawa, M., et al. (2007) Multimodality molecular imaging identifies proteolytic and osteogenic activities in early aortic valve disease. *Circulation* **115**, 377–86.

9. Alencar, H., Mahmood, U., Kawano, Y., Hirata, T., and Weissleder, R. (2005) Novel multiwavelength microscopic scanner for mouse imaging. *Neoplasia* 7, 977–83.
10. Binstadt, B. A., Patel, P. R., Alencar, H., Nigrovic, P. A., Lee, D. M., Mahmood, U., et al. (2006) Particularities of the vasculature can promote the organ specificity of autoimmune attack. *Nat. Immunol.* 7, 284–92.
11. Swirski, F. K., Pittet, M. J., Kircher, M. F., Aikawa, E., Jaffer, F. A., Libby, P., et al. (2006) Monocyte accumulation in mouse atherogenesis is progressive and proportional to extent of disease. *Proc. Natl. Acad. Sci. USA* **103**, 10340–5.

Chapter 10

MR Imaging of Transplanted Stem Cells in Myocardial Infarction

Dara L. Kraitchman, Dorota A. Kedziorek, and Jeff W.M. Bulte

Abstract

Recently, several protocols for labeling of stem cells with superparamagnetic iron oxides (SPIOs) have been developed, leading to an active and growing field aimed at visualizing stem cells using MRI (magnetic resonance imaging), including image-guided stem cell injections. This development occurred simultaneously with a significant rise in the number of cell therapy clinical trials for cardiovascular applications and their preceding pre-clinical studies in animal models. In this chapter, we will describe several labeling strategies that can be used to label cells with SPIO nanoparticles. This is followed by a discussion of current strategies for using MRI to visualize these cells in myocardial infarct.

Key words: Magnetic resonance imaging (MRI), stem cells, superparamagnetic iron oxide (SPIO), cellular labeling, cellular imaging, myocardial infarct.

1. Introduction

Magnetic resonance imaging (MRI) is an ideal technique for precise MR-guided delivery of cells followed by monitoring of their trafficking within the body. On the one hand, MRI offers the interactivity of X-ray interventional techniques without exposing the patient or cells to ionizing radiation. On the other hand, the high spatial resolution and exquisite soft tissue detail of MRI are superior to X-ray cardiac interventional methods, which can only provide information about the lumen of the heart or vessels in combination with iodinated contrast agents. Moreover, MRI allows non-invasive, serial imaging for dynamic tracking of cell migration and engraftment (1–12).

K. Shah (ed.), *Molecular Imaging*, Methods in Molecular Biology 680,
DOI 10.1007/978-1-60761-901-7_10,

There are many magnetic labeling methods to detect cells with MRI. Pre-labeling with superparamagnetic iron oxide (SPIO) contrast agents is currently the most widely used method (13–17). SPIO-labeling methods are relatively simple, fast, and inexpensive. Among the different MR contrast agents that are available, SPIO particles offer currently the highest sensitivity (18). Several clinically approved formulations of SPIO-based contrast agents are available that have been used for cell labeling in a variety of diseases. The toxicity of the magnetic nanoparticles is low, since they are composed of biocompatible iron which can be recycled using endogenous iron metabolic pathways. Compared to gadolinium-based contrast agents, SPIOs become more effective upon cell internalization due to particle clustering and, thereby, create large "blooming" hypointensities on standard clinical MRI scanners (18). While SPIOs are not internalized by non-phagocytic cells without further modification, simple methods to induce internalization and uptake have been developed and tested in a variety of stem cells. One of the most commonly used method is "magnetofection" – a method where transfection agents (TAs) are complexed with SPIOs to provide the formation of SPIO oligomers with a highly positive surface charge (15), which induces macropinocytosis (endocytosis) of the SPIO-TA complexes (13, 14). Concentrations of 2–20 pg iron/cell can be easily achieved after 24–48 h incubation in vitro (13). After magnetic labeling of stem cells, SPIOs are stably maintained in endosomes enabling the imaging of stem cells for several months after delivery to the heart (3, 5, 9, 18).

Magnetoelectroporation (MEP) is another method of SPIO cellular labeling. MEP uses small pulsed voltages to induce intracellular uptake of SPIOs (16, 17, 19). No transfection agents are needed, which may aid in more rapid clinical translation. In addition, millions of cells can be labeled in seconds using MEP, which may be important in certain cell lines that are altered by culturing in vivo due to adhesion to tissue culture plastics leading to morphological changes. Furthermore, for cardiac cellular delivery, MEP may prove to be the method of choice where cellular delivery cannot be delayed by 24–48 h after an acute cardiac event, in particular when using off-the-shelf frozen stem cells within hours after a patient would be brought in.

Both magnetofection and MEP can be used to label cells with a variety of contrast agents, including manganese oxide nanoparticles (19). A recent study performing a head-to-head comparison of magnetofection and MEP demonstrated preserved cell viability and proliferation in embryonic stem cells by both techniques (20). However, cardiac differentiation of embryonic stem cells was most attenuated by MEP and iron uptake was greatest with magnetofection (20). This study has shown the importance of carefully selecting the magnitude and form of the applied electrical pulses. Detailed methods using these techniques to label stem cells for cardiovascular applications using SPIO contrast agents are given below.

2. Materials

2.1. Cell Culture and Preparation

1. Stem cell media, suitable for specific cell type, e.g., MEM alpha supplemented with 10% fetal bovine serum and 1% antibiotic/antimycotic containing penicillin, streptomycin, and amphotericin B for mesenchymal stem cells.
2. Phosphate buffered saline (PBS), 10 mM phosphate, 0.9% NaCl, pH = 7.4.
3. Trypsin (0.5 g/l) with ethylenediaminetetraacetic acid (EDTA 0.2 g/l), prewarmed to 37°C in a water bath before use. Long-term storage of trypsin should be at –80°C.

2.2. Labeling with Transfection Agents

Transfection agents (TAs) are highly charged molecules that will form complexes with iron oxide particles through electrostatic interactions. There are several classes of these agents, but the most convenient and most commonly utilized labeling methods are those based on commercially available TAs that are polycations, including dendrimers, such as Superfect®, poly-L-lysine (PLL), Lipofectamin®, and FUGENE®. SPIOs are used in conjunction with TAs to label cells and can be distinguished primarily based on the size of the nanoparticles. For brevity, we list several formulations that are approved or under development by major pharmaceutical companies.

1. *Iron oxide contrast agents:*
   (a) Commercially available ferumoxides are Feridex® (Berlex Laboratories Inc., Wayne, NJ, USA) or Endorem™ (Guerbet SA, Paris, France). Ferumoxide stock solution contains 11.2 mg Fe/ml with particles approximately 80–150 nm in diameter (21). Ferumoxide stock solution should be stored at 4°C, and should not be frozen. Feridex® is an FDA-approved liver contrast agent since 1996. In Europe, this compound is registered under name Endorem; both are identical. Both agents contain a dextran coating as a stabilizer.

   (b) Ferucarbotran (Resovist, Bayer Schering Pharma AG, Berlin, Germany) is an SPIO composed of nanoparticles coated with carboxydextran. It is currently used for the detection and characterization of focal liver tumor lesions and approved for clinical use in the European, Australian, and Japanese markets (*see* **Note 1**), as well as labeling cells.

(c) Ferumoxtran (Sinerem™, Guerbet SA, Paris, France, or Combidex®, AMAG Pharmaceuticals Inc., Cambridge, MA, USA) is a member of the ultrasmall superparamagnetic iron oxide (USPIO) class of contrast agents with a median diameter <50 nm. Due to the smaller diameter, these particles will not be taken up by the reticuloendothelial system as quickly as SPIOs when injected intravenously. Thus, they tend to accumulate in lymph nodes and are used to distinguish normal from metastatic nodes (*see* **Note 2**). The particles are much less magnetic than SPIOs and also complex less well with TAs and have therefore not been widely used for magnetic labeling.

2. *Transfection agents:*
   (a) Poly-L-lysine (PLL, Sigma, St Louis, MO, USA) as a hydrobromide with a molecular weight of 388,000 Daltons is the most commonly used TA. A stock solution of PLL in sterile water at a concentration of 1.5 mg/ml should be stored in –20°C.
   (b) Protamine sulfate (American Pharmaceuticals Partner, Schaumburg, IL, USA), which is a drug used clinically to reverse the effects of heparin therapy, is another commonly used TA. It is available in bottles at a concentration of 10 mg/ml, and stored at 4°C.

   Both transfection agents may be used (*see* **Note 3**).

2.3. Magnetoelectroporation

1. Ferumoxide stock solution. (*See* **Section 2.2.**)
2. Electroporation cuvettes, 0.4 mm gap (Gene Pulser BioRad, Hercules, CA). It is important to deliver electrical pulses with the proper field strength and duration. The exact pulse delivery will be dependent on the type of cells that will be labeled. Mammalian cells typically require field strengths up to 6.15 kV/cm, which can be obtained using a 0.4-cm cuvette.
3. BTX electroporation system (Harvard Apparatus, Holliston, MA).
4. Culture media and 10 mM PBS as in **Section 2.1**.

2.4. Magnetic Resonance Imaging

1. Clinical MRI scanner equipped with surface coils to image the heart.
2. MRI-compatible ECG leads and monitoring equipment.

3. Methods

3.1. Cell Culture and Preparation

1. Prior to labeling, the cells must be prepared in a clean, sterile environment. The cells can be frozen and thawed immediately prior to labeling. To obtain a high fraction of viable cells, they can be cultured overnight following the removal of dead cells.
2. When stem cells approach confluency in a culture dish/flask, remove the old media and wash the monolayer once or twice with PBS.
3. Remove PBS with a pipette and add a minimal volume (~1 ml for a T-75 flask) of prewarmed trypsin.
4. Incubate the cells in trypsin for at 37°C in humidified, enriched in 5% CO_2 air, then check microscopically to determine whether the monolayer of cells is lifting off the culture dish.
5. When single cell suspension has been obtained, add ~10 ml of complete media and transfer the cell suspension to a sterile 15-ml conical tube and spin the cells on tabletop centrifuge (~ 600×*g* for 10 min).
6. Discard the supernatant carefully, so as not to disturb the cell pellet and resuspend the cells in complete media for counting.
7. Once the number and concentration of cells has been determined, reseed the cells. For example, MSCs typically will be reseeded into a fresh T-75 flask at a concentration of ~2 × 10^5 cells/ml.

3.2. Complexing of SPIO and Labeling Using Transfection Agents

Each combination of TA and (U)SPIOs should be carefully titrated and optimized, since too low concentrations may not lead to sufficient cellular uptake, whereas too high concentrations may induce precipitates or may be cytotoxic. The examples below are given for PLL and protamine sulfate (21). **Figure 10.1** shows a representative example of intracellular labeling with Feridex®-PLL for a variety of cell types.

3.2.1. Poly-L-lysine

1. Use sterile culture medium, specific for the cell type being used, and add 2.2 μl Feridex® stock (11.2 mg Fe/ml, Berlex Laboratories) per ml of medium in order to prepare a medium solution containing 25 μg Fe/ml. Mix well (*see* **Notes 1–4**).
2. Add transfection agent to the Feridex®-medium at the appropriate concentration, i.e. 375 ng/ml (250 nl/ml

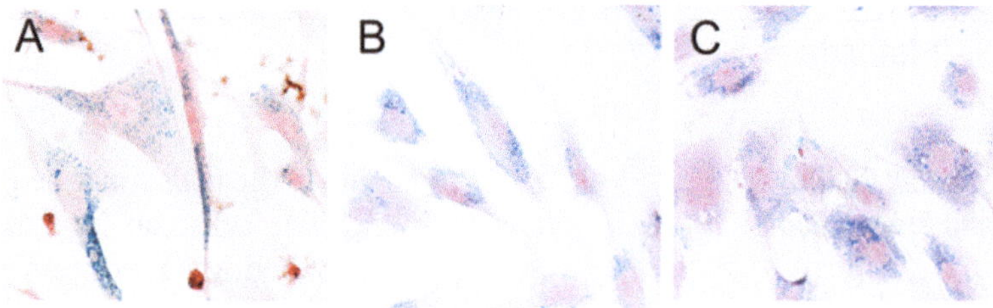

Fig. 10.1. Labeling of cells using Feridex®-PLL complexes. Cells were labeled for 48 h with 25 μg Fe/ml Feridex and 375 ng/ml PLL. Prussian blue staining of labeled human embryonic germ-derived pluripotent stem cells (**a**), human mesenchymal stem cells (**b**), and swine mesenchymal stem cells (**c**) show an efficient intracellular uptake of particles into endosomes that is non-specific across species.

medium using the 1.5 mg/ml stock). Mix well (*see* **Notes 2** and **4**).

3. Incubate the PLL-Feridex® medium for 60 min at room temperature using a rotating shaker. This allows the formation of PLL-Feridex® complexes through electrostatic interactions.
4. For adherent cells, remove the old medium, and add the PLL-Feridex® containing medium. For floating cells, spin the cells down at 400×*g* and resuspend the pellet in the PLL-Feridex® medium. For cells that are very sensitive to (autocrine) growth factors and supplements in the medium, spin the cells down at 400×*g*, resuspend the cells in 50% old medium, and add 50% PLL-Feridex® medium containing 50 μg Fe/ml Feridex® and 750 ng/ml PLL.
5. Incubate cells for 24–48 h. Shorter incubation times will induce less uptake.

3.2.2. Protamine Sulfate

1. Dilute protamine sulfate in distilled water to a concentration of 1 mg/ml just before initiating labeling.
2. Combine (U)SPIOs with appropriate serum-free media based on the cell type to obtain a concentration of 100 μg Fe/ml. For example, add 9 μl of ferumoxide formulation per every 1 ml of media for MSCs.
3. Add protamine sulfate to the (U)SPIO solution to obtain a concentration of 4.5–6 μg/ml (22–24) and mix the solution for 5–10 min.
4. After 5–10 min, add an equal volume of standard cell culture media with a double concentration of serum to create a final ferumoxide concentration of 50 μg/ml.
5. Replace old media in cell culture with newly created media with (U)SPIO–protamine sulfate complexes and incubate with cells overnight.

6. After overnight incubation, remove the media containing (U)SPIO-protamine sulfate complexes, rinse the cells with warm PBS, trypsinize, and collect for counting and administration.

3.3. Magnetoelectroporation

1. Remove media and wash cells with PBS.
2. Trypsinize and count cells. After counting, spin the cells using a tabletop centrifuge (~600×*g* for 10 min for MSCs) and wash with PBS.
3. Resuspend the cells in 10 mM sterile PBS at a density of 1–5 × 10^6 cells/ml (*see* **Note 5**) and transfer to sterile electroporation cuvette(s). While cell suspensions <1 ml/cuvette may be used, care must be taken to ensure that the cuvettes are entirely filled with the cell suspension. For example, using the BTX apparatus and 0.4-mm gap electroporation cuvettes, the total volume of cell suspension mixed with (U)SPIOs cannot be smaller than 700 μl.
4. Add (U)SPIOs to obtain a final concentration (after mixing with cell suspension) of 2 mg Fe/ml. For example, mix 130 μl of ferumoxides with 600 μl of cell suspension to obtain a final cuvette volume equal to 730 μl (*see* **Note 6**).
5. Using the BTX electroporation system (*see* **Fig. 10.2**), electroporate cells using the following conditions: 50 V pulse strength; 5 ms pulse duration; and 20 pulses in intervals of 100 ms.

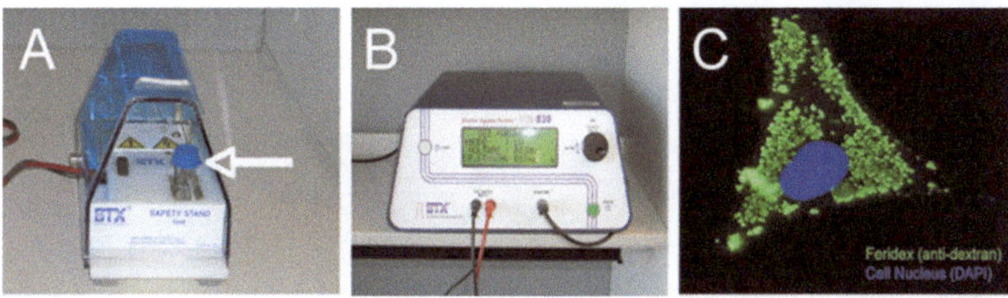

Fig. 10.2. Instant MR labeling of cells using magnetoelectroporation (MEP). **a** Cells are suspended in a sterile electroporation cuvette (*arrow*), mixed with Feridex®, and placed in a cuvette holder. **b** Using the connected electroporator, cells are mildly permeabilized for 10–20 ms. **c** Magnetic labeling is instantaneous, and Feridex clusters are trapped in the cytoplasm as demonstrated by anti-dextran immunofluorescent staining (*green clusters*).

6. Leave the cuvettes in the holder for 1 min, transfer to ice, and let them to rest for 5 min to allow for membrane recovery.
7. Remove the small top layer of foam and transfer cells to 50-ml conical tube containing culture media. Leave the tube with cells on ice for at least 15–20 min.

8. Wash the cells twice with PBS. Spin the cells in media using a tabletop centrifuge (~600×*g* for 10 min).
9. Remove the supernatant, resuspend MSCs in fresh, sterile 10 mM PBS, and spin down again. Repeat Steps 8 and 9 and then proceed to Step 10.
10. Discard the supernatant and resuspend cell pellet in 1 ml (or other desired amount) of PBS. Count the cells and dilute to final concentration for administration.

3.4. Cardiac Magnetic Resonance Imaging

SPIO-labeled stem cells can be delivered several ways including direct visualization during open-chest procedures, intracoronary administration using conventional angiographic catheters, and transmyocardially using specialized catheters for delivery of therapeutics to the myocardium. High spatial resolution T2*-weighted images will depict the labeled cells as hypointensities (*see* **Fig. 10.3**). Because these hypointensities can be hard to distinguish from other hypointensities, such as calcified plaque or metallic objects like stents, off-resonance imaging techniques have been developed to portray the magnetic susceptibilities from iron-labeled cells as hyperintense signal (25–29) (*see* **Fig. 10.4**).

3.4.1. T2*-Weighted Imaging

1. For high-resolution imaging, images are acquired over multiple cardiac cycles using ECG-gating. Motion artifacts from breathing are suppressed using either navigator echo techniques or breath-holding.

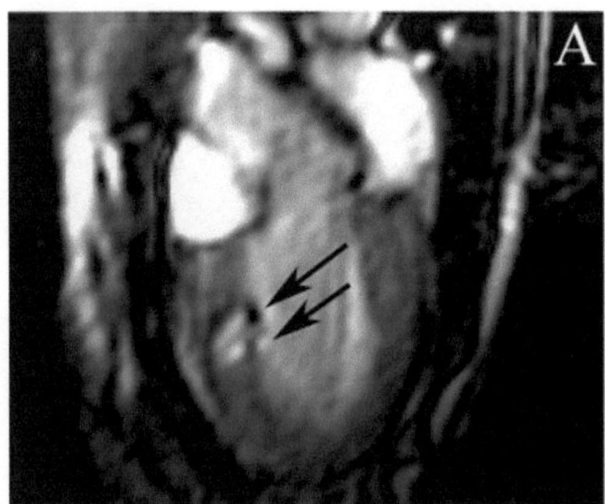

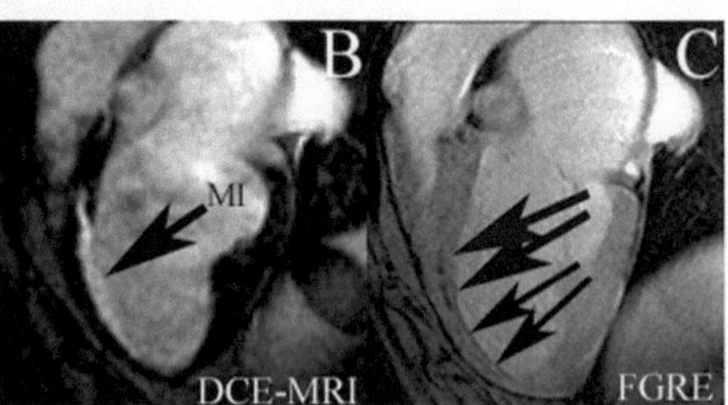

Fig. 10.3. MR-guided real-time injection of Feridex®-labeled MSCs in a dog myocardial infarct model. **a** Still frame long-axis view from real-time MRI demonstrating Feridex®-labeled MSCs as hypo-enhancing artifacts (*arrows*) after initial two injections at 3 days post-infarction (MI). *Top* lesion is 7×10^6 Feridex®-labeled MSCs; *bottom* lesion is 3×10^6 labeled MSC with 4×10^6 unlabeled MSCs. At 8 weeks after injection, initial two injections (**c**, *upper arrows*) are still visible, as well as additional injections (**c**, *lower arrows*) with as low as 1×10^5 labeled MSCs at initial injection in fast gradient echo images (FGRE). Hypo-enhancing artifacts change from round lesions to linear lesions by 8 weeks and align along the edge of the infarct (hyper-enhancing artifact [MI]) on delayed contrast enhanced (DCE) MRI (**b**). (Adapted from Bulte et al. (5), with permission.)

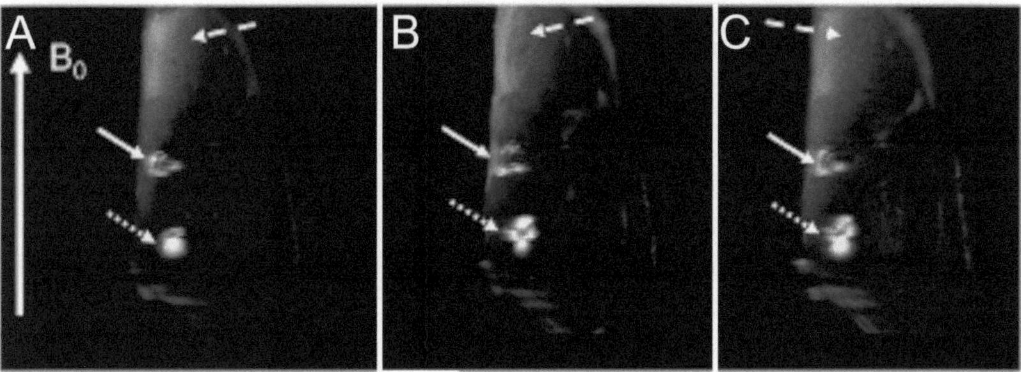

Fig. 10.4. Positive contrast (IRON) imaging of Feridex®-labeled MSCs transplanted in the hindlimb muscle of an ischemic rabbit. Adjacent double-oblique slices (**a–c**) from an in vivo 3T FSE 3D IRON acquisition obtained in an ischemic rabbit hindlimb with two injection sites of SPIO-labeled MSCs (2.5×10^5 cells at *dotted white arrow* and 1.25×10^5 cells at *solid white arrow*). Note the excellent background suppression that leads to clear visualization of the stem cell injection sites with positive contrast and a larger volume of hyperintense signal for the 250,000-cell injection site. (Adapted from Stuber et al. (28), with permission.)

2. While T2*-weighting can be obtained using several imaging techniques, gradient echo imaging with an extended echo time (TE) that does not degrade cardiac images appears to provide the best compromise in image quality on clinical scanners (2).
3. Typical gradient echo imaging parameters are 6 ms repetition time (TR); 1.6 ms TE; 20° flip angle; 512 × 512 image matrix; 5–8 mm slice thickness (ST): 32-kHz bandwidth (BW); and 2–4 number of signal averages (NSA). Images are acquired in the standard short or long axis planes to cover the extent of the left ventricle.

3.4.2. Off-Resonance Imaging

There are several types of off-resonance imaging techniques that have been used to image (U)SPIOs. One method uses a spectral excitation in combination with spin echo imaging, which is probably not well-suited for cardiac applications (26). Another method, GRadient echo Acquisition for Superparamagnetic particles/suscePtibility (GRASP), modifies the refocusing pulses to create positive contrast from iron-labeled cells (27, 30). Background suppression using this technique is excellent. A third method, Inversion-Recovery with ON-resonant water suppression (IRON), uses frequency-selective prepulses to suppress the water signal leaving positive contrast from iron-labeled cells (28). While not providing as much background suppression as the GRASP method, IRON MRI provides the flexibility to be combined with either spin echo or gradient echo techniques as well as two-dimensional single plane or three-dimensional volume acquisitions (*see* **Fig. 10.4**). Recently, it has been demonstrated that these off-resonance imaging techniques will not benefit from field strengths > 4.7T (31). Thus, these techniques are ideal for use on currently available clinical scanners.

1. As with T2*-weighted imaging, ECG-gating and respiratory gating or breath holds are used to suspend cardiac and respiratory motion, respectively.
2. Typical imaging parameters for three dimensional fast spin echo IRON imaging at 3T are 2 ms TR; 11.6 ms TE; 24 echo train length (ETL): 11.6 ms interecho spacing; 170 Hz bandwidth water suppression; 95° iron saturation pulse. In the heart, fat suppression is recommended. Depending on the number of (U)SPIO-labeled cells per voxel and the image resolution, the off-resonant positive contrast will appear as hyperintense areas surrounding the cells and with a typical dipole appearance. The volume of the hyperintensities can be measured to determine a relative concentration of labeled cells.

4. Notes

1. Instead of using complete medium, PLL-Feridex® complex formation may also be carried out in serum-free medium.
2. The amount of TA should be carefully titrated and optimized for each cell type. The suggested concentration of 375 ng/ml is only a guideline; this amount has been found to provide sufficient SPIO endocytosis without affecting cell proliferation or differentiation for most cell types.
3. Either PLL or protamine sulfate works well for cell labeling. For future clinical applications, protamine sulfate may be preferred as it is already clinically used as an anti-heparin product; however, in our experience, PLL labels most cells more effectively than protamine sulfate.
4. It is mandatory to first add the Feridex® to the medium and mix very well before adding the PLL or other TA. If this is not done, formation of large TA-SPIO aggregates and precipitation will occur.
5. If cell density per cuvette exceeds 5 × 10 (6), cell clumping can occur during MEP. Thus, using less than 2 × 10 (6) cells per cuvette is recommended to avoid cell clumping (16).
6. Iron uptake will be determined in part by of the type of cells. Cells with more cytoplasmic volume can be labeled with a larger amount of SPIOs. In addition, increasing the SPIO concentration can enhance intracellular iron uptake during MEP. Walczak et al. have demonstrated a correlation between concentrations ranging from 0.25 to 2 mg Fe/mL and cellular iron uptake (16).

References

1. Weissleder, R., Cheng, H. C., Bogdanova, A., and Bogdanov, A., Jr. (1997) Magnetically labeled cells can be detected by MR imaging. *J. Magn. Reson. Imaging* **7**, 258–63.
2. Kraitchman, D. L., Heldman, A. W., Atalar, E., et al. (2003) In vivo magnetic resonance imaging of mesenchymal stem cells in myocardial infarction. *Circulation* **107**, 2290–3.
3. Hill, J. M., Dick, A. J., Raman, V. K., et al. (2003) Serial cardiac magnetic resonance imaging of injected mesenchymal stem cells. *Circulation* **108**, 1009–14.
4. Garot, J., Unterseeh, T., Teiger, E., et al. (2003) Magnetic resonance imaging of targeted catheter-based implantation of myogenic precursor cells into infarcted left ventricular myocardium. *J. Am. Coll. Cardiol.* **41**, 1841–6.
5. Bulte, J. W. and Kraitchman, D. L. (2004) Monitoring cell therapy using iron oxide MR contrast agents. *Curr. Pharm. Biotechnol.* **5**, 567–84.
6. Rickers, C., Gallegos, R., Seethamraju, R. T., et al. (2004) Applications of magnetic resonance imaging for cardiac stem cell therapy. *J. Interv. Cardiol.* **17**, 37–46.
7. Kustermann, E., Roell, W., Breitbach, M., et al. (2005) Stem cell implantation in ischemic mouse heart: a high-resolution magnetic resonance imaging investigation. *NMR Biomed.* **18**, 362–70.
8. de Vries, I. J., Lesterhuis, W. J., Barentsz, J. O., et al. (2005) Magnetic resonance tracking of dendritic cells in melanoma patients for monitoring of cellular therapy. *Nat. Biotechnol.* **23**, 1407–13.
9. Stuckey, D. J., Carr, C. A., Martin-Rendon, E., et al. (2006) Iron particles for noninvasive monitoring of bone marrow stromal cell engraftment into, and isolation of viable engrafted donor cells from, the heart. *Stem Cells* **24**, 1968–75.
10. Amado, L. C., Schuleri, K. H., Saliaris, A. P., et al. (2006) Multimodality noninvasive imaging demonstrates in vivo cardiac regeneration after mesenchymal stem cell therapy. *J. Am. Coll. Cardiol.* **48**, 2116–24.
11. Ebert, S. N., Taylor, D. G., Nguyen, H. L., et al. (2007) Noninvasive tracking of cardiac embryonic stem cells in vivo using magnetic resonance imaging techniques. *Stem Cells* **25**, 2936–44.
12. Arai, T., Kofidis, T., Bulte, J. W., et al. (2006) Dual in vivo magnetic resonance evaluation of magnetically labeled mouse embryonic stem cells and cardiac function at 1.5 t. *Magn. Reson. Med.* **55**, 203–9.
13. Frank, J. A., Miller, B. R., Arbab, A. S., et al. (2003) Clinically applicable labeling of mammalian and stem cells by combining superparamagnetic iron oxides and transfection agents. *Radiology* **228**, 480–7.
14. Frank, J. A., Zywicke, H., Jordan, E. K., et al. (2002) Magnetic intracellular labeling of mammalian cells by combining (FDA-approved) superparamagnetic iron oxide MR contrast agents and commonly used transfection agents. *Acad. Radiol.* **9**, S484–7.
15. Kalish, H., Arbab, A. S., Miller, B. R., et al. (2003) Combination of transfection agents and magnetic resonance contrast agents for cellular imaging: relationship between relaxivities, electrostatic forces, and chemical composition. *Magn. Reson. Med.* **50**, 275–82.
16. Walczak, P., Kedziorek, D., Gilad, A. A., Lin, S., and Bulte, J. W. (2005) Instant MR labeling of stem cells using magnetoelectroporation. *Magn. Reson. Med.* **54**, 769–74.
17. Walczak, P., Ruiz-Cabello, J., Kedziorek, D. A., et al. (2006) Magnetoelectroporation: improved labeling of neural stem cells and leukocytes for cellular magnetic resonance imaging using a single FDA-approved agent. *Nanomedicine* **2**, 89–94.
18. Bulte, J. W. and Kraitchman, D. L. (2004) Iron oxide MR contrast agents for molecular and cellular imaging. *NMR Biomed.* **17**, 484–99.
19. Gilad, A. A., Walczak, P., McMahon, M. T., et al. (2008) MR tracking of transplanted cells with "positive contrast" using manganese oxide nanoparticles. *Magn. Reson. Med.* **60**, 1–7.
20. Suzuki, Y., Zhang, S., Kundu, P., Yeung, A. C., Robbins, R. C., and Yang, P. C. (2007) In vitro comparison of the biological effects of three transfection methods for magnetically labeling mouse embryonic stem cells with ferumoxides. *Magn. Reson. Med.* **57**, 1173–9.
21. Arbab, A. S., Yocum, G. T., Kalish, H., et al. (2004) Efficient magnetic cell labeling with protamine sulfate complexed to ferumoxides for cellular MRI. *Blood* **104**, 1217–23.
22. Janic, B., Iskander, A. S., Rad, A. M., Soltanian-Zadeh, H., and Arbab, A. S. (2008) Effects of ferumoxides-protamine sulfate labeling on immunomodulatory characteristics of macrophage-like THP-1 cells. *PLoS ONE* **3**, e2499.
23. Rad, A. M., Janic, B., Iskander, A. S., Soltanian-Zadeh, H., and Arbab, A. S.

(2007) Measurement of quantity of iron in magnetically labeled cells: comparison among different UV/VIS spectrometric methods. *Biotechniques* **43**, 627–8.

24. Pawelczyk, E., Arbab, A. S., Pandit, S., Hu, E., and Frank, J. A. (2006) Expression of transferrin receptor and ferritin following ferumoxides-protamine sulfate labeling of cells: implications for cellular magnetic resonance imaging. *NMR Biomed.* **19**, 581–92.
25. Seppenwoolde, J. H., Viergever, M. A., and Bakker, C. J. (2003) Passive tracking exploiting local signal conservation: the white marker phenomenon. *Magn. Reson. Med.* **50**, 784–90.
26. Cunningham, C. H., Arai, T., Yang, P. C., McConnell, M. V., Pauly, J. M., and Conolly, S. M. (2005) Positive contrast magnetic resonance imaging of cells labeled with magnetic nanoparticles. *Magn. Reson. Med.* **53**, 999–1005.
27. Mani, V., Saebo, K. C., Itskovich, V., Samber, D. D., and Fayad, Z. A. (2006) GRadient echo Acquisition for Superparamagnetic particles with Positive contrast (GRASP): sequence characterization in membrane and glass superparamagnetic iron oxide phantoms at 1.5T and 3T. *Magn. Reson. Med.* **55**, 126–35.
28. Stuber, M., Gilson, W. D., Schär, M., et al. (2007) Positive contrast visualization of iron oxide-labeled stem cells using inversion recovery with ON-resonant water suppression (IRON). *Magn. Reson. Med.* **58**, 1072–77.
29. Kraitchman, D. L. and Bulte, J. W. (2008) Imaging of stem cells using MRI. *Basic Res. Cardiol.* **103**, 105–13.
30. Mani, V., Briley-Saebo, K. C., Hyafil, F., Itskovich, V., and Fayad, Z. A. (2006) Positive magnetic resonance signal enhancement from ferritin using a GRASP (GRE acquisition for superparamagnetic particles) sequence: ex vivo and in vivo study. *J. Cardiovasc. Magn. Reson.* **8**, 49–50.
31. Farrar, C. T., Dai, G., Novikov, M., et al. (2008) Impact of field strength and iron oxide nanoparticle concentration on the linearity and diagnostic accuracy of off-resonance imaging. *NMR Biomed.* **21**, 453–63.

Chapter 11

In Vivo Imaging of the Dynamics of Different Variants of EGFR in Glioblastomas

Khalid Shah

Abstract

A number of altered pathways in cancer cells depend on growth factor receptors. The amplification/alteration of the epidermal growth factor receptor (EGFR) has been shown to play a significant role in enhancing tumor burden in a number of tumors, including malignant glioblastomas (GBM). To dissect the role of EGFR expression in tumor progression in mouse models of cancer and ultimately evaluate targeted therapies, it is necessary to visualize the dynamics of EGFR in real time in vivo. Non-invasive imaging based on quantitative and qualitative changes in light emission by fluorescent and bioluminescent markers offers a huge potential to facilitate drug development. Multiple approaches could be used to follow a molecular target or pathway with the fusion of a bioluminescent–fluorescent marker. This unit describes a protocol for simultaneously imaging EGFR activity and progression of GBM in a mouse model. Human glioma cells transduced with lentiviral vectors bearing different combinations of fluorescent and bioluminescent proteins either fused to EGFR or expressed alone can be grown as monolayers and maintained over several passages. The unit begins with a method for transducing glioma cells with lentiviral vectors for stable expression of these fluorescent and bioluminescent markers in vitro, followed by transplantation of engineered glioma cells in mice, and, finally, sequential bioluminescent imaging of EGFR expression and GBM progression in mice. The protocol details characterization of engineered glioma cells in culture, surgical preparation, craniotomy, cell implantation, animal recovery, and imaging procedures to study kinetics of EGFR expression and GBM progression.

Key words: EGFR, glioma and in vivo imaging.

1. Introduction

In primary malignant GBMs, overexpression and amplification of EGFR is found in 40–60% of the cases (1) making this the most frequent oncogenic change in GBMs. In GBMs, EGFR

K. Shah (ed.), *Molecular Imaging*, Methods in Molecular Biology 680,
DOI 10.1007/978-1-60761-901-7_11, © Springer Science+Business Media, LLC 2011

amplifications are often accompanied by gene rearrangements, resulting in seven known variant EGFRs (2) of which the most common rearrangement is an in-frame deletion from exon 2–7, which results in a mutant receptor designated de2-7EGFR (EGFRvIII) (3). Although EGFRvIII has a truncated extracellular domain and is incapable of binding epidermal growth factor (EGF), the receptor is moderately but constitutively active and has been shown to enhance the tumorigenic potential of glioma cells in vivo (4). The fact that EGFR is frequently overexpressed and mutated in GBMs, thereby up-regulating different pro-survival pathways, makes it an excellent target for cancer therapy. However, the lack of non-invasive assessment methods to monitor the intended target (EGFR expression) and its influence on the progression of GBMs in real time in experimental GBM models is a major hindrance to further develop new and efficient targeted therapies.

Non-invasive imaging based on quantitative and qualitative changes in light emission by fluorescent and bioluminescent markers (for example, GFP, DsRed2, and firefly and Renilla luciferase) offers a huge potential to facilitate drug development. A combination of both fluorescent and bioluminescent marker in one transcript would facilitate the study of the expression of the intended target at different spatial resolution scales. Multiple approaches could be used to follow a molecular target or pathway with the fusion of a bioluminescent–fluorescent marker. For example, this reporter could be placed under the control of a transcriptional promoter that is responsive to the molecule or pathway of interest. In another approach, this reporter can be fused directly to the -N or the -C terminus of the mutated or overexpressed protein of interest. This chapter describes the use of engineered glioma cells expressing recombinant EGF receptors fused to fluorescent and bioluminescent markers to simultaneously follow the EGF receptor expression and progression of GBMs both in culture and in vivo in real time.

2. Materials

2.1. Cell Culture and Viral Transduction

1. Gli36 human primary glioma cells provided by Dr. Anthony Capanogni (UCLA, CA)
2. Dulbecco's Modified Eagle's Medium (DMEM) (Gibco/BRL, Bethesda, MD) supplemented with 10% fetal bovine serum (FBS, HyClone, Ogden, UT).
3. Solution of trypsin (0.25%) and ethylenediamine tetraacetic acid (EDTA) (1 mM) from Gibco/BRL.

4. 1× penicillin/streptomycin (from 200× stock, Invitrogen).
5. LV-EGFR-GFP-Rluc, LV-EGFRvIII-GFP-Rluc and LV-Fluc-DsRed2 (5).
6. Polybrene (Fisher Scientific) (8 μg/ml from a stock solution of 8 mg/ml in PBS).

2.2. Fluorescence Microscopy

1. PBS
2. 4% paraformaldehydye solution
3. NH_4Cl
4. Nail varnish

2.3. Bioluminescence Imaging

1. D-Luciferin (firefly luciferase substrate) solution 150 mg/ml in PBS.
2. Coelenterazine (substrate for *Renilla* luciferases) 1 mg/ml stock in EtOH.
3. Bioluminescence imaging system with IVIS-200 or IVIS-100 (Caliper) or similar bioluminescence imaging system.

2.4. Cell Transplantation and Imaging In Vivo

1. Nude mice (6–8 weeks old; Charles River Laboratories, Wilmington, MA)
2. Anesthesia: ketamine, 120 mg/kg; xylazine 16.0 mg/kg
3. Stereotaxic frame (Harvard Apparatus, Cambridge, MA)
4. Hand-held micro-drill (Fine Science tools, Foster city, CA)
5. 0.45-mm Round drill burr (VWR, Willard, OH)
6. Fine scissors (Fine Science tools, Foster city, CA)
7. 1-ml Syringes with 27-gauge needle (Becton and Dickinson, Franklin Lakes, NJ)
8. Cotton-tipped applicators (Scientifics)
9. Forceps, angled and straight and ultrafine angled (Fine Science tools, Foster city, CA)
10. Stereo dissecting microscope – variable magnification ("1–4.5) (Nikon, Melville, NY)
11. 10-μl 26-gauge Hamilton Gastight 1701 syringe (Hamilton, Reno, NV)
12. 70% Isopropyl alcohol (Fisher Scientific, Pittsburgh, PA)
13. Betadyne solution (Bruce Medical, Waltham, MA)
14. Bone wax (Ethicon, Somerville, NJ)
15. Coelenterazine (100 μg/animal in 150 μl saline) (Biotium, Hayward, CA)
16. D-Luciferin (150 μg/g body weight in 150 μl saline) (Biotium, Hayward, CA)

3. Methods

3.1. In Vitro Studies

3.1.1. Cell Culture and Viral Transduction

1. Human glioma cell line, Gli36 is cultured in Dulbecco's Modified Eagle Medium (DMEM) containing and supplemented with 10% heat-incubated fetal bovine, 100 μg/ml penicillin, and 100 μg/ml streptomycin. All cells were incubated at 37°C in a humidified 5% CO_2 incubator. Glioma cells grow as monolayers and are passaged every 4 days by trypsinizing cells in 0.25% trypsin/EDTA. Cells are seeded at 20% density in glioma cell culture medium (*see* **Notes 1** and **2**).
2. Plate Gli36 human glioma cells at 60% confluency in a 5 cm dish and 18 h later, transduce cells with LV-EGFR-GFP-Rluc or LV-EGFRvIII-GFP-Rluc at an M.O.I. of 1 in their culturing medium containing 8 μg/ml polybrene (Fisher Scientific (5)).
3. Forty-eight hours after transduction, wash cells twice in culturing medium. Following expansion in culture, co-transduce Gli36 cells with LV-Fluc-DsRed2 at an M.O.I of 1.
4. Forty-eight hours after second viral transduction, wash cells twice in culturing medium. Following expansion in culture sort cells expressing EGFR-GFP-Rluc or EGFRvIII-GFP-Rluc and DsRed2 by fluorescence activated cell sorting (FACSAria Cell-Sorting System, BD Biosciences, San Jose, CA) to obtain monoclonal cell populations (*see* **Note 3**).
5. Expand sorted cells plated at 20% confluency in 5-cm dishes.
6. Two weeks post-sort, analyze cells by flow cytometry (FACScalibur, BD Biosciences) to confirm that an equal number of cells are GFP and DsRed2-positive in both cell lines.

3.1.2. Fluorescence Confocal Microscopy

1. Glioma cells expressing EGFR-GFP-Rluc or EGFRvIII-GFP-Rluc and Fluc-DsRed2 are passaged as described above, except that the experimental samples are 5-cm dishes containing sterile coverslips. The coverslips must first be sterilized by holding with tweezers, addition of 95% ethanol, and passing through the flame of a Bunsen burner and then placed in the culture dishes to cool.
2. Twenty-four hours later, rinse cells and change medium to serum-free DMEM when cells are still below sub-confluence so that individual cells are clearly visible.

3. Twenty-four hours later, rinse cells rapidly twice with ice-cold PBS and then add paraformaldehyde solution for 10 min at room temperature to fix the cells.
4. Discard paraformaldehyde (into a hazardous waste container) and wash the samples twice for 5 min each with PBS. Residual formaldehyde is quenched by incubation in NH_4Cl for 10 min at room temperature, followed by a further two washes with PBS.
5. The samples are then ready to be mounted. Carefully invert the coverslip into a drop of mounting medium on a microscope slide. Use nail varnish to seal the sample. The sample can be viewed immediately after the varnish is dry, or it can be stored in the dark at 4°C for up to a month.
6. The slides are first viewed under phase contrast microscopy (to locate the cells and identify the focal plane) and finally under confocal microscopy. Excitation at 488 nm induces the green fluorescence for EGFR-GFP expression, while excitation at 510 nm induces red fluorescence for DsRed2 expression. Software can be used to overlay the phase contrast and fluorescence images. Examples of the signals for EGFR-GFP and DsRed2 expression are shown in **Fig. 11.1**.

3.1.3. Dual Bioluminescence Imaging of Transduced Glioma Cells in Culture

1. Using a black-walled, clear bottom 96-well tissue culture plate, seed glioma cells expressing EGFR-GFP-Rluc or EGFRvIII-GFP-Rluc and Fluc-DsRed2 at different densities (1,000–10,000 cells per well) in a 100-μl volume.
2. To visualize the expression of EGFR by *Renilla* luciferase (Rluc) and cell proliferation by firefly luciferase (Fluc) imaging, add substrates for Fluc and Rluc sequentially as described below.
3. 18–24 h after seeding cells add D-luciferin (substrate for Fluc) to the culture medium in 1/10 volume at a final concentration of 0.15 mg/ml using a multichannel pipette.
4. Rock the plate and take images in bioluminescence imager with the appropriate exposure. For firefly luciferase, peak light production from intact cells occurs approximately 10 min after substrate addition.
5. Wash cells 4–5 times with PBS to remove any residual D-luciferin hours and add coelenterazine (substrate for Rluc) for a final concentration of 0.1 μg/ml, using a multichannel pipettor.
6. Rock the plate and take images in bioluminescence imager with the appropriate exposure. For *Renilla* luciferase, peak

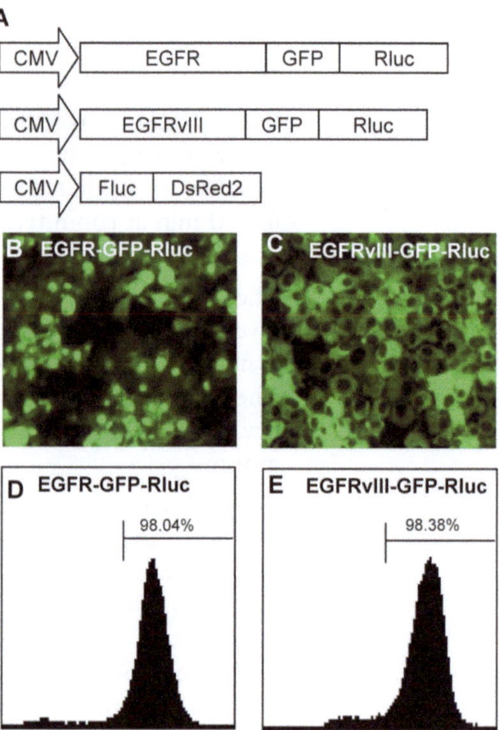

Fig. 11.1. Transduced human glioma cells express functional recombinant EGFR proteins. **a** A self-inactivating lentiviral system based on HIV-1 was used to construct vectors expressing fusions between EGFR and EGFRvIII with a fluorescent (GFP) and a bioluminescent (*Renilla* luciferase) fusion protein-marker cloned in front of a cytomegalovirus (CMV) promoter and designated as LV-EGFR-GFP-Rluc and LV-EGFRvIII-GFP-Rluc. **b** Gli36 human glioma cells were transduced with LV-EGFR-GFP-Rluc or LV-EGFRvIII-GFP-Rluc and visualized for GFP expression by confocal microscopy 24 h after transduction. Magnification: ×20; inserts ×40 (**c** and **d**). Flow cytometry analysis of lentiviral transduced Gli36 cells. (Adapted from Arwert et al. (5), with permission.)

light production from intact cells occurs immediately after substrate addition. Examples of the correlation signals for EGFR-GFP-Rluc/EGFRvIII-GFP-Rluc and Fluc-DsRed2 expression are shown in **Fig. 11.2**.

3.2. In Vivo Studies

3.2.1. Cell Transplantation and Imaging

This protocol is used for transplantation of glioma cells expressing different combinations of bioluminescent and fluorescent markers in mice. This protocol also describes the dual imaging of EGFR expression and tumor progression in mice GBM model.

3.2.1.1. Anesthetizing and Handling the Animal

1. The animal should be grasped firmly with one hand and anesthetized by injecting ketamine and xylazine intraperitoneally. The ideal dosage for each animal will vary primarily based upon the animal's body mass (120 mg/kg ketamine and 16 mg/kg xylazine) (*see* **Notes 4** and **5**).

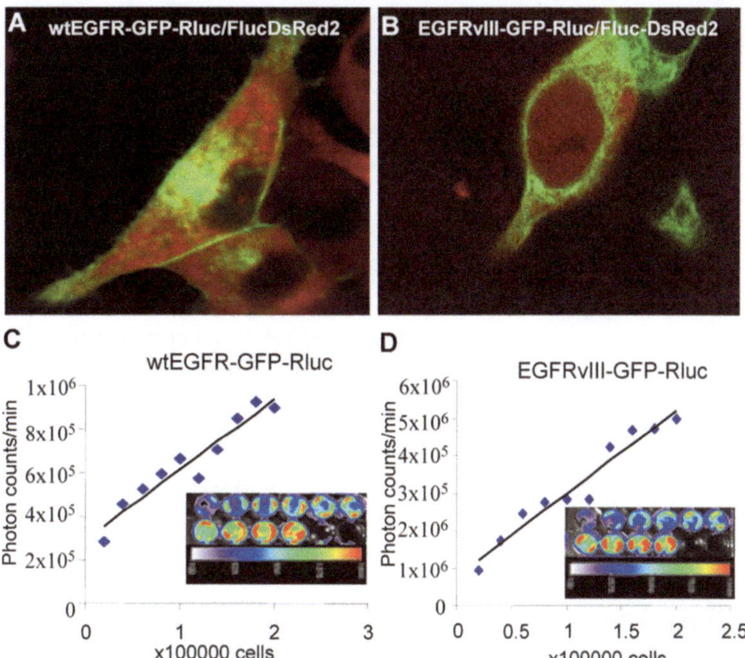

Fig. 11.2. Expression and correlation of recombinant EGFR proteins in vitro: Gli36 glioma cells, transduced with LV-EGFR-GFP-Rluc (**a**) or LV-EGFRvIII-GFP-Rluc (**b**) and co-transduced with LV-Fluc-DsRed2 were subjected to confocal fluorescence microscopy. Magnification: ×80 (**c** and **d**) Gli36 glioma cells, expressing EGFR-GFP-Rluc (**c**) or EGFRvIII-GFP-Rluc (**d**) were plated in different concentrations and 24 h later incubated in a medium containing 1 μg/ml of coelenterazine and imaged with a CCD camera. Correlation between the number of cells and Rluc signal is shown. (Adapted from Arwert et al. (5), with permission.)

2. Secure animal on a stereotactic head frame and trim dorsal surface of the animal's head. Disinfect the shaved area by applying alternating two coats of Betadyne and isopropyl alcohol.
3. Using scissors and forceps, remove the skin from the disinfected region and use a dry cotton swab to completely remove the periosteum membrane from the exposed skull surface. The skull should be kept moist by frequent application of sterile PBS following the removal of the periosteum.
4. Use a handheld micro-drill to drill through the bone at the location of the proposed implantation site until the cortical surface is exposed.

3.2.1.2. Tumor Cell Implantation

1. Trypsinize glioma cells expressing EGFR-GFP-Rluc or EGFRvIII-GFP-Rluc and Fluc-DsRed2 0.25% trypsin/EDTA.
2. Centrifuge cells at 300×*g* for 10 min and wash cells twice in PBS and centrifuge at 300×*g* for 10 min. Prepare cells

for transplantation by adding PBS to the cell pellet (1×10^6 cells in 50 μl voulume).

3. Place 5-μl of Gli36-Rluc-DsRed2 glioma cells (100,000 cells) in a 10-μl 26-gauge Hamilton Gastight 1701 syringe needle and insert the needle to a specified depth into the left frontal lobe. In our experiments we used the following stereotactic co-ordinates (2.5 mm lateral and 2.0 mm caudal to bregma; depth 2.5 mm from dura).
4. Implant cells over a period of 4 min with 30-s intervals. Care should be taken to consistently implant tumors at the same location and depth to facilitate bioluminescence interpretation from within this relative point source.
5. After implantation is complete, wait for 5 min and remove needle over a period of 10 min with an interval of 1 min.
6. Seal the burrow hole with bone wax and close the wound with 4.0 vicryl or surgical staples.

3.2.2. In Vivo Tumor Cell Bioluminescence Imaging

1. Imaging can be performed 24 h after cell implantation. Anesthetize mouse by injecting ketamine and xylazine intraperitoneally. First, acquire a surface image of each animal using dim polychromatic illumination. The spatial distribution of luciferase activity within the mouse brain can then be measured by photon count recording in a CCD camera with no illumination (*see* **Note 6**).
2. Image mice for Rluc activity by injecting coelenterazine intravenously via the tail vein and record photon counts 5 min later over a 5-min period using IVIS-200 or IVIS-100 (Caliper) or similar bioluminescence imaging system.
3. Twenty-four hours post Rluc imaging, image mice for Fluc activity by injecting the mice intraperitoneally with D-luciferin (Biotium, Inc, Hayward, CA, 150 μg/g body weight) and acquire images 10 min after D-luciferin administration over a period of 5 min using IVIS-200 or IVIS-100 (Caliper) or similar bioluminescence imaging system (*see* **Notes 7** and **8**).
4. Measure the spatial distribution of luciferase activity within the brain of the animal by recording photon counts in the CCD with no illumination. Mice can be imaged every day for Fluc and Rluc activity.
5. There should be at least a 24-h period between imaging sessions to make sure there's no residual luciferase activity of the previous session. Examples of dual bioluminescence imaging EGFR activity and cell proliferation are shown in **Fig. 11.3**.

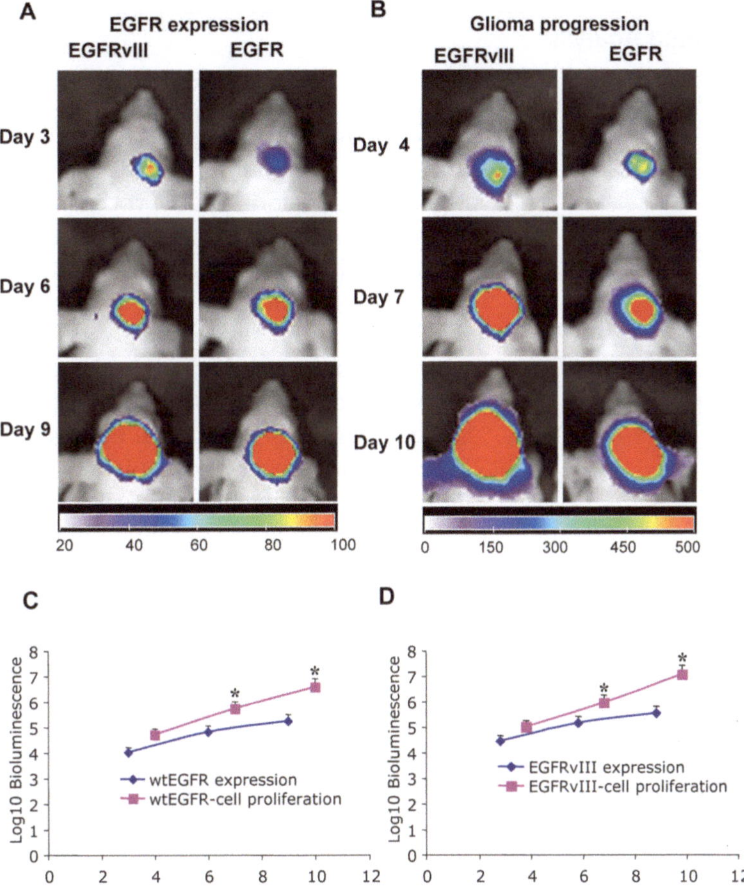

Fig. 11.3. Real-time imaging of EGFR expression and GBM burden in vivo: Gli36 glioma cells expressing EGFR-GFP-Rluc or EGFRvIII-GFP-Rluc and Fluc-DsRed were implanted into the frontal lobe of nude mice and mice were followed for 12 days by bioluminescence imaging. **a** Rluc imaging; mice injected with coelenterazine via tail vain were imaged for EGFR expression by Rluc activity on days 3, 6, and 9 after glioma cell implantation. **b** Fluc imaging: mice injected with D-luciferin i.p. and imaged for GBM proliferation by Fluc activity on days 4, 7, and 10 after glioma cell implantation. The images are a merge from the pseudocolor Rluc or Fluc activity image and the white light image of the mouse. The log 10 bioluminescence intensities of wtEGFR (**c**) and EGFRvIII (**d**) expression and cell proliferation are plotted. (Adapted from Arwert et al. (5), with permission.)

3.3. Animal Recovery

For the most part, the animal should survive the procedure despite the absence of an external heat source. Make certain the animal is restrained and when the animal is maintaining its own normal body temperature and has a reflexive response to toe-pinch stimulation, it is ready to be returned to a clean and un-occupied cage. The usual recovery time for this procedure can range from 2 to 12 h. If the animal has not resumed normal grooming and eating behavior beyond this time frame, it may require additional medical attention or euthanasia.

4. Data Analysis

Software accompanying the imaging equipment is used to perform the region of interest (ROI) analysis. In our studies, following data acquisition, post-processing and visualization was performed using a home written program with image display and analysis suite developed in IDL (Research Systems Inc., Boulder, CO). Regions of interest were defined using an automatic intensity contour procedure to identify bioluminescence signals with intensities significantly greater than the background. The mean, standard deviation, and sum of the photon counts in these regions were then calculated. For visualization purposes, the bioluminescence images were fused with the corresponding white light surface images as a transparent pseudocolor overlay, permitting correlation of areas of bioluminescence activity with anatomy. Maintaining a standard region of interest within an experiment (or series of experiments) is important to facilitate comparison of mouse imaging data.

5. Notes

1. All solutions and equipment coming into contact with live cells must be sterile.
2. All culture incubations should be performed in a humidified 37°C, 5%, CO_2 incubator unless otherwise specified.
3. An efficient and robust way to follow cells both in culture and in vivo is to transduce them with lentiviral vectors expressing fusions of bioluminescent and fluorescent marker genes. Viral transductions on human stem cells and glioma cells and cell culture procedures are performed in a biosafety level (BL)-2 facility in a laminar-flow hood.
4. All protocols involving live animals must be reviewed and approved by an Institutional Committee for Ethical Animal Care and Use (IACUC) and must conform to government regulations for the care and use of laboratory animals.
5. Mouse surgical procedures are performed in a surgical room designated for animal surgeries. Proper aseptic techniques should be used accordingly.
6. Knowing the depth and optical properties of the tissue through which the light will pass is essential in calculating numbers of cells needed to obtain a detectable signal. Generally, firefly luciferase light will be attenuated approximately tenfold for each centimeter of tissue, but optically

dense tissues such as liver will attenuate light much more than skin, bone, or lung. Thus the number of luciferase expressing cells and their localization within the body is critical to obtain a detectable signal to follow fate of cells in vivo; the deeper the tumors within the body or intracranial tumors, the greater the signal attenuation. For example, in subcutaneous tumors, cell number as low as 1,000 firefly luciferase expressing cells can be detected. Also, D-Luciferin has more favorable biodistribution than coelenterazine and an i.p. injection of luciferin is much more reproducible than tail vein injection that is required for delivering coelenterazine.

7. Transplanting cells expressing Fluc and Rluc in various sites, using various gene delivery vectors, and transgenic models the high accessibility of D-luciferin (Fluc substrate) to various tissues, including the brain. On the other hand, coelenterazine is also accessible to many tissues because of its diffusable nature (6) but its distribution in the intact brain, is limited by drug transport proteins, which can hinder in vivo imaging of *Renilla* luciferase (7). This problem may be overcome by injecting mice with blood brain barrier (BBB) disrupter, e.g., mannitol. Also, mouse fur attenuates and scatters light, and this effect is most pronounced in black mice. This problem may be overcome by using nude mice or shaving animals over the region(s) of interest for imaging.

8. Luciferase imaging in mice offers the possibility of imaging mice serially. To perform repetitive imaging of mice, the user should take into account that luciferase levels in mice peak approximately 10 min after i.p. injection, then decline slowly to background levels by 6–8 h post injection (8). Coelenterazine has a more rapid kinetic course in mice. Therefore, maximum imaging signal for *Renilla* luciferases is obtained immediately after injecting coelenterazine through intravenous or intra-cardiac routes (9). For imaging two different molecular events simultaneously, for example, stem cell fate and GBM volumes in the same mouse, it is advisable to image *Renilla* luciferase activity first and then image firefly luciferase activity.

References

1. Watanabe, K., Tachibana, O., Sata, K., Yonekawa, Y., Kleihues, P., and Ohgaki, H. (1996) Overexpression of the EGF receptor and p53 mutations are mutually exclusive in the evolution of primary and secondary glioblastomas. *Brain Pathol.* 6, 217–23; discussion 23–4.
2. Rasheed, B. K., Wiltshire, R. N., Bigner, S. H., and Bigner, D. D. (1999) Molecular pathogenesis of malignant gliomas. *Curr. Opin. Oncol.* **11**, 162–7.
3. Wikstrand, C. J., Reist, C. J., Archer, G. E., Zalutsky, M. R., and Bigner, D. D. (1998) The class III variant of the epidermal growth

factor receptor (EGFRvIII): characterization and utilization as an immunotherapeutic target. *J. Neurovirol.* **4**, 148–58.

4. Nishikawa, R., Ji, X. D., Harmon, R. C., Lazar, C. S., Gill, G. N., Cavenee, W. K., and Huang, H. J. (1994) A mutant epidermal growth factor receptor common in human glioma confers enhanced tumorigenicity. *Proc. Natl. Acad. Sci. USA* **91**, 7727–31.
5. Arwert, E., Hingtgen, S., Figueiredo, J. L., Bergquist, H., Mahmood, U., Weissleder, R., and Shah, K. (2007) Visualizing the dynamics of EGFR activity and antiglioma therapies in vivo. *Cancer Res.* **67**, 7335–42.
6. Lorenz, W. W., Cormier, M. J., O'Kane, D. J., Hua, D., Escher, A. A., and Szalay, A. A. (1996) Expression of the Renilla reniformis luciferase gene in mammalian cells. *J. Biolumin. Chemilumin.* **11**, 31–7.
7. Pichler, A., Prior, J. L., and Piwnica-Worms, D. (2004) Imaging reversal of multidrug resistance in living mice with bioluminescence: MDR1 P-glycoprotein transports coelenterazine. *Proc. Natl. Acad. Sci. USA* **101**, 1702–7.
8. Paroo, Z., Bollinger, R. A., Braasch, D. A., Richer, E., Corey, D. R., Antich, P. P., and Mason, R. P. (2004) Validating bioluminescence imaging as a high-throughput, quantitative modality for assessing tumor burden. *Mol. Imaging* **3**, 117–24.
9. Bhaumik, S. and Gambhir, S. S. (2002) Optical imaging of Renilla luciferase reporter gene expression in living mice. *Proc. Natl. Acad. Sci. USA* **99**, 377–82.

Chapter 12

Fluorescence Lifetime-Based Optical Molecular Imaging

Anand T.N. Kumar

Abstract

Fluorescence lifetime is a powerful contrast mechanism for in vivo molecular imaging. In this chapter, we describe instrumentation and methods to optimally exploit lifetime contrast using a time domain fluorescence tomography system. The key features of the system are the use of point excitation in free-space using ultrashort laser pulses and non-contact detection using a gated, intensified CCD camera. The surface boundaries of the imaging volume are acquired using a photogrammetric camera integrated with the imaging system, and implemented in theoretical models of light propagation in biological tissue. The time domain data are optimally analyzed using a lifetime-based tomography approach, which is based on extracting a tomographic set of lifetimes and decay amplitudes from the long time decay portion of the time domain data. This approach improves the ability to locate in vivo targets with a resolution better than conventional optical methods. The application of time domain lifetime multiplexing and tomography are illustrated using phantoms and tumor bearing mouse model of breast adenocarcinoma. In the latter application, the time domain approach allows an improved detection of fluorescent protein signals from intact nude mice in the presence of background autofluorescence. This feature has potential applications for longitudinal pre-clinical evaluation of drug treatment response as well as to address fundamental questions related to tumor physiology and metastasis.

Key words: Fluorescence, lifetime, fluorescent proteins, optical tomography, tissue optics.

1. Introduction

Optical molecular imaging offers several advantages over conventional techniques such as positron emission tomography (PET) and magnetic resonance imaging (MRI). Foremost among these is cost effectiveness, portability, and the lack of radiation damage. In addition, a wide range of optical probes have been synthesized that allow the ability to multiplex based on fluorescence

K. Shah (ed.), *Molecular Imaging*, Methods in Molecular Biology 680,
DOI 10.1007/978-1-60761-901-7_12,

spectrum and lifetime. In addition to extrinsic targeting of disease using conjugated fluorophores, intrinsic contrast can also be achieved using fluorescent proteins (FPs). FPs are powerful tools for imaging gene expression and tracking disease progression such as metastasis (1, 2). While multi-spectral techniques have been employed to enhance deep tissue fluorescence imaging (3, 4), the application of fluorescence lifetime has been restricted mainly to microscopy techniques (5). For example, a major confound for deep tissue, whole-body imaging of fluorescent proteins is that their excitation wavelength is in the visible region (400–650 nm), and can overlap strongly with tissue autofluorescence (AF) (6). While multi-spectral techniques can be used to alleviate this problem to some extent (4), fluorescence lifetime contrast is an additional mechanism that can improve the separation of the FP signal from background AF using their distinct temporal responses on the nanosecond timescales. More general applications of whole-body lifetime-based molecular imaging are only beginning to emerge in recent years (7, 8). A major challenge for lifetime imaging for deep tissue applications is the technical complexity involved in time domain (TD) instrumentation and in the interpretation of the data. In this chapter, we describe the experimental and theoretical steps involved in obtaining three-dimensional in vivo distributions of multiple lifetimes present within an imaging sample from TD fluorescence measurements.

2. Materials

2.1. Tomography System

A schematic of a free-space, non-contact small animal fluorescence molecular imaging system is shown in **Fig. 12.1**. The main components of the tomography system are an excitation source, detection apparatus, and a 3D camera for surface boundary acquisition. In the non-contact geometry, the sample to be imaged (animal or subject) is placed on a transparent plate directly below the camera and is excited either from below or above using a fiber that delivers the light output of the laser. The individual components are detailed below.

2.2. Excitation and Detection

1. For time domain measurements, a pulsed laser source (<50 ps pulse duration) is necessary. The most versatile excitation sources for NIR measurements are based on Ti:Sapphire lasers for excitation in the near infrared (such as the Mai Tai, Newport-Spectra Physics, Mountain View CA, ~150 fs pulse width, 80 MHz repetition rate, 690–1,020 nm tuning range) or fiber lasers for visible to

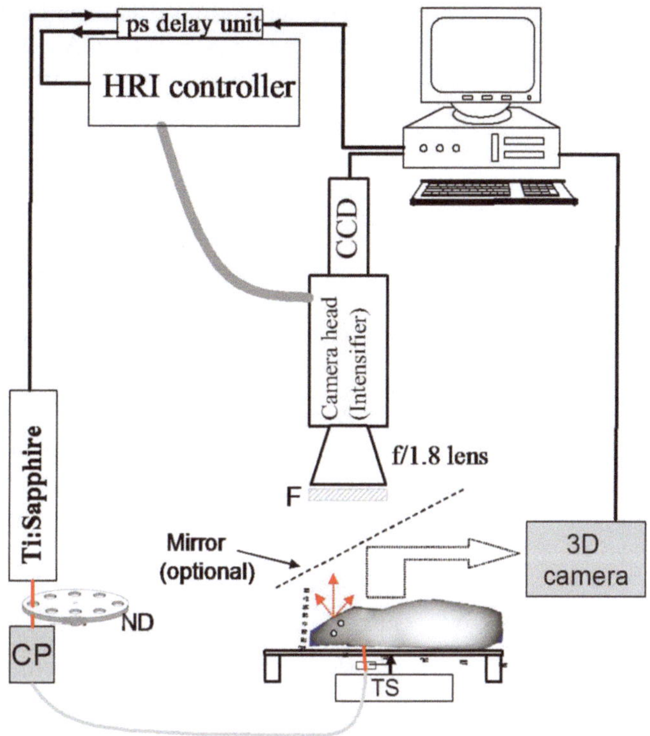

Fig. 12.1. Schematic of the free space TD fluorescence tomography system. The source consists of a Ti:Sapphire laser (750–850 nm), the output of which is collimated using a collimation package (CP) and launched into a 200-μm step-index fiber. The other end of the fiber is connected to a collimation package, to allow for a tight focus spot (1 mm) on the sample surface, and mounted on a translation stage (TS) for scanning over the surface of the imaging subject (*see* **Note 1**). Detection is performed using an intensifier in conjunction with a CCD camera mounted on a manually adjustable rail system. The other symbols are as follows – F: filter (optional); ND: Neutral density filter wheel.

infrared excitation (such as the Fianum, from Fianium Inc., Southampton UK).

2. The light output from the pulsed source is attenuated to about 10 mW depending on the sample thickness, and launched into an SMA connectorized fiber using a fiber collimation package (FC) (Thorlabs Inc.).
3. Using a second collimation package, the light at the output end of the fiber is focused to a fine spot on the imaging surface, resulting in an approximately point excitation source.
4. For tomographic scanning, the second collimation package system is mounted on a computer-controlled, micrometer precision XY translation stage system (Velmex Inc., Bloomfeld NY).

5. The detection is performed in free space using a CCD camera (Picostar HR-12 CAM 2, LaVision GmbH, Goettingen, Germany, quantum efficiency of 65%).
6. A time gated image intensifier (Picostar HR-12, LaVision GmbH, Goettingen, Germany), with a 200 ps minimum gate width, provides nanosecond time resolution.
7. A fast delay unit (Picostar HRI, 1 ms switching, 25 ps minimum steps) is used to delay the trigger output from that of the laser, across one duty cycle of 12.5 ns (80 MHz).
8. The output of the delay unit is in-turn used to trigger the intensifier unit.
9. A camera lens (AF Nikkor, f2.8, Nikon) mounted on the CCD camera is used to obtain a well-focused image of the entire surface of the mouse head on the CCD image plane.
10. A 2 in. interference filter can optionally be mounted to the front of the camera lens to allow excitation or emission measurements (*see* below).
11. Since the scanning speed of the stepper motor is much slower than the delay switching time, the full temporal signal can be collected for one source position at a time (*see* **Note 2**).

2.3. Surface Boundary Acquisition

For accurate forward modeling of the light propagation, the boundary information of the phantom or animal is necessary. Photogrammetric 3D camera systems (such as the 3D Facecam 100, Technest Holdings Inc., Bethesda MD) may be employed to acquire the surface image. The 3D image is acquired by sliding a mirror in front of the camera lens as shown in **Fig. 12.1**. Further details on processing the 3D camera image and co-registration with the CCD image are presented in Section **3** below.

3. Methods

The tomographic reconstruction of fluorescence distribution is achieved using several steps as shown schematically in **Fig. 12.2** (*see* **Note 6**).

1. The TD data comprise of the full temporal profile for multiple sources and detectors (CCD camera pixels) on the surface of the imaging subject. A typical measurement set includes two wavelengths, λ_x and λ_m, which correspond to the absorption and emission maxima of the fluorophore employed for contrast enhancement. Excitation measurements, denoted as $U^{(x,x)}$ and $U^{(m,m)}$, correspond to the

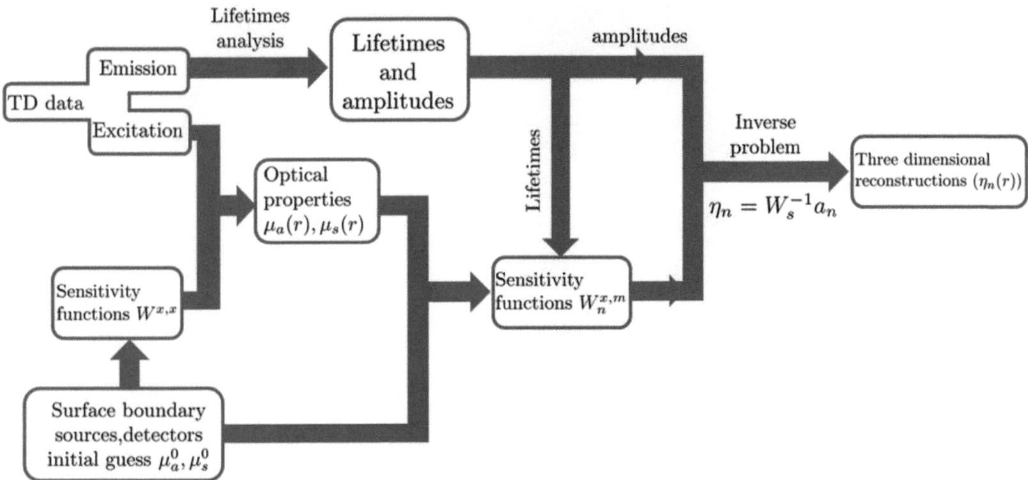

Fig. 12.2. Schematic representation of the steps involved in processing time domain fluorescence data for tomographic reconstructions.

direct detection of light transmitted through the sample at wavelengths λ_x and λ_m and are first acquired with the filter wavelength matching the laser excitation.

2. Emission data (denoted as $U^{(x,m)}$) refer to purely fluorescence emission and are collected with the laser tuned to λ_x, whereas the filter is tuned to λ_m.
3. The excitation and emission data are processed along independent paths. The excitation data are used to determine the background optical property distribution of the sample and to generate sensitivity functions for reconstructing the fluorescence. In parallel, the emission data are analyzed using multi-exponential analysis to recover the amplitudes of all the lifetime components present in the sample.
4. Finally, these amplitudes are used along with the sensitivity functions to invert the 3D yield distribution for each lifetime component. The individual steps are further detailed below.

3.1. Measuring the Impulse Response, Time Origin, and Source Positions

1. The system impulse response function (IRF) is defined as the signal at the detector in the absence of any sample. The IRF can be readily measured by placing a thin, non-scattering absorber, such as a piece of paper on the imaging plate (without the sample). The signal collected at the camera then directly gives the IRF. The IRF provides information for the initial time t_0 when the excitation pulse is incident on surface of the imaging medium. A correct estimate of t_0 ensures that the relative amplitudes of the multiple lifetime components are correct, and is crucial for estimating the optical properties using TD data.

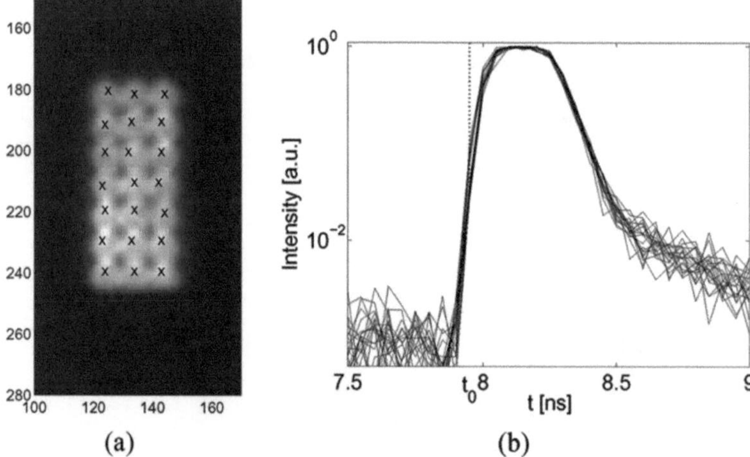

Fig. 12.3. Measurement of IRF and time origin. **a** Direct CCD image of the source illumination, obtained by focusing the fiber output on a thin sheet of paper placed on the imaging plate (without the imaging subject present). The image shown is the integrated TD signal for 21 source positions, used for the phantom measurements reported in the text. The source coordinates were obtained as the points of maximum intensity. **b** Normalized TD Impulse response curves for all the 21 sources. The *vertical dotted line* indicates the time origin t_0, estimated as the time at 1% of the peak intensity. The time t_0 corresponds to the initial time of excitation at the boundary of a subject placed on the plate, assuming the subject surface is approximately flat. Reproduced from Kumar et al., with permission from IEEE (© 2008, IEEE) (13).

2. **Figure 12.3a** shows the time integrated, i.e., continuous wave (CW) IRFs for a grid of 21 source positions spaced 2 mm along the X and Y translation directions. The source grid image in **Fig. 12.3a** also serves to determine the coordinates of the sources for forward modeling. These are obtained as the points of maximum intensity, after the image for each source position is median-filtered.
3. **Figure 12.3b** shows the corresponding IRF's for all source positions. The width of the IRF is ideally nearly equal to the gate width setting of the intensifier unit. Since the variation between the IRF is minimal across the sources (<10 ps), the initial time t_0 can be assumed to be identical for all source positions and estimated from the mean of the impulse response as the time at 1% of the peak. This value can be assumed to be the excitation time at the surface of the imaging medium provided the boundary of the imaging volume is approximately flat (*see* **Note 3**).
4. The measured IRF can be directly forward convolved into the model before tomographic inversion. (This procedure is superior to a de-convolution of the IRF from the raw fluorescence data, which is a highly ill-posed problem.)

3.2. Surface Boundary and Co-registration

1. The imaging subject is placed on the imaging plate and its boundary secured using additional restraints for repeatability in positioning.
2. The 3D image surface is then acquired with the optional mirror in place (**Fig. 12.1**).
3. The 3D camera captures a surface image of the mouse as triangulated vertex data with a resolution of 100 μm. This high-density data are first reduced to a set of unique surface mesh points, which are then interpolated using the Matlab (The Mathworks, Natick, MA) function "ndgrid," to provide a surface on a uniform mesh.
4. The surface image is then co-registered with the planar image of the CCD camera with which the fluorescence data are acquired. The transformation can be effected as a 2D affine transformation between the CCD image and the 3D surface image, using four fiducial points in the form of metal screws placed on the subject plate at points identifiable both in the 3D camera and the CCD field-of-view (indicated by a "+" sign in **Fig. 12.4**).
5. Once the affine transformation matrix between the 3D camera image and the CCD image has been determined, the source and detector locations are transformed to the reference frame of the 3D camera image. The surface data are next converted into an indexed volume image and used in numerical modeling of light transport (*see* **Note 4**).
6. A single 3D image thus acquired along with the fiducials can be used as the reference image for any optical measurement using the same subject provided that the fiducial points are visible on the CCD image and the subject is placed at the same relative position with respect to the fiducials.

Figure 12.4 shows the co-registration results for a mouse shaped phantom. **Figure 12.4a** shows the CCD image with the mouse phantom, the fiducials, and a grid of 93 detector positions arranged on the camera image. **Figure 12.4b** shows the planar image of the 3D surface used for the co-registration, along with source and detector coordinates mapped on the surface image using the affine transformation.

3.3. Multi-exponential Fits

We envisage a scenario where a single or multiple fluorophore(s) are injected into an animal and the in vivo distribution of each lifetime component of the fluorophore(s) can reveal potential information about the disease target. To proceed with the analysis, a key step is the extraction of the lifetimes and the decay amplitudes as measured on the surface. As shown in **Fig. 12.2**, this proceeds independently of the optical property estimation.

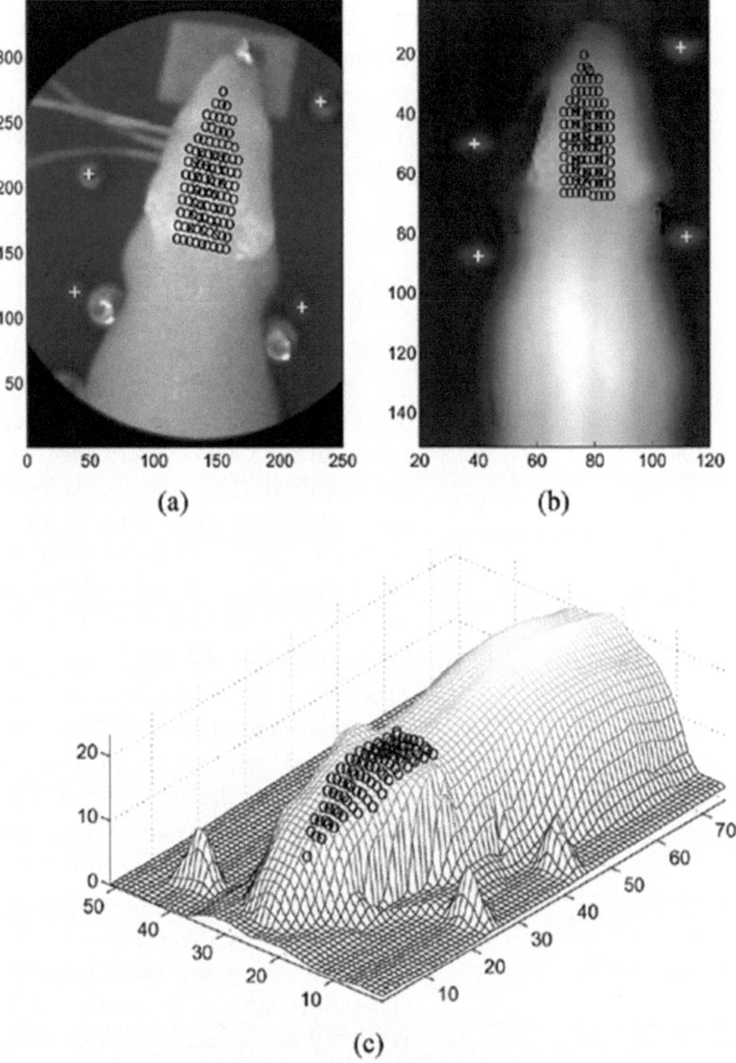

Fig. 12.4. Coregistration of CCD camera image with 3D camera surface image. **a** Room light illuminated image of the mouse phantom placed on the imaging plate. The + symbols indicate the fiducial points used for co-registration. The sources (x) determined from the impulse response (*see* **Fig. 12.3**) and detectors (o) assigned on the camera image also shown. **b** *Top-down* view of the 3D surface of the mouse phantom, also showing the fiducials (+) and the mapped sources and detectors, whose coordinates were determined from the affine transformation (**Section 3.2**). **c** 3D view of the surface image of the phantom shown along with the transformed detectors from the CCD image. Reproduced from Kumar et al., with permission from IEEE (© 2008, IEEE) (13).

1. According to the asymptotic model (9), the measured fluorescence signal, $U(x,m)$, can be expressed in the asymptotic limit as a sum of discretized exponential decays with lifetime components, τ_n, which are independent of the measurements locations (i.e., the S-D coordinates):

$$U^{(x,m)}(\mathbf{r}_s, \mathbf{r}_d, t) \rightarrow \sum_n a_n(\mathbf{r}_s, \mathbf{r}_d) e^{-t/\tau_n} \qquad [1]$$

where $\mathbf{r}_s$ and $\mathbf{r}_d$ are the coordinates of the source and detector. The amplitudes, a_n, which can be recovered simply by fitting the decay portion of the time domain data, are directly related to the spatial distribution of the fluorophore corresponding to that lifetime, labeled as $\eta_n(r)$. The nonlinear fits to recover the lifetimes and amplitudes are numerically implemented using built-in Matlab functions such as "fminsearch," which employs an unconstrained nonlinear optimization using the Nelder-Mead simplex approach (*see* **Note 5**).

2. In some applications (such as autofluorescence and other complex fluorophores), the fluorescent target of interest may exhibit non-exponential behavior, i.e., cannot be described by a single exponential decay function. In this case it is more appropriate to analyze the fluorophore in terms of basis functions that have been pre-determined. One example is tissue autofluorescence (*see* equation [4] and related discussion in **Section 3.9**).

3.4. Optical Property Estimation and Sensitivity Functions

With a knowledge of source-detector locations in the reference frame of the 3D digitized volume of the imaging subject, the next step is the computation of the "forward problem," which involves modeling the light propagation within the tissue volume. This can be carried out either using a transport equation-based approach, numerically implemented using the Monte-Carlo (MC) method (10, 11) or a diffusion-equation based approach implemented using the finite element method (FEM) (12).

1. The forward problem is calculated with an initial assumption for the optical absorption, μ^0 and scattering, μ^0 coefficients, usually assumed to be homogeneous throughout the sample volume.
2. The computational prediction from the model is then matched with the measured excitation measurements ($U^{(x,x)}$ and $U^{(m,m)}$) using iterative fitting procedures to obtain heterogeneous distributions of the absorption and scattering $\mu_a(r)$ and $\mu_s(r)$, at λ_x and λ_m, where r denotes the position within the imaging sample.
3. The continuous-wave fluorescence sensitivity functions for each lifetime component, $W^{(x,m)}$, are then calculated using the heterogeneous absorption reduced by $1/v\tau_n$, i.e., $\mu_a(r) - 1/v\tau_n$, where v denotes the velocity of light in the medium (13). These sensitivity functions will be later used to recover the fluorescence distribution for each lifetime component as detailed below.

3.5. Inverse Problem and Tomographic Reconstruction

The amplitudes recovered from the asymptotic approach (**Section 3.3**) are directly related to the fluorescence sensitivity profiles $W^{(x,m)}$ (**Section 3.4**) and the fluorescence distributions for each lifetime $\eta_n\,(r)$ as follows:

$$a_n(\mathbf{r}_s, \mathbf{r}_d) = \int d^3 r W_n^{(x,m)}(\mathbf{r}_s, \mathbf{r}_d, \mathbf{r})\eta_n(\mathbf{r}). \qquad [2]$$

The above equation needs to be solved for the unknown fluorescence yield distributions $\eta_n(\mathrm{r})$. Denoting $W_n^{(x,m)}$ as W for simplicity, the inverse solution is written as $\eta_n = W_s^{-1} a_n$, where the pseudo-inverse of the sensitivity function defined as

$$W_s^{-1} = W^T (WW^T + \alpha\lambda I)^{-1} \qquad [3]$$

where $\alpha = \max(\mathrm{diag}(WW^T))$. Various conditioning techniques may be employed to improve the quality of the reconstruction (12).

3.6. Mouse Phantoms

1. Mouse shaped phantoms are prepared using the negative mold made from a sacrificed mouse. The mold for the phantom consists of a two-part epoxy resin (7132) and hardener (2001) mixture, from Douglas & Sturgess Inc. (San Francisco, CA).
2. First, calculate the net volume of the mold to be filled. Then weigh two parts of the resin and one-part hardener by weight in separate containers, and mix them thoroughly.
3. Next, add a combination of TiO_2 (paint) and ink to the epoxy-resin mixture, to achieve approximate background optical properties of $\mu_s = 10\ \mathrm{cm}^{-1}$ and $\mu_a = 0.1\ \mathrm{cm}^{-1}$. Mix thoroughly.
4. Inclusions (cavities) can be created inside the phantom by positioning low-melting-point agar beads (5 mm diameter) using pairs of syringe needles. The agar beads can be cast in a spherical negative mold.
5. Pour the epoxy mixture into the negative mold and let it cure for about 12 h.
6. Once the mold is cured, remove the needles and the negative mold. Next, attach fresh needles along with polypropylene tubing, to enable dynamic injection of fluorophores into the inclusions. **Figure 12.5a** shows a photograph of the mouse phantom along with the injection tubes.

3.7. Cell Culture Preparation and Tumor Mice Models

1. Tumor bearing mouse models were derived from the human breast cancer cell line, MDA-MB-231, which expressed both enhanced green fluorescent protein (EGFP) and cyan fluorescent protein (CFP).

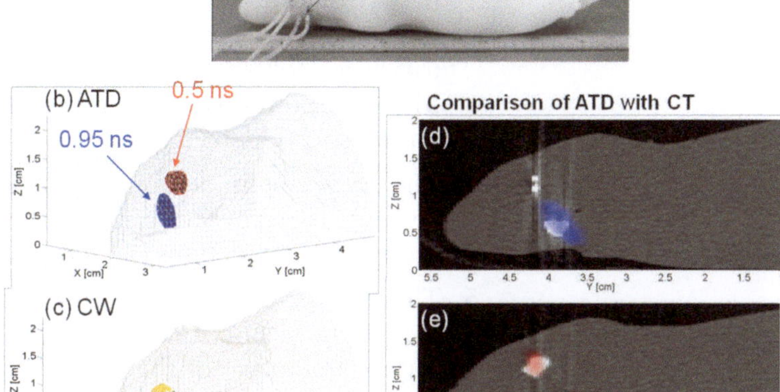

Fig. 12.5. Phantom validation of lifetime based tomography. **a** The phantom (epoxy+Ti02+ink combination) had two inclusions (*A* and *B*) for fluorophore injection. **b** TD reconstruction of data collected with the two inclusions filled with a NIR dye in water (0.5 ns) and glycerol (0.95 ns). The reconstructed yields are shown for 0.5 ns (*red*) and 0.95 ns (*blue*) as iso-surfaces at 95% the maximum intensity. The gray mesh is the 3D surface (from the 3D camera) used for the forward modeling. **c** The CW reconstruction does not resolve the two inclusions separately. The ATD reconstruction are shown **d** for the 0.95 ns component (*blue*) and **e** for the 0.5 ns component (*red*), co-registered with the CT images of the phantom (*grayscale*, with inclusions seen as *white*). The images in (d) and (**e**) show sagittal planes containing the centroid of the two inclusions. (The two tubes feeding inclusion *A* are visible in (d).)

2. Cells are first grown in a humidified atmosphere under 5% CO_2. The cells ($\approx 2 \times 10^6$) are then suspended in 50 μl of Hanks' Balanced Salt Solution (Invitrogen, New York).
3. For in vitro studies, the cells are placed in eppendorf tubes and imaged in a reflectance model with the TD system.
4. For in vivo imaging, the tumor cells are injected directly into the mammary fat pads of 6- to 8-week-old female nude mice.
5. The mice are imaged 3–4 weeks post implantation, when the tumor is 7–8 mm in diameter.

3.8. Tomography with Mouse Phantoms

1. **Figure 12.5** shows a demonstration of lifetime-based tomography in a mouse shaped phantom. The phantom had two approximately spherical inclusions (**Fig. 12.5a**), filled with a NIR dye (3,3′-diethylthiatricarbo-cyanine) with absorption and emission maxima near 755 and 790 nm.
2. To achieve lifetime contrast, two solutions were prepared with the dye dissolved in distilled water and glycerol solutions, which resulted in intrinsic lifetimes of 0.5 and 0.95 ns, respectively (13).

3. The longer lived dye solution in glycerol was injected in inclusion B and the shorter lived aqueous dye solution of the dye in inclusion A (*see* **Fig. 12.5a**). The mouse phantom was placed in the imaging setup shown in **Fig. 12.1** and the data were collected in the trans-illumination geometry for 21 source positions and 93 assigned detectors on the camera image (source-detector arrangement shown in **Fig. 12.4**).
4. The decay amplitudes for the two lifetime components were inverted to recover the fluorescence yield localizations as prescribed in equations [2] and [3].
5. The reconstruction results using the lifetime-based approach are shown in **Fig. 12.5b** as 3D images overlayed with the surface boundary of the phantom. The images shown are isosurface maps at 95% peak intensity.
6. The regularization parameter λ (equation [3]) was near unity for the reconstructions shown and was chosen based on an empirical assessment of image quality.
7. The yield reconstruction for the shorter lifetime of 0.5 ns is seen to have a shallower depth than that for the longer lifetime of 0.95 ns, as expected.
8. Also shown in **Fig. 12.5c** is the reconstruction of the two inclusions using the CW component of the data, which is unable to resolve the two axially located inclusions. (Further details regarding the accuracy of the reconstructions can be found in reference (12).)
9. The TD reconstructions were compared with CT images of the mouse phantom, to verify accuracy. As seen from **Fig. 12.5d, e**, the asymptotic yield reconstructions match the true locations of the inclusions as recovered by the CT image reasonably well.

3.9. Imaging of Fluorescent Protein Expression in Tumor Bearing Mice

1. **Figure 12.6** shows an example application of lifetime multiplexing for imaging fluorescent protein expressing tumors in a mouse model of breast adenocarcinoma. **Figure 12.6b** shows the CW (intensity only) reflectance image for area illumination across the torso of the mouse placed in supine position, for 488 nm (10 nm width) excitation and 515 nm (long pass) emission. The CW image is overlaid on the white light image of the mouse. While the location of the tumor is apparent from the intensity image, the AF component is significant across the whole illumination area and effectively reduces the contrast of the FP signal.
2. The AF decay is highly non-exponential and has lifetime components overlapping with the FP lifetime, making the two indistinguishable in a multi-exponential analysis approach. Thus, rather than fit the surface TD

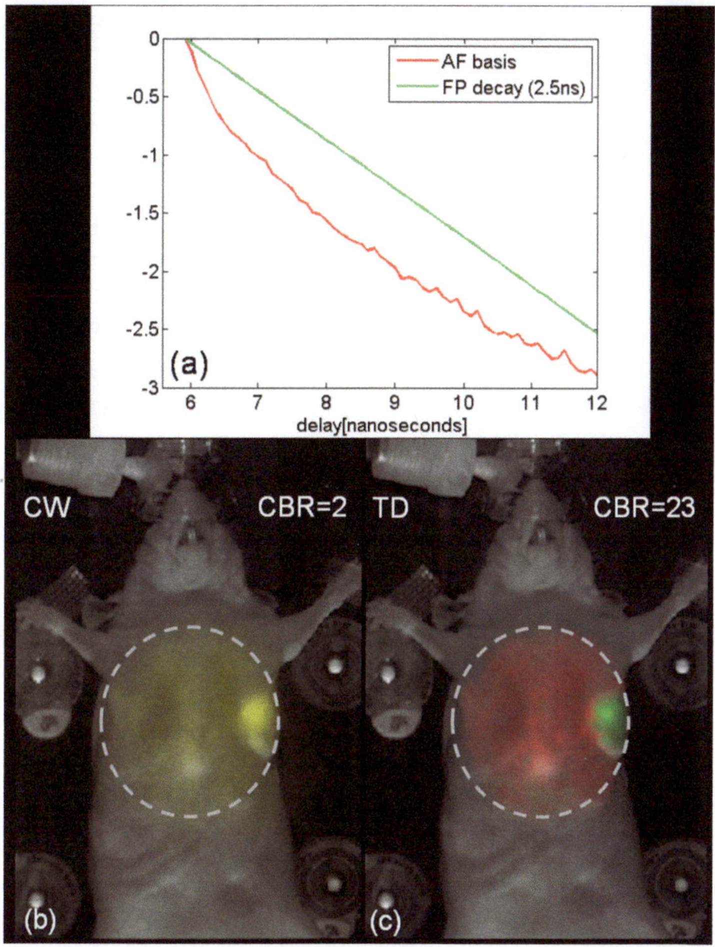

Fig. 12.6. Whole-body fluorescence lifetime measurements with FP expressing tumor mouse models. **a** Temporal responses of the autofluorescence and the dual EGFP/CFP expressing tumor cell lines. The AF decay is non-exponential, described by a basis function $B(t)$ while the FP decay is exponential with a lifetime of 2.5 ns. **b** CW component (*yellow*) of the reflectance TD fluorescence measurement (exc:488 nm, em:515 nm longpass) of an anesthetized nude mouse placed in supine position. 2×10^6 EGFP/CFP expressing breast tumor cell lines (MDA-MB-231) were implanted in the mammary fat pad. The images shown were obtained 3 weeks post implantation. **c** The amplitude components of the AF (*red*) and FP (*green*) decays, *a*AF and *a*FP, obtained by fitting equation [4] to the raw TD fluorescence data are shown as a single RGB image. The *dashed lines* indicate the illumination area ($\approx$2.5 cm^2). The background image of the mouse is shown in *grayscale*.

decays to a sum of exponentials, more robust results can be obtained using a "basis function" approach that performs a linear fit for the decay amplitudes, using a priori knowledge of the decay profiles of the AF and FP.

3. First, the FP lifetimes can be easily measured in vitro using the tumor cells prior to injection into the mice. The lifetime

of the dual EGFP/CFP expressing cells used here was found to be 2.5 ns.

4. Second, the AF basis function was formed as the average AF response (for 488 nm excitation/515 nm long pass detection, corresponding to the FP excitation and emission) across the torso of three mice. **Figure 12.6a** shows the decay profiles of the AF and the FP fluorescence used as basis functions. Using the known FP lifetime and the AF basis $B(t)$, a simple bi-functional linear model was used to fit the asymptotic portion (8) of the raw TD data:

$$U(\mathbf{r}_d, t) = a_{\mathrm{AF}}(\mathbf{r}_d)B(t) + a_{\mathrm{FP}}(\mathbf{r}_d)\exp(-t/\tau_{\mathrm{FP}}), \quad [4]$$

where τ_{FP} is the lifetime of the FP and r_d is the location of an image pixel. **Figure 12.6c** shows the decoupled AF (red) and FP (green) amplitudes as the red and green components of a single RGB image matrix. The error of the fit was less than 5% across the entire illumination area. The TD approach (**Fig. 12.6c**) confirms the presence of the tumor and provides a superior delineation of the tumor from the background AF, as compared to the CW intensity image (**Fig. 12.6a**).

5. The contrast-to-background ratio (CBR) was estimated for the CW (TD) approaches as the ratio of the net intensity (decay amplitude) within the tumor region and corresponding value outside the tumor region. The CBR was near 23 for the TD approach, compared to near 2 for the CW case, suggesting a > tenfold improvement.

6. While this example shows that planar lifetime imaging can by itself enable longitudinal quantification of tumor growth, angiogenesis and therapeutic response in a single animal, the FP amplitudes, a_{FP}, could also be employed in lifetime-based tomography techniques as detailed in earlier in **Section 3** for recovering 3D distributions of FP expression.

4. Notes

1. Reflectance measurements could also be readily performed, if needed, by mounting the fiber above the phantom plate (not shown in **Fig. 12.1**).

2. An alternative approach to stepper motor based scanning is the use of gavanometers with millisecond switching times. This will allow whole body scans for each time step.

3. The measured time at the detector pixels is offset from the actual t_0 by the time for free space propagation of light from the source to the camera. When an imaging medium of small thickness, such as a mouse, is placed on the source plate, the corresponding offset for fluorescence emitted on the surface will very nearly equal the offset from the source. A small correction factor can be applied to account for the propagation time in free space corresponding to the thickness of the mouse (e.g., for a 2-cm-thick mouse, the time offset is ≈ 50 ps).
4. If the heterogeneous tissue structure of the animal is available from either MRI or CT scans, these can be employed directly in the approach presented here with appropriate fiducials and co-registration.
5. The recovery of lifetimes from decay data is a non-linear problem that can be computationally challenging, especially for more than two lifetimes. The best-case scenario is when the in vivo lifetimes are known in advance. Alternatively, the multi-exponential analysis can be performed in two stages for robust fitting results. First, an integrated decay function is formed by summing the decays from all S-D pair measurements, to obtain a high signal-to-noise ratio (SNR) temporal data set. This "global" signal is composed of all the lifetime components present in the system, and allows a more robust determination of the lifetimes through a non-linear analysis. In the second step, the lifetimes determined from the surface-integrated time domain data are used in a *linear* fit of the DFTR for each individual S-D pair. Besides improving the robustness of the fitting procedure for the lifetimes and decay amplitudes, the global analysis is computationally much less cumbersome than performing a non-linear fit for every S-D measurement.
6. Other approaches for analyzing time domain fluorescence data have also been presented particularly based on using the early arriving photons for improved resolution (14). This chapter is concerned with fluorescence lifetime contrast which involves the late arriving photons, and provides complementary information regarding the in vivo fluorescence distribution.

Acknowledgement

This research was supported by the National Institutes of Health grant NIH AG026240.

References

1. Jain, R. K., Munn, L. L., and Fukumura, D. (2002) Dissecting tumor pathophysiology using intravital microscopy. *Nat. Rev. Cancer* **2**, 266.
2. Yang, M., et al. (2003) Dual-color fluorescence imaging distinguishes tumor cells from induced host angiogenic vessels and stromal cells. *Proc. Nat. Acad. Sci. USA* **100**, 14259.
3. Gao, X., Cui, Y., Levenson, R. M., Chung, L. W. K., and Nie, S. (2004) In vivo cancer targeting and imaging with semiconductor quantum dots. *Nat. Biotech.* **22**, 969.
4. Tam, J. M., Upadhyay, R., Pittet, M. J., Weissleder, R., and Mahmood, U. (2007) Improved in vivo whole-animal detection limits of green fluorescent protein-expressing tumor lines by spectral fluorescence imaging. *Mol. Imaging* **6**, 269–76.
5. Bastiaens, P. I. H. and Squire, A. (1999) Fluorescence lifetime imaging microscopy: spatial resolution of biochemical processes in the cell. *Trends Cell. Biol.* **9**, 48.
6. Deliolanis, N. C., Kasmieh, R., Wurdinger, T., Tannous, B. A., Shah, K., and Ntziachristos, V. (2008) Performance of the red-shifted fluorescent proteins in deep-tissue molecular imaging applications. *J. Biomed. Opt.* **13**, 044008.
7. Bloch, S., Lesage, F., Mackintosh, L., Gandjbakche, A., Liang, K., and Achilefu, S. (2005) Whole-body fluorescence lifetime imaging of a tumor-targeted near-infrared molecular probe in mice. *J. Biomed. Opt.* **10**, 054003.
8. Kumar, A. T. N., Chung, E., Raymond, S. B., Van de Water, J., Shah, K., Fukumura, D., Jain, R. K., Bacskai, B. J., and Boas, D. A. (2009) Feasibility of in vivo imaging of fluorescent proteins using lifetime contrast. *Opt. Lett.* **34**, 2067.
9. Kumar, A. T. N., Raymond, S. B., Boverman, G., Boas, D. A., and Bacskai, B. J. (2006) Time resolved fluorescence tomography based on lifetime contrast. *Opt. Exp.* **14**, 12255–70.
10. Wang, L., Jacques, S. L., and Zheng, L. (1995) MCML-Monte Carlo modeling of light transport in multi-layered tissues. *Comput. Methods Programs Biomed.* **47**, 131–46.
11. Boas, D. A., Culver, J. P., Stott, J. J., and Dunn, A. K. (2002) Three dimensional Monte Carlo code for photon migration through complex heterogeneous media including the adult human head. *Opt. Exp.* **10**, 159–70.
12. Arridge, S. R. (1999) Optical tomography in medical imaging. *Inverse Probl.* **15**, R41–93.
13. Kumar, A. T. N., Raymond, S. B., Dunn, A. K., Bacskai, B. J., and Boas, D. A. (2008) A time domain fluorescence tomography system for small animal imaging. *IEEE Trans. Med. Imaging* **27**, 1152.
14. Niedre, M. J., de Kleine, R. H., Aikawa, E., Kirsch, D. G., Weissleder, R., and Ntziachristos, V. (2008) Early photon tomography allows fluorescence detection of lung carcinomas and disease progression in mice in vivo. *Proc. Natl. Acad. Sci. USA* **105**, 19126–31.

Section III

Imaging in Clinical Settings

Chapter 13

PET Imaging of $\alpha v\beta 3$ Expression in Cancer Patients

Ambros J. Beer and Markus Schwaiger

Abstract

Imaging of $\alpha v\beta 3$ expression in malignant diseases has been extensively studied in the last years, mainly because the level of integrin $\alpha v\beta 3$ expression might be a surrogate parameter of angiogenic activity. Most studies have been performed using preclinical tumor models but recently first results if imaging $\alpha v\beta 3$ expression in patients have been published. The first approach used was the radiotracer approach with tracers for positron emission tomography (PET) like [^{18}F]Galacto-RGD or tracers for single photon emission computed tomography (SPECT) like [^{99m}Tc]NC100692. In this article we will focus on the experimental design and methodology of PET imaging of $\alpha v\beta 3$ expression with the tracer [^{18}F]Galacto-RGD. Common difficulties and pitfalls in image acquisition and interpretation will be discussed. Finally, the performance of PET will be compared to other methods of imaging of $\alpha v\beta 3$ expression, like magnetic resonance imaging, ultrasound, or optical imaging.

Key words: PET, integrin alpha v beta 3, molecular imaging, angiogenesis, RGD, [^{18}F]Galacto-RGD.

1. Introduction

Integrins are heterodimeric transmembrane glycoproteins, which play an important role in cell–cell and cell–matrixinteractions and are involved in angiogenesis and tumor metastasis (1). Integrins are cell adhesion molecules consisting of two non-covalently bound transmembrane subunits with large extracellular segments that bind to create heterodimers with distinct adhesive capabilities (2). Up to now, 18 α and 8 β subunits have been described, which assemble into 24 different receptors. Integrins are on the one hand expressed on tumor cells and facilitate metastasis by mediating tumor cell invasion and movement across blood vessels.

K. Shah (ed.), *Molecular Imaging*, Methods in Molecular Biology 680,
DOI 10.1007/978-1-60761-901-7_13,

However, integrins are also expressed on activated endothelial cells and modulate cell migration and survival during angiogenesis. Especially well examined in this respect is the integrin αvβ3. The αvβ3 integrin is significantly up-regulated on activated endothelial cells during angiogenesis but not on quiescent endothelial cells (2, 3). A common feature of many integrins like αvβ3 is that they bind to extracellular matrix proteins via the 3 amino acid sequence arginine-glycine-aspartic acid (RGD). The importance of αvβ3 for angiogenesis is further supported by the fact, that inhibition of αvβ3 integrin activity by cyclic RGD peptides, peptidomimetics, and monoclonal antibodies, can induce endothelial cell apoptosis and inhibits angiogenesis (4). However, the exact role of αvβ3 expression in the context of angiogenesis is still a matter of debate. Experiments in knock-out mice lacking the integrin αvβ3 led to a reevaluation of the role of αvβ3 concerning angiogenesis because the knock-out mice showed normal developmental angiogenesis and even excessive tumor angiogenesis (5). Nowadays, αvβ3 is assumed to have a positive and a negative regulatory role in angiogenesis depending on the respective biological context. Among all 24 integrins discovered to date, the integrin αvβ3 is still the most extensively examined factor of angiogenesis concerning imaging strategies which aim at finding a surrogate parameter of angiogenic activity. Molecular imaging for non-invasive assessment of angiogenesis is of great interest for clinicians as well as the pharmaceutical industry because antiangiogenic drugs recently have been successfully used in cancer patients like the VEGF (vascular endothelial growth factor) antibody bevacizumab in combination with standard cytotoxic chemotherapy first in metastasized colorectal cancer, and subsequently in breast cancer and non-small cell lung cancer (6, 7). Imaging of αvβ3 expression could potentially be used as a biomarker and an early indicator of effectiveness of antiangiogenic therapy at a molecular level. It has been found that several extracellular matrix (ECM) proteins like vitronectin, fibrinogen, and fibronectin interact with integrins via the amino acid sequence arginine-glycine-aspartic acid or RGD in the single letter code (8). Kessler and co-workers developed the pentapeptide cyclo(-Arg-Gly-Asp-DPhe-Val-), which shows high affinity and selectivity for αvβ3 (9). For the first evaluation of this approach, Haubner et al. have synthesized radioiodinated RGD peptides, which showed comparable affinity and selectivity to the lead structure. In vivo they revealed receptor-specific tumor uptake but also predominantly hepatobiliary elimination, resulting in high activity concentration in liver and intestine, which is unfavorable for patient studies (10). Consequently, several strategies to improve the pharmacokinetics of radiohalogenated peptides have been developed. The glycosylation approach is based on the introduction of sugar derivatives which are conjugated to the ε-amino function of a corresponding lysine in the peptide sequence. By conjugating the RGD containing cyclic pentapeptide cyclo(-Arg-Gly-Asp-DPhe-Val-) with galactose-based sugar amino acids, [^{18}F]Galacto-RGD has been developed for PET imaging of αvβ3 expression. In this review, we will discuss the methodology of positron emission tomography (PET) imaging of αvβ3 expression in cancer patients with a focus on [^{18}F]Galacto-RGD. Potential pitfalls and the performance of PET compared to alternative strategies of imaging αvβ3 expression will be addressed as well.

2. Materials

2.1. Radiotracers for PET Imaging of Integrin αvβ3 Expression in Clinical Studies

1. [^{18}F]Galacto-RGD
   [^{18}F]Galacto-RGD was the first substance applied in patients for PET imaging. For details on the synthesis of [^{18}F]Galacto-RGD, please refer to reference (11). Final RP-HPLC with a semipreparative column allows preparation of [^{18}F]Galacto-RGD with radiochemical purities >98% and with specific activities ranging from 40 to 100 TBq/mmol. The total radiochemical yield was 29.5 ± 5.1% (EOB) with a total reaction time of 200 ± 18 min including final HPLC purification (calculation based on 1.0 mg of peptide, 70°C, and 10 min reaction time). Typically, starting with 2,200 MBq of [^{18}F]F-, 185 MBq of [^{18}F]Galacto-RGD was prepared in a synthesis time compatible with the half-life of [^{18}F]-fluorine. Usually we decide to prepare ~600 MBq [^{18}F]Galacto-RGD per synthesis. For application in patients, high performance liquid chromatography (HPLC) eluent is completely removed by evaporation and 0.5 ml absolute ethanol and 10 ml phosphate buffered saline (PBS, pH 7.4) are added and passed through a Millex GV filter (Millipore GmbH, Eschborn, Germany) prior to injection. Starting with the synthesis in the morning, this allows for imaging of up to three patients, starting at noon with PET imaging. However, as the yield might vary, we usually decide to scan only two patients per synthesis. Usually, enough tracer is left for small animal studies, which can be performed in parallel. As the procedure is technically challenging and might result in relevant radiation exposure especially to the hands of the radiochemist, well-trained personnel routinely involved in [^{18}F]Galacto-RGD synthesis is mandatory. We usually do not synthesize [^{18}F]Galacto-RGD more than once per week for patient studies. For small animal studies requiring

substantial less amounts of tracer, a higher frequency of synthesis is feasible.

2. [^{18}F]AH111585
   Another αvβ3 and αvβ5 specific PET radiotracer which has recently been used in clinical trials is [^{18}F]AH111585 (12). The chemical synthesis of the precursor for ^{18}F-AH111585 has previously been described (13). Radiosynthesis was performed on an automated module (TRACERlab FX F-N; GE Healthcare) by coupling an aminooxy-functionalized precursor of [^{18}F]AH111585 with 4-18F-fluorobenzaldehyde at pH 3.5 to form the oxime [^{18}F]AH111585. A full description of the synthesis has been published elsewhere (13). The specific activity of the injectate, determined by high-performance liquid chromatography (HPLC), ranged between 76 and 170 GBq/mmol, which is substantially less compared to [^{18}F]Galacto-RGD. As we do not have experience with this tracer and only limited amount of data on its clinical use is available up to now, this paper will focus on the use of [^{18}F]Galacto-RGD.

3. Methods

3.1. Imaging Protocols

Imaging can be performed on stand-alone PET scanners, as well as on PET/CT scanners. We usually use the ECAT EXACT PET scanner (Siemens/CTI, Knoxville, TN, USA) for research purposes. A transmission scan is acquired for 5 min per bed position (five bed positions) using three rotating [^{68}Ge] rod sources (each with approximately 90 MBq [^{68}Ge]). Static emission scans are acquired in two-dimensional mode in the caudocranial direction (5–7 bed positions, 8 min per bed position). Positron emission data are corrected for randoms, dead time, and attenuation and are reconstructed using the ordered-subsets expectation maximization (OSEM) algorithm using eight iterations and four subsets. The images are corrected for attenuation using the collected transmission data. OSEM images underwent a 5-mm FWHM Gaussian post smoothing and are zoomed with a factor of 1.2. For image analysis, the CAPP software, version 7.1 (CTI/Siemens) is used.

No special patient preparation is necessary for imaging of αvβ3 expression with [^{18}F]Galacto-RGD. After acquiring written and informed consent, an i.v. line is inserted. The calculated effective dose found in our first studies was approximately 19 μSv/MBq, which is very similar to an [^{18}F]FDG scan (14). However, as the dose can be substantially reduced by decreasing the voiding interval and lowering the concentration of tracer in the urogenital tract, we decided to routinely administer a diuretic agent for static emission scans, unless contraindicated. We use furosemide in a dose of 20 mg, which is injected directly before tracer administration. The patient is asked to void directly before positioning him in the scanner. This protocol only applies to static emissions scans. In case of dynamic scans, no diuretic agent is used because the urge to void during the examination would be too uncomfortable for most patients. We first performed dynamic imaging studies to evaluate the optimum imaging time point after tracer injection for static emission scans. Distribution volume (D_v) values, which are supposed to reflect the receptor concentration in the tissue, were on average four times higher for tumor tissue than for muscle tissue, suggesting specific tracer binding. In a recent study we performed dynamic emissions scans over 60 min and kinetic modeling studies using the aorta as arterial input function in patients with invasive ductal breast cancer. We compared SUVs derived from the last nine time frames with the D_v values measured in normal tissue (breast, muscle) and in the tumors. The correlation between both parameters increased continuously over time with an optimum at ~55 min p.i. with $r = 0.92$ (15). This suggests that standardized uptake values (SUVs) derived from static emission scans at ~60 min. p.i. can be used for assessment of αvβ3 receptor density with reasonable accuracy. Scans should not be started much earlier, as unspecific effects like tracer activity in the blood pool are likely to affect the SUVs. However, it should be kept in mind that starting a scan at 60 min p.i. at the pelvis could result in substantial later imaging time points at the more cranial bed positions, e.g., up to 40 min time interval between the first and last bed position for five bed positions with 8 min each. Therefore, the scan protocol including the scanning direction should not be changed to allow for comparison of the results from different studies. As most of the tracer is excreted via the urogenital tract, we also advice to perform scanning in the caudocranial direction, as activity in the bladder is less at the beginning of the scan and too much activity in the bladder might deteriorate image quality in the pelvis. As the dynamics of [^{18}F]AH111585 seem to be similar to [^{18}F]Galacto-RGD, a similar protocol is recommended by the authors, with a starting point 40–60 min. p.i. for static emission scans (12).

3.2. Data Analysis

A variety of software tools can be used for data analysis. Concerning analysis of dynamic scans, the selection of time-activity curves (TACs) and subsequent kinetic analyses were performed using the PMOD Medical Imaging Program version 2.5 (PMOD Group, Zurich Switzerland). A ROI approach was applied to the dynamic images in order to obtain TACs for lesions as well as background tissue. In the case of tumor tissue, polygonal ROIs were drawn over the whole tumor in all slices with visible tumor uptake. Circular ROIs with a diameter of 15 mm were drawn over background tissue in the whole volume of interest and oral mucosa at the height of the palate. The last frame of the dynamic image series was used to define the ROIs for the different tissues. In order to derive an image-based input function, freehand ROIs were placed over artery in the field of view in every slice where the artery could be identified on the frames acquired 40 s p.i. The diameter of the ROIs was adapted to the visible lumen of the vessel and always chosen smaller then the apparent vessel diameter to minimize partial volume effects. All ROIs were then projected onto the complete dynamic dataset and TACs were subsequently derived. Individual rate constants were generated by non-linear regression analysis using the Marquardt-Levenberg least squares minimization algorithm as implemented in PMOD. Various compartment models were fitted to the data and kinetic constants were estimated by minimizing the sum of squared differences between the tissue TACs and the model predicted curves. The model with the lowest Akaike information criterion (AIC) value was chosen. The AIC is calculated as follows:

$$\mathrm{AIC} = n^* \sum w(y - y_1)^2 + 2^* p$$

with $n =$ number of observations (image frames);

$w =$ weighting factor (Gaussian);

$y =$ calculated data; $y_1 =$ measured data;

$p =$ number of constants.

A two-tissue compartment (2 TC) model best characterized the tumor data. In muscle tissue, it was difficult to resolve the second compartment; therefore, a one-tissue (1 TC) compartment model was used for further analysis of this tissue. The total distribution volume (DV_{tot}) was calculated for all ROIs based on the directly estimated kinetic rate constants ($K_1 - k_4$) and the estimated fraction of blood volume V_B according to the formula:

$$DV_{\mathrm{tot}} = \frac{K_1}{k_2}^* \left(1 + \frac{k_3}{k_4}\right) \text{ (2 TC model) or}$$

$$DV = \frac{K_1}{k_2} \text{ (1 TC model)}$$

A more detailed description of the compartment models can be found elsewhere (16–18).

The advantage of the dynamic approach is that quantitative information can be derived from the dataset instead of merely semiquantitative SUV measurements. However, there are many disadvantages for use in daily routine. First only a limited field of view of one bed position is available for image analysis. This is major limitation in cancer patients, were often multiple lesions in different parts of the body have to be assessed. Moreover, if no large artery is within the field of view, arterial blood sampling would probably be necessary for a correct arterial input function. This procedure is not without complications and an additional burden to the patient. We therefore prefer the approach of using static emissions cans of the whole torso and SUVs for further analysis. As mentioned before, SUVs in a study on breast cancer correlated well with the results from dynamic imaging studies and kinetic modeling.

We routinely use the CAPP software, version 7.1 (CTI/Siemens) for analysis of SUVs in static emission scans; however, any software capable of creating ROIs and volume of interest (VOIs), and of calculating SUVs can be used. Usually, a VOI is placed around the lesion to be analyzed and a 60% isocontour is used to define the hottest pixels inside the volume. Up to now, there is no "gold standard" in image analysis and the optimum way of analysis of PET imaging of αvβ3 expression has still to be further evaluated in future studies. For simple qualitative analysis of images for lesion identification, we use attenuation corrected PET images in the transaxial, coronal, and sagittal plane. We prefer an inverted black and white color scale. The range of SUV is usually set to 0–5 or 0–4. For analysis of lung lesions, non-attenuation corrected images are sometimes helpful, if tracer uptake is only faint. Consequently the image analysis is quite similar to the analysis of an [^{18}F]FDG PET scan in daily routine.

4. Notes

4.1. Image Quality

We could successfully image αvβ3 expression in human tumors with good tumor/background ratios using PET with SUVs ranging from background levels up to a maximum of ~10. In our patients, rapid, predominantly renal tracer elimination was observed, resulting in low background activity in most regions of the body (19). Further biodistribution and dosimetry studies confirmed rapid clearance of [^{18}F]Galacto-RGD from the blood pool and primarily renal excretion. Background activity in lung and muscle tissue was low. Currently, due to regulatory issues from the local radioprotection agency, we are not allowed to inject more than 200 MBq [^{18}F]Galacto-RGD per patient. In our experience this amount is sufficient in most cases and generally results in good image quality like mentioned before. However, in heavier patients (> 90 kg body weight), there is usually substantially impaired image quality. Therefore for more widespread clinical use in the future, a higher dose, maybe similar to [^{18}F]FDG of ~300–400 MBq would be advisable, adapted to body weight.

Concerning the biodistribution of [^{18}F]Galacto-RGD, its predominantly renal tracer elimination impairs analysis of lesions of the urogenital tract. Therefore tumors like kidney cancer, transitional cell carcinoma of bladder and ureter, and localized prostate cancer cannot be adequately visualized using [^{18}F]Galacto-RGD. To a lesser amount this also applies to the liver, spleen and intestine. Usually intermediate to high tracer uptake is notable in these organs as well with SUVs ranging from 2.5 to 4.0. As this is also in the range of tracer accumulation of many malignant lesions, they often cannot be differentiated from background when located inside or near these organs. Organ systems with low background tracer uptake which are consequently well suited for PET imaging of αvβ3 expression are the extremities, the skeletal system in general, the lungs, mediastinum, and thorax including the breast and the head-and-neck area (**Fig. 13.1**). Concerning the brain, our results suggest that [^{18}F]Galacto-RGD does not cross the blood–brain barrier, as tracer uptake in normal brain tissue is even lower than in

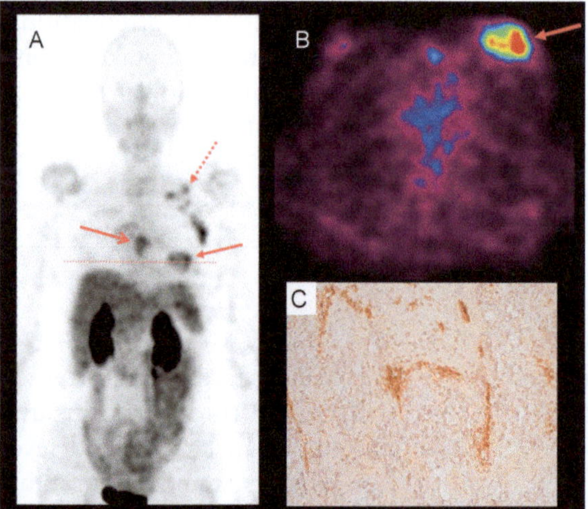

Fig. 13.1. Maximum intensity projection (MIP) of a [^{18}F]Galacto-RGD PET (**a**) of a patient with invasive ductal breast cancer on the *left side* (*arrow closed tip*) and multiple lymph node metastases on the *left side* (*arrow dotted line*) and an osseuous metastasis to the sternum (*arrow open tip*). Physiological tracer accumulation can be seen in the MIP in the liver, spleen, and intestine and mostly in the kidneys and bladder, due to predominantly renal tracer elimination. Image **b** shows a transaxial slice of the primary tumor of the [^{18}F]Galacto-RGD PET at the level of the *dotted red line* in the MIP. Note good tumor to background contrast in the area of the thorax, whereas there is more background activity in the abdomen and pelvis. Image **c** shows the immunohistochemistry of avb3 expression with staining of the microvessels using the αvβ3-specific antibody LM609.

background tissue like muscle or the galea. Consequently, tumor-to-background ratios are generally excellent in the brain. However, we noted that absolute tracer uptake in malignant brain tumors is generally lower than in lesions of the body stem, although receptor αvβ3 expression in malignant brain tumors can be demonstrated in substantial quantities (20). Although malignant brain tumors show a disruption of the normal blood-brain-barrier to some extent, as can be demonstrated by gadolinium enhanced MRI scans, we cannot exclude that there is at least some influence on tracer uptake in the central nervous system (CNS), which is different from the rest of the body. Until further examined in more detail, we recommend cautious interpretation of PET imaging studies of αvβ3 expression in the CNS, especially when results are compared to tumors outside the CNS.

4.2. Expression Patterns of Integrin αvβ3

High inter- and intraindividual variance in tracer accumulation in tumor lesions was noted in our studies, suggesting great diversity of αvβ3 expression in different tumor lesions. We could also demonstrate that tracer uptake [^{18}F]Galacto-RGD in fact correlates with the intensity of αvβ3 expression. In 19 patients with solid tumors (musculoskeletal system $n = 10$, melanoma $n = 4$, head and neck cancer $n = 2$, glioblastoma $n = 2$, breast cancer $n = 1$) SUVs and tumor/blood ratios were found to correlate significantly with the intensity of immunohistochemical staining as well as with the microvessel density. Moreover, immunohistochemistry confirmed lack of αvβ3 expression in normal tissue and in the two tumors without tracer uptake (21). These findings emphasize the potential value of non-invasive techniques for appropriate selection of patients entering clinical trials with αvβ3-tagreted therapies. However, αvβ3 is not only expressed on activated endothelial cells during angiogenesis, but also on a variety of cells like malignant tumor cells, macrophages, and osteoclasts. Consequently, this has to be kept in mind if imaging of αvβ3 expression was to be used as a surrogate parameter of angiogenesis. We are now systematically examining different tumor entities with respect to their αvβ3 expression patterns as shown by [^{18}F]Galacto-RGD PET. In squamous cell carcinoma of the head and neck (SCCHN), we could demonstrate good tumor/background ratios with [^{18}F]Galacto-RGD PET. Immunohistochemistry demonstrated predominantly vascular αvβ3 expression; thus in SCCHN, [^{18}F]Galacto-RGD PET might be used as a surrogate parameter of angiogenesis (22). On the other hand, in malignant melanoma, it might not be optimal as a parameter of angiogenesis, as αvβ3 expression can be found in substantial amounts on tumor cells as well. Consequently the interpretation of imaging results of αvβ3 specific tracers depends strongly on the tumor type which is under investigation (**Fig. 13.2**).

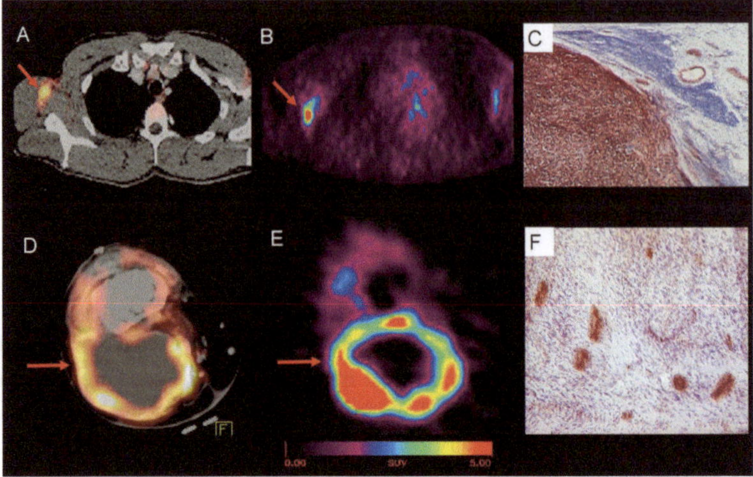

Fig. 13.2. In the *upper row* (**a–c**) [^{18}F]Galacto-RGD PET images from a patient with a lymph node metastasis to the right axilla. Note intense tracer uptake in the lymph node (**a**: PET/CT image fusion; **b**: transaxial PET image). Immunohistochemistry demonstrates αvβ3 expression predominantly on the tumor cells. Consequently, [^{18}F]Galacto-RGD PET is probably not an ideal marker of angiogenesis in this case. In the *lower row* (**d–f**) [^{18}F]Galacto-RGD PET images from a patient with soft tissue sarcoma of the knee are shown (**c**: PET/CT image fusion; **d**: transaxial PET image). Immunohistochemistry demonstrates αvβ3 expression predominantly on the neovasculature. In this case, [^{18}F]Galacto-RGD PET might be used as a potential marker of angiogenesis.

4.3. PET Imaging of αvβ3 Expression for Identification of Malignant Lesions and Tumor Staging

As angiogenesis is a hallmark of malignancies, imaging of angiogenesis is potentially interesting for identification of tumors and tumor staging. As αvβ3 is supposed to be a key player in angiogenesis, PET imaging of αvβ3 expression is sometimes advocated for tumor identification, like with commonly used tracers like [^{18}F]FDG or [^{11}C]Choline. However, in our experience, for most tumor entities, PET imaging of αvβ3 expression is not superior to conventional imaging methods like [^{18}F]FDG PET. We have compared the tracer uptake of [^{18}F]FDG and [^{18}F]Galacto-RGD in patients with non-small cell lung cancer (NSCLC, $n = 10$) and various other tumors ($n = 8$). The results showed no correlation between the two tracers when all lesions were included ($r = 0.157$). For the subgroup of [^{18}F]FDG-avid lesions and lesions in patients with NSCLC, there was a slight trend toward a higher [^{18}F]Galacto-RGD uptake in more [^{18}F]FDG-avid lesions ($r = 0.337$). However, the correlation coefficient was very low. Our results suggests that αvβ3 expression and glucose metabolism are not closely correlated in tumor lesions and that consequently [^{18}F]FDG and [^{18}F]Galacto-RGD provide different information (23). The results also showed that conventional staging including contrast enhanced CT and [^{18}F]FDG PET identified substantially more lesions than [^{18}F]Galacto-RGD PET. Lesion identification in [^{18}F]Galacto-RGD PET was particularly difficult in the liver, as already mentioned before, due to the relatively high background activity. Therefore assessment of $\alpha v\beta 3$ expression with $[^{18}F]$Galacto-RGD PET in liver lesions with only moderate or low tracer uptake is problematic. This also illustrates that tumors in which $[^{18}F]$FDG PET has already demonstrated good results for staging, $[^{18}F]$Galacto-RGD PET is unlikely to produce better results. However, in one patient with a bronchial carcinoid, tracer uptake in the $[^{18}F]$Galacto-RGD PET was substantially higher than in the $[^{18}F]$FDG PET in the primary tumor as well as in the metastases. Therefore it cannot be excluded that in tumors with low or intermediate $[^{18}F]$FDG uptake, like prostate cancer or carcinoid tumors, imaging of $\alpha v\beta 3$ expression might produce better results for lesion identification and tumor staging than $[^{18}F]$FDG PET (**Fig. 13.3**). This, however, is only a hypothesis and has to be proven in future prospective studies. Variations in tracer design are supposed to further improve the performance of $\alpha v\beta 3$ imaging, e.g., using multimeric RGD peptides (24).

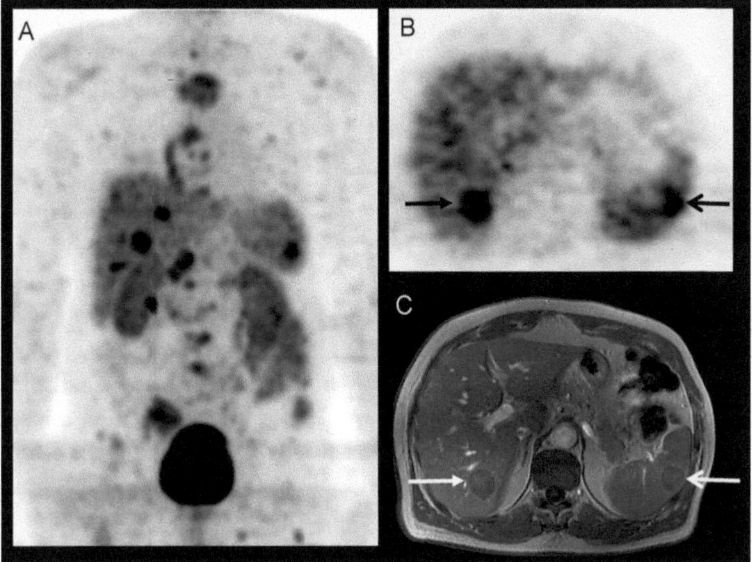

Fig. 13.3. $[^{18}F]$Galacto-RGD PET images from a patient with multiple metastases from a bronchial carcinoid to the bones, liver (*arrow closed tip*), spleen (*arrow open tip*) and abdominal lymph nodes. In the maximum intensity projection (MIP; **a**), the lesions are depicted with good tumor to background contrast due to very intense tracer uptake. Even in organs like liver and spleen with relatively high background activity due to physiological tracer uptake, lesions can be delineated (**b**: contrast enhanced MRI of the liver and spleen; **c**: corresponding transaxial slice of the $[^{18}F]$Galacto-RGD PET).

Another problem in the context of tumor staging/identification of malignant lesions is the specificity of the signal derived by $[^{18}F]$Galacto-RGD PET or other $\alpha v\beta 3$ targeting tracers. Benign conditions can also show substantial $\alpha v\beta 3$ expression on a variety of cells, like macrophages, osteoclasts, and smooth muscle cells. This has been demonstrated by our group and others preclinically and clinically, e.g., in myocardial infarction and carotid plaques (25). Inflammatory lesions also show increased angiogenesis and can sometimes not be differentiated from malignancies according to the [^{18}F]Galacto-RGD PET signal (26, 27). Consequently, similar problems in image interpretation are expected with αvβ3 specific PET tracers as with [^{18}F]FDG. In summary, routine clinical staging with currently available αvβ3 specific PET tracers should not be performed uncritically or outside well-defined clinical studies.

4.4. Comparison of Pet and Other Methods of Imaging αvβ3 Expression

1. SPECT Imaging
   Recently, the SPECT tracer [^{99m}Tc]NC100692 was introduced by GE healthcare for imaging αvβ3 expression in humans and was first evaluated in breast cancer. Nineteen of twenty-two tumors could be detected with this agent, which was safe and well tolerated by the patients (28). It is therefore expected that commercial agents for SPECT imaging of αvβ3 expression will soon be available. Both PET and SPECT imaging have the advantage of being very sensitive to low concentrations of tracer molecules and having unlimited depth penetration. An advantage of SPECT imaging is its much wider availability than PET imaging. Moreover, the radionuclides used for SPECT are easier to prepare and usually have a longer half-life than those used for PET (6 h for [^{99m}Tc], 67 h for [^{111}In], and 13.2 h for [^{123}I]). However, PET is approximately ten times more sensitive than SPECT and is able to detect picomolar concentrations of tracer (29). Moreover, data quantification is easier accomplished with PET data compared to SPECT data, which is a major advantage when it comes to serial studies, e.g., for response evaluation of antiangiogenic therapies. However, with the rising use of SPECT/CT including attenuation correction, quantitative imaging might be feasible with SPECT as well (30).
2. Magnetic Resonance Imaging
   MRI is widely used clinically to identify tumor lesions, to assess tumor growth, and for response evaluation. However, no reports about clinical imaging of αvβ3 expression with MRI techniques are available up to now, although many preclinical imaging studies have demonstrated the potential of MRI for molecular imaging of αvβ3 expression. By using Gd^{3+}-containing paramagnetic liposomes with a diameter of 300–350 nm and the αvβ3 specific antibody LM609 as a ligand, MRI of squamous cell carcinomas in a rabbit model was successfully achieved (31). Peptidomimetic integrin αvβ3 antagonist conjugated magnetic nanoparticles were also used for MRI in a Vx-2 squamous cell carcinoma model with a common clinical MRI scanner at 1.5 T (32). By the same

group, nude mice with human melanoma tumor xenografts were successfully imaged using αvβ3 integrin-targeted paramagnetic nanoparticles (33). A startup company named "Kereos" (www.kereos.de) is planning to use this approach commercially and in patient trials in the future. However, Gd^{3+} for enhancing the T1 contrast can only be reliably detected at millimolar levels. Superparamagnetic iron oxide (SPIO) nanoparticles can be detected at a much lower concentration because of the high susceptibility induced by this particles, which leads to a decrease of the signal in T2 and especially T2* weighted sequences ("negative contrast") (34). In a recent study, αvβ3 integrin-targeted ultrasmall SPIO (USPIO) nanoparticles were used for non-invasive differentiation of tumors with high and lower area fractions of αvβ3-positive tumor vessels (35).

An advantage compared to radiotracer techniques is that MRI does not use ionizing radiation and generally is more widely available than PET. MRI also offers good depth penetration and its resolution is usually higher than that of clinical PET scanners, although this depends on the exact protocol applied. A major disadvantage of MRI compared to radiotracer techniques is its lower sensitivity for the detection of targeted agents. Therefore, targeted molecular imaging agents for MRI have not entered clinical trials yet, except for the fibrin specific contrast agent EP2140R (36). However, the problem of limited sensitivity might be overcome in the future by signal amplification strategies that generate higher target to background contrast (37). Another disadvantage of MRI is that it is not a fully quantitative method because the changes in signal strength in MRI are not linear over the range of concentrations of gadolinium. Moreover, MRI protocols and instrument performance have substantial effects on signal strength, making it difficult to compare data obtained with different instruments at different institutions.

3. Ultrasound

Targeted ultrasound imaging of integrin αvβ3 during tumor angiogenesis has been successfully achieved preclinically (38). Rats with orthotopic U87MG human glioma tumors were scanned at 2 or 4 weeks after implantation with contrast-enhanced ultrasound (CEU) using microbubbles coated with echistatin, a RGD-containing disintegrin which binds specifically to integrin αvβ3 (39). CEU perfusion imaging using non-targeted microbubbles was also performed to determine the tumor microvascular blood volume and blood velocity. The maximum CEU signal was obtained at the periphery of tumors where integrin expression was most prominent based on immunohistochemistry, correlating well with tumor microvascular blood volume. Moreover, detection of tumor neovasculature in athymic nude mice has also been achieved using a research ultrasound scanner after injection of targeted perfluorocarbon nanoparticles (40). Recent results suggest that a quantification of CEU is also possible by acoustic means (41). However, no reports about clinical use of αvβ3-targeted microbubbles are available up to now.

Ultrasound (US) has relatively high spatial resolution (50–500 μm) and does not use ionizing radiation, yet it also has some disadvantages such as the relatively poor depth penetration (usually a few centimeters depending on the frequency used) and limited sensitivity. Further limitations of US are the dependence on the skill of the operator and the fact that not all regions of the body are assessable with US (lung, bone, and brain in adults). Moreover, adequate documentation for comparison of examinations at different time points is still problematic in a clinical setting. However, the complete non-invasiveness of the method makes it ideally suited for repeat exams for assessment of therapeutic response. Additionally, since most contrast-enhanced ultrasound imaging uses microbubbles that are at least several micrometers in diameter, only the tumor endothelium is be targeted as these microbubbles are too large to extravasate (42). Therefore it has the potential of truly measuring integrin αvβ3 expression on the neovasculature independent of the amount of αvβ3 on other cells. This might be advantageous compared to PET imaging using [^{18}F]Galacto-RGD.

4. Optical Imaging

Many sensitive molecular imaging probes associated with angiogenesis specific targets have been developed for Optical Imaging (OI), such as agents sensitive for matrix metalloproteases or αvβ3 (43). The simplest technique is the use of cyanine dyes like Cy5.5 coupled to RGD-peptides. This approach has been successfully used for imaging of U87MG tumor xenografts in mice using NIRF (44). Analogous to the radiotracer approach, multimeric compounds like Cy5-RAFT-c(-RGDfK-)4 demonstrated increased binding affinity compared to the monomeric compound (45). Finally, the use of FMT allows for quantification of fluorochrome concentrations in living subjects, therefore potentially allowing for quantification of αvβ3 expression by RGD-specific cyanine dyes. The principle of FMT using Cy5.5-RGD has recently been successfully demonstrated by the group of Bremer et al. (46). However, no reports are available about the use of OI of αvβ3 expression in the clinical arena. This is mainly due to its limited depth penetration. Therefore it is mostly applied in preclinical animal studies and in superficial tissues or in combination with endoscopy. Moreover, conventional optical imaging does not allow for quantitative measurements. However, this has changed with the introduction of fluorescence mediated tomography (FMT), which allows for quantitative measurements of fluorochrome concentrations at different tissue depths (47). On the other hand, OI has the advantage of being relatively inexpensive, highly sensitive and non-invasive. This approach is therefore well suited for high-throughput studies and a potential alternative to radiotracer studies in the preclinical setting. In the clinical setting, it will probably not be an alternative to PET imaging of αvβ3 expression in the near future.

5. Outlook

Variations in tracer design are supposed to further improve the performance of αvβ3 imaging, e.g., using multimeric RGD peptides. A series of RGD peptides have been labeled with [^{18}F] for PET imaging by various groups, e.g., using PEGylation and polyvalency to improve the tumor-targeting efficacy and pharmacokinetics. [^{18}F]FB-E[c(RGDyK)]2 (abbreviated as [^{18}F]FRGD2) showed predominant renal excretion and almost twice as much tumor uptake in the same animal model compared with the monomeric tracer [^{18}F]FB-c(RGDyK) (48, 49). Overall, the multimerization approach leads to increased binding affinity and tumor uptake as well as retention and might improve the performance of αvβ3 imaging in the clinical arena.

Concerning the optimum imaging technique, the PET approach of imaging αvβ3 expression will probably be the first to be used on a wider scale in patients in the intermediate term, due to its high sensitivity and low amounts of tracer which have to be used. Therefore toxicity issues are of less importance compared to MRI or Ultrasound imaging probes. In the long term, MRI might be an alternative, due to its lack of ionizing radiation and high spatial resolution. Independent of the technique or specific tracer used, the most important next step has to be a clinical trial using imaging of αvβ3 expression for response assessment of antiangiogenic or combined cytotoxic/antiangiogenic therapies. Only the results of such a trial will tell us if imaging of αvβ3 expression really can keep up to its expectations in the clinical routine. Hopefully, by imaging of αvβ3 expression, we will have a new tool at hand for tailoring and guiding antiangiogenic therapies within the concept of "individualized medicine."

References

1. Hood, J. D. and Cheresh, D. A. (2002) Role of integrins in cell invasion and migration. *Nat. Rev. Cancer* **2**, 91–100.
2. Ruoslahti, E. (1996) RGD and other recognition sequences for integrins. *Annu. Rev. Cell Dev. Biol.* **12**, 697–715.
3. Xiong, J. P., Stehle, T., Zhang, R., et al. (2002) Crystal structure of the extracellular segment of integrin αvβ3 in complex with an Arg-Gly-Asp ligand. *Science* **296**, 151–5.
4. Cai, W. and Chen, X. (2006) Anti-angiogenic cancer therapy based on integrin αvβ3 antagonism. *Anti-Cancer Agents Med. Chem.* **6**, 407–28.
5. Hynes, R. O. (2002) A reevaluation of integrins as regulators of angiogenesis. *Nat. Med.* **8**, 918–21.
6. Kerbel, R. S. (2006) Antiangiogenic therapy: a universal chemosensitization strategy for cancer? *Science* **312**, 1171–5.
7. Hurwitz, H., Fehrenbacher, L., Novotny, W., et al. (2004) Bevacizumab plus irinotecan, fluorouracil, and leucovorin for metastatic colorectal cancer. *N. Engl. J. Med.* **350**, 2335–42.
8. Ruoslahti, E. and Pierschbacher, M. D. (1987) New perspectives in cell adhesion: RGD and integrins. *Science* **238**, 491–7.
9. Haubner, R., Finsinger, D., and Kessler, H. (1997) Stereoisomeric peptide libraries and peptidomimetics for designing selective inhibitors of the αvβ3 integrin for a new cancer therapy. *Angew. Chem. Int. Ed. Engl.* **36**, 1374–89.
10. Haubner, R., Wester, H. J., Reuning, U., et al. (1999) Radiolabeled αvβ3 integrin antagonists: a new class of tracers for tumor targeting. *J. Nucl. Med.* **40**, 1061–71.
11. Haubner, R., Kuhnast, B., Mang, C., Weber, W. A., Kessler, H., Wester, H. J., and Schwaiger, M. (2004, Jan-Feb) [^{18}F]Galacto-RGD: synthesis, radiolabeling, metabolic stability, and radiation dose estimates. *Bioconjug. Chem.* **15**(1), 61–9.
12. Kenny, L. M., Coombes, R. C., Oulie, I., Contractor, K. B., Miller, M., Spinks, T. J., McParland., B., Cohen, P. S., Hui, A. M., Palmieri, C., Osman, S., Glaser, M., Turton, D., Al-Nahhas, A., and Aboagye, E. O. (2008, Jun) Phase I trial of the positron-emitting Arg-Gly-Asp (RGD) peptide radioligand 18F-AH111585 in breast cancer patients. *J. Nucl. Med.* **49**(6), 879–86.
13. Glaser, M., Morrison, M., Solbakken, M., Arukwe, J., Karlsen, H., Wiggen, U., Champion, S., Kindberg, G. M., and Cuthbertson, A. (2008, Apr) Radiosynthesis and biodistribution of cyclic RGD peptides conjugated with novel [^{18}F]fluorinated aldehyde-containing prosthetic groups. *Bioconjug. Chem.* **19**(4), 951–7.
14. Beer, A. J., Haubner, R., Wolf, I., et al. (2006) PET-based human dosimetry of ^{18}F-galacto-RGD, a new radiotracer for imaging αvβ3 expression. *J. Nucl. Med.* **47**, 763–9.
15. Stangier, I., Wester, H. J., Schwaiger, M., and Beer, A. J. (2007) Comparison of standardised uptake values and distribution volume for imaging of αvβ3 expression in breast cancer patients with [^{18}F]Galacto-RGD PET. *J. Nucl. Med.* **48**(S2), 406 (abstract).
16. Carson, R. E. (2003) Tracer kinetic modelling in PET. In Positron emission tomography – basic science and clinical practice, Valk, P. E., Bailey, D. L., Townsend, D. W., and Maisey, M. N., (Eds.), 2nd ed. Springer, London, pp. 147–80.
17. Slifstein, M. and Laruelle, M. (2001) Models and methods for derivation of in vivo neuroreceptor parameters with PET and SPECT reversible radiotracers. *Nucl. Med. Biol.* **28**, 595–608.
18. Spilker, M. E., Sprenger, T., Valet, M., Henriksen, G., Wagner, K., Wester, H. J., et al. (2004) Quantification of [^{18}F]diprenorphine kinetics in the human brain with compartmental and non-compartmental modeling approaches. *Neuroimage* **22**, 1523–33.
19. Beer, A. J., Haubner, R., Goebel, M., et al. (2005) Biodistribution and pharmacokinetics of the αvβ3 selective tracer 18F Galacto-RGD in cancer patients. *J. Nucl. Med.* **46**, 1333–41.
20. Schnell, O., Krebs, B., Wagner, E., Romagna, A., Beer, A. J., Grau, S. J., Thon, N., Goetz, C., Kretzschmar, H. A., Tonn, J. C., and Goldbrunner, R. H. (2008, Jul) Expression of integrin αvβ3 in gliomas correlates with tumor grade and is not restricted to tumor vasculature. *Brain Pathol.* **18**(3), 378–86.
21. Beer, A. J., Haubner, R., Sarbia, M., Goebel, M., Luderschmidt, S., Grosu, A. L., Schnell, O., Niemeyer, M., Kessler, H., Wester, H. J., Weber, W. A., and Schwaiger, M. (2006) Positron emission tomography using [^{18}F]Galacto-RGD identifies the level of integrin αvβ3 expresssion in man. *Clin. Cancer Res.* **12**, 3942–9.
22. Beer, A. J., Grosu, A. L., Carlsen, J., Kolk, A., Sarbia, M., Stangier, I., Watzlowik, P., Wester, H. J., Haubner, R., and Schwaiger, M. (2007, Nov 15) [^{18}F]Galacto-RGD PET

for imaging of αvβ3 expression on neovasculature in patients with squamous cell carcinoma of the head and neck. *Clin. Cancer Res.* **13**(22 Pt 1), 6610–6.

23. Beer, A. J., Lorenzen, S., Metz, S., Herrmann, K., Watzlowik, P., Wester, H. J., Peschel, C., Lordick, F., and Schwaiger, M. (2008, Jan) Comparison of integrin αvβ3 expression and glucose metabolism in primary and metastatic lesions in cancer patients: a PET study using 18F-galacto-RGD and 18F-FDG. *J. Nucl. Med.* **49**(1), 22–9.
24. Beer, A. J. and Schwaiger, M. (2008, Jun 4) Imaging of integrin αvβ3 expression. *Cancer Metastasis Rev.* **27**, 631–44.
25. Makowski, M. R., Ebersberger, U., Nekolla, S., and Schwaiger, M. (2008, Mar 27) In vivo molecular imaging of angiogenesis, targeting αvβ3 integrin expression, in a patient after acute myocardial infarction. *Eur. Heart J.* **29**, 2201.
26. Haubner, R., Weber, W. A., Beer, A. J., Vabuliene, E., Reim, D., Sarbia, M., Becker, K. F., Goebel, M., Hein, R., Wester, H. J., Kessler, H., and Schwaiger, M. (2005, Mar) Noninvasive visualization of the activated αvβ3 integrin in cancer patients by positron emission tomography and [^{18}F]Galacto-RGD. *PLoS Med.* **2**(3), e70.
27. Pichler, B. J., Kneilling, M., Haubner, R., Braumüller, H., Schwaiger, M., Röcken, M., and Weber, W. A. (2005, Jan) Imaging of delayed-type hypersensitivity reaction by PET and 18F-galacto-RGD. *J. Nucl. Med.* **46**(1), 184–9.
28. Bach-Gansmo, T., Danielsson, R., Saracco, A., Wilczek, B., Bogsrud, T. V., Fangberget, A., Tangerud, A., and Tobin, D. (2006, Sep) Integrin receptor imaging of breast cancer: a proof-of-concept study to evaluate 99mTc-NC100692. *J. Nucl. Med.* **47**(9), 1434–9.
29. Weber, W. A. (2006) Positron emission tomography as an imaging biomarker. *J. Clin. Oncol.* **24**(20), 3282–92.
30. Buck, A. K., Nekolla, S., Ziegler, S., Beer, A., Krause, B. J., Herrmann, K., Scheidhauer, K., Wester, H. J., Rummeny, E. J., Schwaiger, M., and Drzezga, A. (2008, Aug) Spect/Ct. *J. Nucl. Med.* **49**(8), 1305–19.
31. Sipkins, D. A., Cheresh, D. A., Kazemi, M. R., Nevin, L. M., Bednarski, M. D., and Li, K. C. (1998) Detection of tumor angiogenesis in vivo by αvβ3-targeted magnetic resonance imaging. *Nat. Med.* **4**, 623–6.
32. Winter, P. M., Caruthers, S. D., Kassner, A., et al. (2003) Molecular imaging of angiogenesis in nascent Vx-2 rabbit tumors using a novel αvβ3-targeted nanoparticle and 1.5 tesla magnetic resonance imaging. *Cancer Res.* **63**, 5838–43.
33. Schmieder, A. H., Winter, P. M., Caruthers, S. D., et al. (2005) Molecular MR imaging of melanoma angiogenesis with αvβ3-targeted paramagnetic nanoparticles. *Magn. Reson. Med.* **53**, 621–7.
34. Thorek, D. L., Chen, A. K., Czupryna, J., and Tsourkas, A. (2006) Superparamagnetic iron oxide nanoparticle probes for molecular imaging. *Ann. Biomed. Eng.* **34**, 23–38.
35. Zhang, C., Jugold, M., Woenne, E. C., et al. (2007) Specific targeting of tumor angiogenesis by RGD-conjugated ultrasmall superparamagnetic iron oxide particles using a clinical 1.5-T magnetic resonance scanner. *Cancer Res.* **67**, 1555–62.
36. Spuentrup, E. and Botnar, R. M. (2006) Coronary magnetic resonance imaging: visualization of vessel lumen and the vessel wall and molecular imaging of arteriotrombosis. *Eur. Radiol.* **16**, 1–14.
37. Jaffer, F. A. and Weissleder, R. (2004) Seeing within: molecular imaging of the cardiovascular system. *Circ. Res.* **94**, 433–45.
38. Ellegala, D. B., Leong-Poi, H., Carpenter, J. E., et al. (2003) Imaging tumor angiogenesis with contrast ultrasound and microbubbles targeted to αvβ3. *Circulation* **108**, 336–41.
39. Kumar, C. C., Nie, H., Rogers, C. P., et al. (1997) Biochemical characterization of the binding of echistatin to integrin αvβ3 receptor. *J. Pharmacol. Exp. Ther.* **283**, 843–53.
40. Hughes, M. S., Marsh, J. N., Zhang, H., et al. (2006) Characterization of digital waveforms using thermodynamic analogs: detection of contrast-targeted tissue in vivo. *IEEE Trans. Ultrason. Ferroelectr. Freq. Control* **53**, 1609–16.
41. Marsh, J. N., Partlow, K. C., Abendschein, D. R., Scott, M. J., Lanza, G. M., and Wickline, S. A. (2007) Molecular imaging with targeted perfluorocarbon nanoparticles: quantification of the concentration dependence of contrast enhancement for binding to sparse cellular epitopes. *Ultrasound Med. Biol.* **33**(6), 950–8.
42. Bloch, S. H., Dayton, P. A., and Ferrara, K. W. (2004) Targeted imaging using ultrasound contrast agents. Progess and opportunities for clinical and research applications. *IEEE Eng. Med. Biol. Mag.* **23**, 18–29.
43. Bremer, C., Bredow, S., Mahmood, U., et al. (2001) Optical imaging of matrix metalloproteinase-2 activity in tumors: feasibility study in a mouse model. *Radiology* **221**, 523–9.

44. Chen, X., Conti, P. S., and Moats, R. A. (2004) In vivo near-infrared fluorescence imaging of integrin αvβ3 in brain tumor xenografts. *Cancer Res.* **64**(21), 8009–14.
45. Jin, Z. H., Josserand, V., Foillard, S., Boturyn, D., Dumy, P., Favrot, M. C., and Coll, J. L. (2007) In vivo optical imaging of integrin αvβ3 in mice using multivalent or monovalent cRGD targeting vectors. *Mol. Cancer* **6**, 41.
46. von Wallbrunn, A., Holtke, C., Zuhlsdorf, M., Heindel, W., Schafers, M., and Bremer, C. (2007) In vivo imaging of integrin αvβ3 expression using fluorescence-mediated tomography. *Eur. J. Nucl. Med. Mol. Imaging* **34**(5), 745–54 (Epub 2006 Nov 28).
47. Jaffer, F. A. and Weissleder, R. (2005) Molecular imaging in the clinical arena. *JAMA* **293**, 855–62.
48. Chen, X., Tohme, M., Park, R., Hou, Y., Bading, J. R., and Conti, P. S. (2004) Micro-PET imaging of αvβ3-integrin expression with ^{18}F-labeled dimeric RGD peptide. *Mol. Imaging* **3**, 96–104.
49. Zhang, X., Xiong, Z., Wu, X., et al. (2006) Quantitative PET imaging of tumor integrin αvβ3 expression with ^{18}F-FRGD2. *J. Nucl. Med.* **47**, 113–21.

Chapter 14

Quantitative Approaches to Amyloid Imaging

Victor L. Villemagne, Graeme O'Keefe, Rachel S. Mulligan, and Christopher C. Rowe

Abstract

Alzheimer's disease (AD), an irreversible, progressive neurodegenerative disorder clinically characterized by memory loss and cognitive decline, is the leading cause of dementia in the elderly, leading invariably to death within 7–10 years after diagnosis. In vivo amyloid imaging with positron emission tomography (PET) is allowing new insights into β-amyloid (Aβ) deposition in the brain, facilitating research into the causes, diagnosis, and future treatment of dementias, where Aβ may play a role. Non-invasive quantification of Aβ burden in the brain with PET has proven useful in the early and differential diagnosis of dementias, showing significantly higher retention in grey matter of AD patients when compared with healthy controls (HC) or patients with frontotemporal lobe degeneration (FTLD). With the advent of new therapeutic strategies aimed at reducing Aβ burden in the brain to potentially prevent or delay functional and irreversible cognitive loss, there is increased interest in developing agents that allow assessment of Aβ burden in vivo. A key aspect for Aβ burden quantification is the application of compartmental or graphical analyses to the kinetic data in order to obtain quantitative and reproducible statements that allow comparison with other nosological groups, correlation with cognitive or biological parameters, and selection, monitoring, and follow-up of individuals in disease modifying therapeutic trials. It is also a necessary step in the validation of simplified approaches that could be applied in routine clinical settings. With the availability of novel amyloid imaging agents radiolabeled with either ^{11}C (half-life 20 min) or ^{18}F (half-life 110 min), a description of different image acquisition approaches is provided.

Key words: Alzheimer's disease, amyloid, Aβ, PiB, positron emission tomography, neurodegenerative disorders, brain imaging.

1. Introduction

Alzheimer's disease (AD), the leading cause of dementia in the elderly, is an irreversible, progressive neurodegenerative disorder clinically characterized by memory loss and cognitive decline (1).

K. Shah (ed.), *Molecular Imaging*, Methods in Molecular Biology 680,
DOI 10.1007/978-1-60761-901-7_14, © Springer Science+Business Media, LLC 2011

It leads invariably to death, usually within 7–10 years after diagnosis. AD not only has devastating effects on the sufferers and their caregivers, but it also has a tremendous socioeconomic impact on families and the health system, a burden which will only increase in the upcoming years (2–4). Age is the dominant risk factor in sporadic AD. The progressive nature of neurodegeneration suggests an age-dependent process that ultimately leads to synaptic failure and neuronal damage in cortical areas of the brain essential for memory and higher mental functions (5, 6). At this point there is no cure for AD. A deeper understanding of the molecular mechanism of Aβ formation, degradation and neurotoxicity is being translated into new therapeutic approaches (1). In the absence of biological markers, direct pathologic examination of brain tissue remains the only definitive method for establishing a diagnosis of AD (6, 8). The typical macroscopic picture is gross cortical atrophy. Microscopically, there is widespread cellular degeneration and diffuse synaptic and neuronal loss, accompanied by reactive gliosis and the presence of the pathological hallmarks of the disease: intracellular neurofibrillary tangles (NFT) and extracellular amyloid plaques (6, 8, 9). While NFTs are intraneuronal bundles of paired helical filaments mainly composed of the aggregates of an abnormally phosphorylated form of tau protein (10, 11), senile plaques consist of extracellular aggregates of amyloid β-peptide (Aβ) (12). Aβ is a 4-kDa, 39–43 amino acid metalloprotein product derived from the proteolytic cleavage of the amyloid precursor protein (APP) by β and γ-secretases (13). To date, all evidential analysis strongly supports the notion that the breakdown of Aβ economy is central to AD pathogenesis (14). Soluble oligomeric forms of Aβ (15–18) in equilibrium with insoluble Aβ in the plaques are thought to be neurotoxic through a number of possible mechanisms including oxidative stress, excitotoxicity, energy depletion, toxic oxidative interaction with various metal species, inflammatory response, and apoptosis. Nevertheless, the exact mechanism by which Aβ might produce synaptic loss and neuronal death is still controversial (1, 18, 19). The presence of extracellular Aβ plaques in highly specialized cortical brain regions implicated in memory and cognition precede the other pathognomonic pathological features of AD, indicating that increases in Aβ are involved in the early presymptomatic stages of the disease. Furthermore, a period of up to 5 years of prodromal decline in cognition, known as Mild Cognitive Impairment (MCI), usually precedes the formal diagnosis of AD (20–22). Compelling genetic data further support the Aβ theory (24–26). To date four genes have been linked to autosomal dominant, early onset familial AD: APP, PS1, PS2 and ApoE, all of which lead to an increase in Aβ production and deposition.

Currently, the clinical diagnosis of AD is based on progressive impairment of memory, decline in at least one other cognitive domain, and the exclusion of other diseases (27). This approach, along with current structural neuroimaging techniques (CT or MRI) is sufficiently sensitive and specific for the diagnosis of AD only at the mid or late stages of the disease. As new disease modifying treatments aimed at preventing or slowing Aβ generation or deposition undergo clinical trials (28, 29), the role of quantifying Aβ burden in vivo is becoming increasingly crucial, being acknowledged as part of the diagnostic evaluation of dementia (30).

Insights into the molecular mechanisms of AD pathogenesis enabled the development of new neuroimaging approaches (1, 31–33), allowing early diagnosis at presymptomatic stages, more accurate differential diagnosis, as well as allowing monitoring of disease-modifying therapy (1, 33) (**Table 14.1**).

Table 14.1
Potential roles for Aβ imaging

• Accurate diagnosis of Alzheimer's disease
• Early diagnosis of Alzheimer's disease, allowing intervention when minimally impaired
• Subject selection for anti-Aβ trials
• Monitor the effectiveness of anti-Aβ therapy
• Investigate the spatial and temporal pattern of Aβ deposition and its relation to disease progression, cognitive decline, and other disease biomarkers

Since Aβ is at the centre of AD pathogenesis, efforts have focused on developing radiotracers or agents that allow Aβ imaging in vivo (34, 35). For a radioligand to be useful as a neuroimaging probe for Aβ, a number of key general properties must be present. These ideal Aβ probes must be lipophilic molecules that cross the blood brain barrier, are preferably not metabolized or metabolized to polar metabolites that cannot cross the blood brain barrier, and reversibly bind to Aβ in a specific and selective fashion (**Table 14.2**). Quantitative imaging of Aβ burden in vivo is allowing the relationship between Aβ burden and clinical and neuropsychological characteristics in AD to be defined. Several compounds have been evaluated as potential Aβ probes: derivatives of histopathological dyes such as Congo red, Chrysamine-G, thioflavin S and T (36–44), NSAID derivatives (45–49), as well as self-associating Aβ fragments (50, 51), anti-Aβ antibodies or antibodies' fragments (52, 53), serum amyloid P, and basic fibroblast growth factor (54).

^{11}C-PiB, the most successful of the currently available amyloid tracers, is a derivative of thioflavin T that has been shown to possess high affinity and high specificity for Aβ fibrils (55–58).

Table 14.2
Ideal Aβ radiotracer

• Easily labeled with ^{18}F, ^{99m}Tc, ^{123}I
• Lipid soluble (crosses BBB)
• High affinity and selectivity for Aβ plaques
• Slow dissociation from binding site
• Rapidly cleared from blood
• Not metabolized
• Provide quantitative and reproducible information about Aβ burden in the brain

PET studies showed that ^{11}C-PiB binding was reversible, clearing fastest from cerebellum and slowest from white matter (59, 60). PET studies have shown a robust difference between the retention pattern in AD patients and healthy controls, with AD cases showing significantly higher retention of ^{11}C-PiB in neocortical areas of the brain affected by Aβ deposition (59, 61–65). Human PET studies have also demonstrated a correlation between ^{11}C-PiB binding and the rate of cerebral atrophy in AD subjects (66), and with decreased cerebrospinal fluid (CSF) $A\beta_{1-42}$ in both demented and non-demented subjects (67). Approximately 30% of HC subjects exhibited ^{11}C-PiB cortical binding, with some of them displaying the same degree of PiB retention as observed in AD subjects (61, 68). These observations suggest that Aβ deposition is not part of normal ageing, supporting the post mortem observations that Aβ deposition occurs well before the onset of symptoms and is likely to represent preclinical AD (61, 65, 68–71). While there is no cortical PiB retention in FTLD patients (61, 72–74), subjects classified as MCI present either an "AD-like" (60–65%) or "HC-like" (35–40%) pattern of cortical ^{11}C-PiB retention. Interestingly, all MCI subjects classified as non-amnestic single-domain MCI were ^{11}C-PiB-negative (75). While Aβ burden, as assessed by PET, does not correlate with measures of cognitive decline in AD, it does correlate with memory impairment and rate of memory decline in MCI and healthy older subjects (76, 77). Aβ burden, as assessed by molecular imaging, matches histopathological reports of Aβ plaque distribution in aging and dementia and appears more accurate than FDG for the diagnosis of AD (65, 78).

Unfortunately, the 20-min radioactive decay half-life of carbon-11 (^{11}C) limits the use of ^{11}C-PiB to centers with an on-site cyclotron and ^{11}C radiochemistry expertise. Consequently, access to ^{11}C-PiB PET is restricted and the high cost of studies is prohibitive for routine clinical use. To overcome these limitations, a tracer for imaging Aβ with characteristics similar to those of ^{11}C-PiB that can be labeled with fluorine-18 (^{18}F) is essential (39). The 110-min radioactive decay half-life of ^{18}F permits centralized production and regional distribution as currently practiced world-wide in the supply of ^{18}F-FDG for clinical use. Novel ^{18}F ligands, such as ^{18}F-BAY94-9172 (Florbetaben®) have been successfully tested in Phase I clinical studies (79). ^{18}F-BAY94-9172 has been shown to clearly distinguish AD patients not only from healthy controls but also from FTLD patients (79).

To illustrate the similarities and differences associated with these molecular imaging approaches, a detailed description of amyloid imaging techniques with ^{11}C-PiB and ^{18}F-BAY94-9172 is provided.

2. Materials

2.1. Radiotracer Synthesis

2.1.1. 0.1 M Lithium Aluminium Hydride in THF (1-ml vials) and the PiB precursor (2-(4′-aminophenyl)-6-hydroxy-benzothiazole) were purchased from ABX Advanced biochemical compounds, Radeberg, Germany.

2.1.2. Bayer Schering Pharna, Berlin, Germany, provided the precursor for production of ^{18}F-BAY94-9172 and reference standard (^{19}F-BAY94-9172).

2.2. PET Scanner

2.2.1. All PET scans at the Austin Health Centre for PET are performed on a Philips-ADAC Allegro (Philips Medical Systems, Cleveland, OH, USA) full-ring 3D PET System with PIXELAR™ GSO crystal detectors in 3D mode, using a 256-mm transverse field of view (FOV) and having a 180-mm axial FOV made up of 90 image slices each of 2 mm thickness and a central transaxial spatial resolution of 5 mm full width half maximum (FWHM).

2.2.2. A transmission scan is acquired prior to the emission scan using a rotating 740 MBq ^{137}Cs rotating point source.

2.3. MRI Scanner

All high resolution structural T1 MRI scans are acquired on a 3.0 Tesla GE Signa Horizon LX scanner (GE Medical Systems, Milwaukee, WI, USA) in a transaxial orientation with 128 matrices of size 256 × 256, a pixel size of 0.977 mm, and a slice thickness of 1.3 mm.

2.4. Image Analysis Software

2.4.1. Wasabi (v2)

2.4.1.a. Wasabi is an in-house image analysis and visualization package developed by Tim Saunder at the Austin Heath Centre for PE (http://wasabi.petnm.unimelb.edu.au).

2.4.1.b. Volumes of interest (VOI) are defined and time–activity curves (TAC) generated for subsequent Logan Plot and kinetic analysis as well as voxel-based Logan Plot analysis.

2.4.2. SPM

2.4.2.a. The Statistical Parametric Mapping (SPM) software was developed by Friston and colleagues at University College of London (80).

2.4.2.b. SPM5 is used to co-register PET and MR images, motion correct individual frames, and to spatially normalize the PET image data for subsequent standardized template analysis as well as individualized VOI analysis.

2.4.3. Neurostat

2.4.3.a. Neurostat, also known as 3D stereotaxic surface projection (3D SSP) mapping, is a statistical parametric mapping software developed by Minoshima and colleagues at the University of Michigan, Ann Arbor (81).

2.4.3.b. PET images are spatially normalized and global normalization of PET images are displayed to allow a statistical comparison through Z-score maps against either existing or in-house definable PET databases.

2.4.4. PMOD

2.4.4.a. PMOD is a commercial biomedical image quantification and kinetic modeling software developed initially at the Zurich University, Switzerland (http://www.pmod.com).

2.4.4.b. Compartment model analysis was performed using the TAC generated by Wasabi VOI processing of PET studies and the VOI Kinetic Analysis module of PMOD.

2.5. AAL ROI Template

2.5.1. The Automated Anatomical Labeling template (AAL) developed by Tzourio-Mazoyer and colleagues (82) allows regional sampling of spatially normalized brain images.

2.5.2. There are 90 anatomical VOI, covering the cortical and subcortical grey matter structures (*see* **Notes 1** and **2**).

3. Methods

To illustrate the similarities and differences associated with the aforementioned molecular imaging approaches, a detailed description of tracer radiosynthesis, image acquisition, reconstruction and analysis, as well as quantitative and semiquantitative approaches for amyloid imaging with ^{11}C-PiB and ^{18}F-BAY94-9172 is provided.

3.1. ^{11}C-PiB

3.1.1. Subjects

1. Healthy elderly individuals with well-documented normal cognitive function are recruited by advertisement in the community.
2. All patients are recruited from the Austin Health Memory Disorders and Neurobehavioural Clinics.
3. All subjects are over 60 years of age, speak fluent English and had completed at least 7 years of education. No subjects with a history or physical or imaging findings of other neurological or psychiatric illness, current or recent drug or alcohol abuse/dependence, or any significant other disease or unstable medical condition is allowed into the study.
4. AD patients meeting NINCDS-ADRDA criteria for probable AD (27).
5. DLB patients meeting consensus criteria – cognitive fluctuation, visual hallucinations, and Parkinsonism – for probable DLB (83).
6. FTLD patients with characteristic clinical presentations (84) plus frontal lobe or temporal lobe atrophy on MRI with concordant hypometabolism on FDG PET.
7. MCI subjects meeting Petersen criteria of subjective and objective cognitive difficulties, predominantly affecting memory, in the absence of dementia or significant functional loss (85).
8. Written informed consent for participation in this study is obtained from all subjects prior to participation and also from the next of kin or carer for the subjects with dementia. Approval for the study was obtained from the Austin Health Human Research Ethics Committee.
9. All subjects are administered a neuropsychological test battery within 1 week of the amyloid PET scan, Mini Mental State Examination (MMSE) (86), and Clinical Dementia Rating (87) to ensure subjects fulfilled diagnostic criteria for

AD or normality. Neuropsychological examination, including evaluation of different domains, included the administration of the California Verbal Learning Test (CVLT II), Rey figure, Logical Memory, verbal and categorical fluency, Boston Naming Task, and digit span. HC are excluded if any score falls below one standard deviation (SD) of the published mean for that test. All probable AD subjects have episodic memory scores below 2 SD of the published mean.

3.1.2. MRI

1. All subjects undergo a 3D T1 MPRAGE and a T2 turbospin echo sequence acquisition for screening, subsequent co-registration with the PET images, and volumetric analysis of grey and white matter, as well as ventricular volumes.

3.1.3. Radiotracer Synthesis

1. $[^{11}C]CO_2$ is produced using the IBA Cyclone 10/5 cyclotron at Austin Health via the $^{14}N(p,a)^{11}C$ nuclear reaction. The target gas consists of 98.02% nitrogen and 1.98% oxygen.
2. Synthesis of ^{11}C-PiB is performed using the one step ^{11}C-methyl triflate approach (88), as described in detail elsewhere (41, 60).
3. After a synthesis time of 30 min, an average radiochemical yield of 20% (non decay corrected) is achieved.
4. Radiochemical purity and specific activity are determined by analytical HPLC using a Luna C18 column (75 mm × 4.8 mm, 5 μm, Phenomenex Inc., Torrence, CA, USA) eluted with 50/50 acetonitrile/0.1 M ammonium formate at a flow rate of 1 ml/min. PiB eluted off this system with a retention time of 2.5 min.
5. The final product has an average specific activity of 55 GBq/μmol at EOS and radiochemical purity >95%.

3.1.4. Positioning/ Mask/Transmission

1. All subjects are positioned in the PET scanner, so to encompass the whole brain within the field of view.
2. An individual thermoplastic mask ensures a stable position of the head during the transmission and emission scans.
3. A rotation transmission sinogram acquisition in 3D mode with a 740 MBq rotating ^{137}Cs transmission point source is performed before the injection of the radiotracer for attenuation correction purposes.

3.1.5. Blood Sampling

1. Before the PET scan, a catheter is inserted into either the radial artery or antecubital vein for arterial or venous blood sampling.

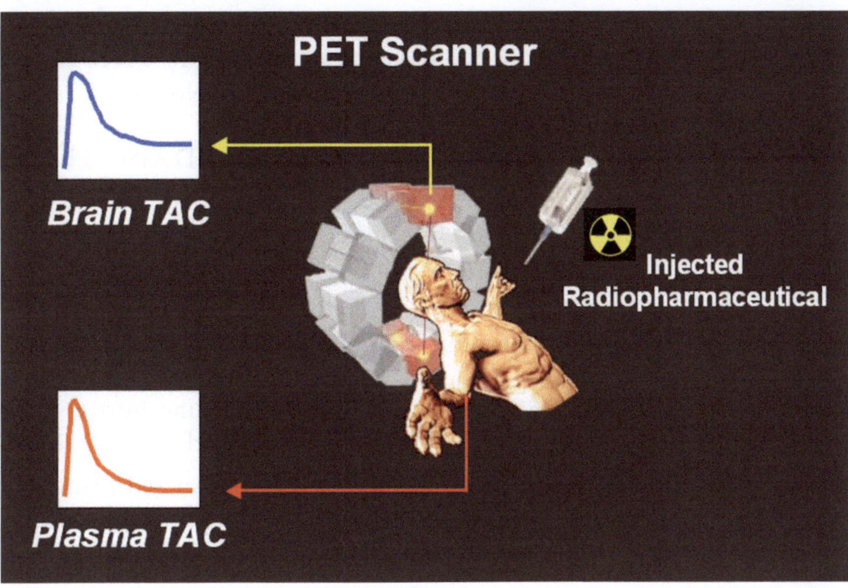

Fig. 14.1. PET acquisition. Schematic representation of a PET scan acquisition. After injection of the radiotracer, radioactivity is measured simultaneously in the brain and blood. Radioactivity is then used to generate brain and blood time-activity curves (TAC), respectively.

2. Approximately 35 hand-drawn samples (0.5 ml) are collected over 90 min (20 collected during first 2 min) in heparinized vials (**Fig. 14.1**).
3. Discrete blood samples (3–7 ml) are obtained after the radiotracer injection to determine plasma metabolites.
4. Plasma samples are measured in an automatic gamma counter.

3.1.6. Metabolite Analysis

1. As previously reported by Drs Mathis and Price from the University of Pittsburgh (60, 89), discrete blood samples (3–7 ml) are collected in heparinized vials at 5, 10, 15, 30, 60, and 90 min after injection of the radiotracer to determine the unmetabolized fraction of ^{11}C-PiB in plasma.
2. Blood is centrifuged for 2 min at 12,900×*g*.
3. The resulting plasma supernatant (500–1,000 l) is then added to an equivalent volume of acetonitrile.
4. This mixture is vortexed for 2 min and centrifuged for 2 min at 12,900×*g*.
5. The supernatant is injected onto an analytical HPLC column (Prodigy ODS-Prep C18, Phenomenex Inc., Torrence, CA, USA) eluted with 45% CH_3CN at a flow rate of 2 ml/min.
6. An on-line radio-HPLC detector (Raytest Corp., GABI system) is used to quantitate radiolabeled peaks.

7. Because there is no difference in the unmetabolized fraction in HC or AD patients, a "population" curve can be applied to correct the plasma samples (*see* **Note 6**).

3.1.7. PET Acquisition

1. PET scans are acquired using a 3D GSO Phillips Allegro scanner in the Austin Health Centre for PET (**Fig. 14.1**).
2. Each subject receives 370 MBq ^{11}C-PiB by intravenous injection over 1 min.
3. A 90-min list-mode emission acquisition is performed in 3D mode after injection of ^{11}C-PiB.

3.1.8. Reconstruction

1. List-mode raw data is sorted off line into 4 × 30-s, 9 × 1-min, 3 × 3-min, 10 × 5-min, and 2 × 10-min frames.
2. The sorted sinograms are reconstructed using a 3D row-action maximum likelihood algorithm (RAMLA) (90) in units of standardized uptake values (SUV).

3.1.9. Co-registration/ Normalization

1. Co-registration of the PET images with each individual's MRI is performed with SPM5 (Statistical Parametric Mapping, MRC Cognition and Brain Sciences Unit) (80) (**Fig. 14.2**).
2. To perform partial volume correction of the PET images, MRI is segmented into grey matter, white matter, and cerebrospinal fluid (CSF).
3. For registration purposes the initial frames of the dynamic PET studies are summed. The early frames of the study reflect regional blood flow allowing an easy co-registration with the MRI.
4. Using the grey matter information obtained from the MR images, PET images are corrected for partial volume.
5. The individual MRI is then spatially normalized into standard (Taliarach) space.
6. Using the same transformation matrix, the co-registered partial volume corrected PET image is spatially normalized (*see* **Notes 3** and **4**).
7. VOI are then drawn on the individual MRI, and transferred to the PET to generate TAC.

3.1.10. Volumes of Interest

1. Mean radioactivity values are obtained from VOI for cortical, subcortical, and cerebellar regions.
2. VOI analysis is conducted by applying the previously described AAL template (82) to the spatially normalized individual MRI and then transferred to the individual PET images.

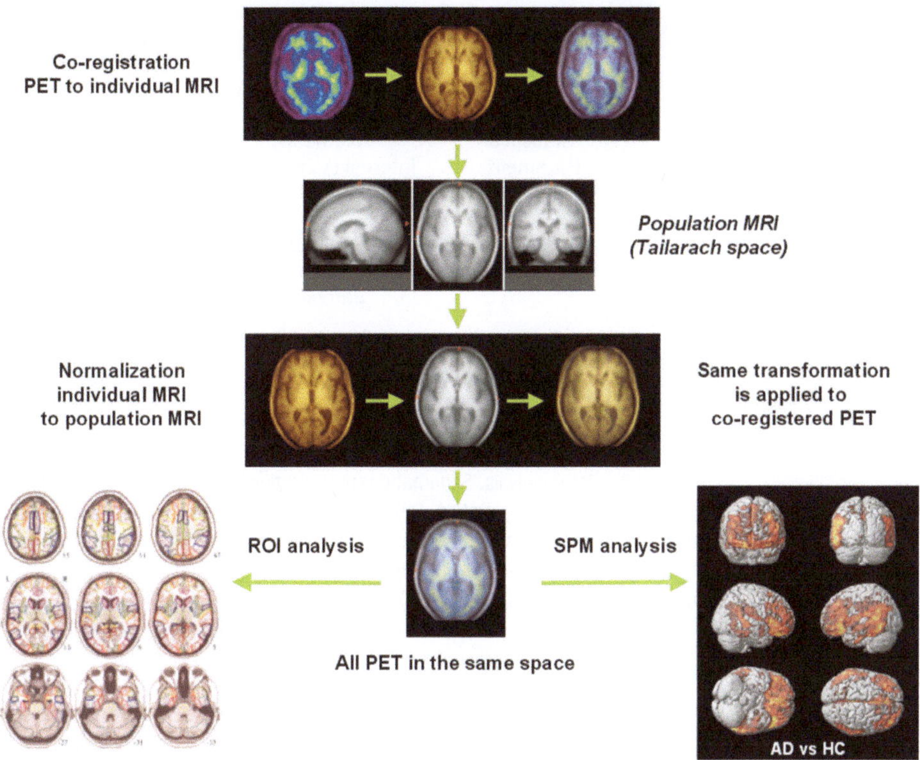

Fig. 14.2. Image analysis. Diagram displaying the PET-MR co-registration and spatial normalization processes. PET images are co-registered to the individual MR. The individual MR is then spatially normalized to standard (Talairach) space. The same transformation matrix is then applied to the co-registered PET images. The spatially normalized PET images can then be analyzed with Statistical Parametric Mapping (SPM), or used for regional VOI analysis, using the Automated Anatomical Labelling (AAL) template.

3. Additional white matter VOIs – placed at the centrum semiovale, pons, and midbrain – as well as cerebellar regions are placed over the cerebellar cortex taking care to avoid cerebellar white matter (*see* **Note 1**).
4. Decay-corrected time–activity curves (TAC) are generated over 90 min from the 28 frames (*see* **Note 7**).

3.1.11. Kinetic Analysis

- Standardized uptake values (SUV), defined as the decay-corrected brain radioactivity concentration, normalized for injected dose and body weight, is calculated for all regions. Given the reversible nature of the radioligand kinetics, distribution volume (DV) and distribution volume ratios (DVR) are determined through graphical analysis (91) (**Fig. 14.3**). Graphical analysis methods, using metabolite-corrected plasma as input function, are applied to the brain dynamic data. Graphical analysis methods are appropriate

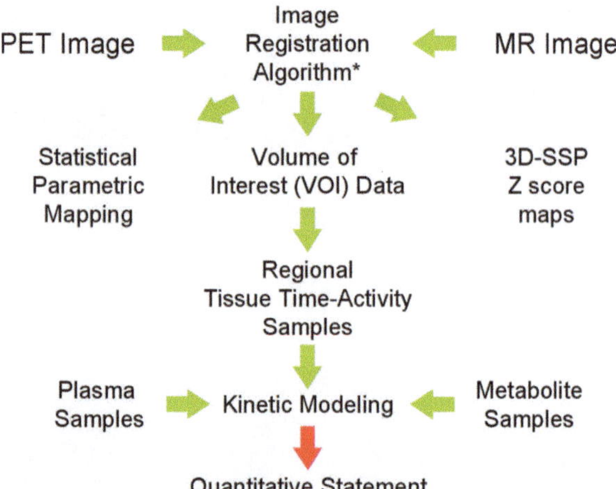

Fig. 14.3. Data analysis. Schematic representation of the analysis of amyloid imaging PET data. After co-registration, PET images can be analyzed and displayed as Z scores using 3D stereotaxic surface projection (3D SSP) mapping (3D SSP), analyzed with Statistical Parametric Mapping (SPM), or used for the estimation of binding parameters using regional volume of interest (VOI) kinetic data.

for reversible ligand-binding kinetics (60) yielding outcome measures of DV (ml/ml) and binding potential (BP, unitless). The DV and BP measures are directly related to the total number of available binding sites (Bmax') and the radiotracer affinity for the binding site expressed as dissociation constant (Kd) (92) (*see* **Notes 8** and **9**).

3.1.11.1. Plasma-Based Arterial Input Function

Radioactive counts obtained from the plasma samples are corrected for percentage of unchanged parent compound (60). Details associated with PiB input function determination have been previously described in detail (60).

3.1.11.2. Image-Based (Carotid) Arterial Input Function

- Summed PET images from the first minute after injection when intravascular radioactivity is highest and best visualized are used for the drawing of VOIs over the internal carotid arteries (89).
- The resulting VOIs are then used to sample the dynamic PET data and to generate carotid TAC.
- Metabolite correction of the carotid TAC data is performed in a manner analogous to that described for **Section 3.1.11.1**, where the unchanged fraction of PiB is determined from blood sampling.

3.1.11.3. Image-Based (Cerebellar Cortex) Input Function

- To avoid arterial blood sampling a simplified reference tissue method (SRTM) is applied using the cerebellar cortex, a region relatively unaffected by amyloid deposition, as input function (59, 60, 91).

- The cerebellar cortex has been shown to contain negligible levels of fibrillar amyloid (93) and similarly low levels of PiB binding in postmortem studies of normal, severe AD, and non-AD demented subjects (42, 59). To further validate the selection of the reference region, SUV are calculated for the cerebellar cortex late in the scan when PiB binding reaches apparent steady state (60, 89) and comparison of the binding in the reference region with age, diagnosis, and cognitive status, shows no differences between groups.
- The SRTM approach, appropriate for reversible ligand-binding kinetics (60) is then applied to yield outcome measures of DVR (unitless), and binding potential (BP, unitless).
- DVR are calculated through graphical analysis using dynamic data acquired for 90 min and using the cerebellum as reference region (60, 61, 91), thus minimizing the influence of non-specific effects (*see* **Notes 10–14**).
- The DVR is closely related to the BP and can be computed from DV estimates for a region (DV_{ROI}) and reference tissue (DV_{REF}), where $DVR = DV_{ROI}/DV_{REF} = BP+1$. *see* **Notes 15–21** for additional simplified Aβ quantification approaches.

3.2. ^{18}F-BAY94-9172

3.2.1. Subjects (Same as Section **3.1.1**)

3.2.2. MRI

1. All subjects undergo a 3D T1 MPRAGE and a T2 turbospin echo sequence acquisition for screening, subsequent co-registration with the PET images, and volumetric analysis of grey and white matter, as well as ventricular volumes.

3.2.3. Radiotracer Synthesis

1. Radiolabeling of ^{18}F-BAY94-9172 (*trans*-4-(*N*-methyl-amino)-4′-{2-[2-(2-[^{18}F]fluoro-ethoxy)-ethoxy]-ethoxy}-stilbene) is performed at the Centre for PET, Austin Health, immediately prior to radiotracer administration, following previously described procedures (79).
2. [^{18}F] Fluoride is produced using the IBA Cyclone 10/5 cyclotron at Austin Health, using a ^{18}O (p,n) ^{18}F reaction. At end of bombardment the [^{18}F] Fluoride is trapped on a conditioned Sep-Pak Light QMA cartridge allowing recovery of the [^{18}O]-enriched water.
3. Radiolabeling was achieved by an automated synthesis process using [^{18}F] potassium fluoride Kryptofix complex followed by acid hydrolysis and semi-preparative HPLC for purification. Standard Sep-pak reformulation produced the injectable product.

4. After a 65-min synthesis, the radiochemical yield ranges from 20 to 30% (non decay corrected).
5. The radiochemical purity and specific activity are determined by analytical HPLC using a LiChrosorb RP Select B-5 column (250 mm × 4.6 mm, 5 μm, Phenomenex Inc., Torrence, CA, USA) eluted with CH_3CN/10 mM disodium hydrogen phosphate at 1 ml/min. On this system ^{18}F-BAY94-9172 elutes with a retention time of 7.5 min.
6. The final product has an average specific activity of 170 GBq/μmol and a radiochemical purity of >95% (79).

3.2.4. Positioning/ Mask/Transmission

1. All subjects are positioned in the PET scanner, so to encompass the whole brain within the field of view.
2. An individual thermoplastic mask ensures a stable position of the head during the transmission and emission scans.
3. A rotation transmission sinogram acquisition in 3D mode with a 740 MBq rotating ^{137}Cs transmission point source is performed before the injection of the radiotracer for attenuation correction purposes.

3.2.5. Blood Sampling

1. Before the PET scan, a catheter is inserted into either the radial artery or antecubital vein for venous blood sampling.
2. Approximately 38 hand-drawn samples (0.5 ml) are collected over 120 min (20 collected during first 2 min) in heparanized vials (**Fig. 14.1**).
3. Discrete blood samples (3–7 ml) at 5, 15, 30, 60, and 90 min after the radiotracer injection are obtained to determine plasma metabolites.
4. Plasma radioactivity is measured in an automatic gamma well counter.

3.2.6. Metabolite Analysis

1. Five 10-ml venous blood samples are taken 5–90 min post injection to determine the unmetabolized fraction of ^{18}F-BAY94-9172 in plasma.
2. Blood is centrifuged for 2 min at 12,900×*g*.
3. The resulting plasma supernatant (500–1,000 l) is treated with MeCN (8 ml) and the supernatant is concentrated prior to injection onto a semi-prep μ-Bondapak C18 column (7.8 mm × 300 mm, 10 μm, Waters, Milford, MA, USA).
4. The column was eluted with a gradient system (20–80% MeCN:H_2O).
5. Total run time is 18 min with ^{18}F-BAY94-9172 eluting with a retention time of 14.5 min.

6. The radioactivity in the ^{18}F-BAY94-9172 peak is then expressed as a percentage of the total injected activity.
7. Because there is no difference in the unmetabolized fraction in HC, FTLD or AD patients, a "population" curve can be applied to correct the plasma samples (*see* **Notes 5** and **6**).

3.2.7. PET Acquisition

1. PET scans are acquired using a 3D GSO Phillips Allegro scanner in the Austin Health Centre for PET (**Fig. 14.1**).
2. A slow i.v. bolus over 30 s of 300 MBq of ^{18}F-BAY94-9172 is given followed by a 60-min list-mode emission acquisition in 3D mode.
3. Further imaging is then performed at 90–120 and 135–165 min post injection using 10-min frames.

3.2.8. Reconstruction

1. List-mode raw data is sorted off line into 4 × 30-s, 9 × 1-min, 3 × 3-min, 10 × 5-min, and 2 × 10-min frames.
2. The images and the sorted sinograms are reconstructed using a 3D RAMLA (90) and reconstructed in units of SUV.

3.2.9. Co-registration/ Normalization

1. Co-registration of the PET images with each individual's MRI is performed with SPM5 (Statistical Parametric Mapping, MRC Cognition and Brain Sciences Unit) (80) (**Fig. 14.2**).
2. To perform partial volume correction of the PET images, MRI is segmented into grey matter, white matter, and cerebrospinal fluid (CSF).
3. For registration purposes the initial frames of the dynamic PET studies are summed. The early frames of the study reflect regional blood flow allowing an easy co-registration with the MRI.
4. Using the grey matter information obtained from the MR images, PET images are corrected for partial volume.
5. The individual MRI is then spatially normalized into standard (Taliarach) space.
6. Using the same transformation matrix, the co-registered partial volume corrected PET image is spatially normalized.
7. VOI are then drawn on the individual MRI and transferred to the PET to generate TAC.

3.2.10. Volumes of Interest

1. Mean radioactivity values are obtained from VOI for cortical, subcortical, and cerebellar regions.
2. VOI analysis is conducted by applying the previously described AAL template (82) to the spatially normalized individual MRI and then transferred to the individual PET images (**Fig. 14.2**).

3. Additional white matter VOI – placed at the centrum semiovale, pons and midbrain – as well as cerebellar regions were placed over the cerebellar cortex taking care to avoid white matter.
4. Decay-corrected TAC are generated over 165 min.

3.2.11. Kinetic Analysis

1. Calculation of binding parameters using metabolite-corrected arterial plasma as input function is described in **Section 3.1.11** (**Fig. 14.3**).
2. To avoid arterial blood sampling, DVR can be calculated using either metabolite-corrected venous plasma, and the cerebellar cortex, a region relatively unaffected by amyloid deposition in early AD, as input function. *see* **Notes 15–21** for additional simplified Aβ quantification approaches.
3. Distribution volume ratios (DVR) are determined through graphical analysis of the 165 min TAC (28 data points) (60, 79, 91) (*see* **Notes 8** and **9**).
4. DVR calculated using metabolite-corrected venous plasma and cerebellar cortex as input functions yield similar results (79) (*see* **Notes 10–14**).
5. This approach has not been validated against a metabolite corrected arterial plasma input curve for ^{18}F-BAY94-9172 but it has provided good distinction between AD and HC, as well as with FTLD (79).

4. Notes

1. Because some regions, crucial for the quantification of Aβ burden in the brain, such as cerebellar cortex, as well as pons, midbrain, and subcortical white matter areas, are not present in the original AAL VOI (82); they have to be added to the template.
2. The segmented grey matter from the MRI is used to restrict the sampling to grey matter areas within the VOI of the AAL template.
3. In those subjects where MRI could not be obtained or is contraindicated, as is the case in subjects suffering from claustrophobia or subjects with intracranial aneurysm clips, intra-orbital metal fragments or electrically, magnetically or mechanically activated implants, VOI can be drawn directly onto the PET images by an expert operator blind to the clinical status of the subjects. Preferably the VOI are placed over the summed initial frames of the dynamic PET study

are summed which reflect regional blood flow instead of amyloid deposition.

4. Another available option is to try to spatially normalize the PET images to the Montreal Neurological Institute (MNI) MRI (94), and then applied the AAL VOI template.
5. To further characterize ^{18}F-BAY94-9172 metabolism, two potential metabolites resulting from *O*-desalkylation of ^{18}F-BAY94-9172 are radiolabeled via nucleophilic substitution of mesylate precursors followed by hydrolysis to form ^{18}F-PEGn3-OH or ^{18}F-PEGn2-OH. ^{18}F-Fluoroethanol was synthesized via ring opening of 1,3,2-dioxathiolane 2,2-dioxide followed by hydrolysis. Coelution studies with patient plasma are then performed with either ^{18}F-PEGn3-OH or ^{18}F-PEGn2-OH or ^{18}F-Fluoroethanol to identify radioactive metabolites formed in vivo.
6. To assess if these radiolabeled metabolites cross the blood brain barrier they are injected into mice via the tail vain and animals are euthanized at sequential intervals and brains removed and counted.
7. VOI analyses are applied to the dynamic PET images to obtain decay-corrected, time–radioactivity curves. To quantify regional radioligand binding, DV and DVR values are determined through graphical analysis.
8. DV, BP, and DVR, the main outcome parameters calculated through these methods, can be estimated with much higher accuracy than using compartmental analysis of radioligand binding kinetics (95).
9. The graphical method described by Logan postulates that at a certain time after the administration of a radioligand, the relationship between the radioligand concentration in tissue and metabolite corrected plasma can be described as a straight line (96). The slope of this line corresponds to total DV, a parameter that reflects how many times the concentration of radioligand in tissue exceeds the concentration of free radioligand in plasma at equilibrium.
10. For regions devoid of specific binding, the concentration of radioactivity in tissue represents the sum of the unbound (free) and non-specifically bound fractions of radioligand.
11. To avoid arterial blood sampling, a simplified approach using a non-specific binding region as input functions can be used to calculate binding parameters through graphical analysis (91).
12. The slope of this line corresponds to DVR, a parameter that reflects the ratio of DV between the specific and non-specific binding regions, respectively. This later approach is also referred to as a reference tissue model.

13. For amyloid imaging studies in sporadic AD, the cerebellum is the most suitable reference tissue, being devoid of neuritic plaques (42, 93) and large enough to permit VOI placement far from tissues of high radioligand retention.
14. Using the graphical analysis approach, we are able to calculate DVR in both 11C-PiB and 18F-BAY94-9712 studies.
15. Simplified methods, aimed to shorten PET scan duration time and use of image-derived estimates of radioactivity concentration in cerebellar cortex as normalizing reference tissue can be applied to obtain semiquantitative statements of Aβ deposition in the brain.
16. Aβ burden is usually assessed through standardized uptake value ratios (SUVR). The SUVR is closely related to the DVR and can be computed from SUV estimates for a region (SUV_{ROI}) and reference tissue (SUV_{REF}), where $SUVR = SUV_{ROI}/SUV_{REF}$.
17. SUVR in amyloid imaging with ^{11}C-PiB are defined as the region to cerebellum ratio after 40–50 min after injection, a time when the ratio of binding in cortical and subcortical grey matter regions to that in plasma (60, 97) or the cerebellar cortex reach apparent steady state (60, 61, 89).
18. A strong correlation is observed between SUVR and DVR for all regions ($r = 0.75$–0.94), with the strongest correlations between SUVR and DVR observed in cortical and subcortical gray matter regions ($r = 0.95$–0.98) and the lowest correlations in midbrain and pons ($r = 0.75$ and 0.78, respectively).
19. PET centers around the world use different approaches to simplified amyloid imaging, all aimed at obtaining valid SUVR measures that yield the best compromise between accuracy, reliability, and feasibility as a routine clinical application. Some PET centers use SUVR derived from images obtained between 40 and 60 min after ^{11}C-PiB injection (89). While providing high count rate images, it can be argued that the radiotracer has not fully reached steady state; therefore, this approach might lead to underestimation of Aβ burden, while being subjected to temporal instability. On the other hand, multicenter strategies such as the Alzheimer's Disease Neuroimaging Initiative (ADNI) (98) are estimating SUVR from images obtained between 50 and 70 min after ^{11}C-PiB injection. While the images' count rate is lower, reflected in poorer image quality, this approach is closer to reflect equilibrium imaging providing a better temporal stability in longitudinal studies (99, 100).

Other PET centers calculate SUVR from images obtained between 60 and 90 min after ^{11}C-PiB injection (101).

20. Overall, SUVR values provide reliable and reproducible semiquantitative statements of Aβ burden and can be obtained from a single 20-to 30-min ^{11}C-PiB PET scan, making it a much more suitable approach for clinical studies, particularly in the elderly and cognitively impaired who may not be able to tolerate a prolonged scan.
21. As with ^{11}C-PiB PET studies, simplified approaches aimed at shortening the duration of PET scans and using image-derived estimates of radioactivity concentration in cerebellar cortex as normalizing reference tissue can also be applied to ^{18}F-BAY94-9172 studies.
22. SUVR for ^{18}F-BAY94-9172 is defined as the region to cerebellum ratio at 90–120 min post injection, a time after the ratio of binding in cortical and subcortical grey matter regions to that in the cerebellar cortex reach apparent steady state (79).
23. A strong correlation is observed between ^{18}F-BAY94-9172 SUVR and DVR for all regions ($r = 0.71$–0.98), with the strongest correlations between SUVR and DVR observed in cortical and subcortical gray matter regions ($r = 0.93$–0.98) and the lowest correlations in white matter and pons ($r = 0.82$ and 0.71, respectively).
24. As with ^{11}C-PiB, SUVR values calculated from ^{18}F-BAY94-9172 images provide reproducible and reliable statements of Aβ burden and can be obtained from a single 20–30 min PET scan, making it a much more suitable approach to Aβ imaging in clinical studies, particularly in the elderly and cognitively impaired who may not be able to tolerate a prolonged scan.

Acknowledgments

Supported in part by funds from the NHMRC Grant #509166, Austin Hospital Medical Research Foundation, Neurosciences Victoria, and the University of Melbourne.

We thank Dr. Henri Tochon-Danguy, Dr. Gordon Chan, Dr. Uwe Ackermann, Dr. Kerryn Pike, Dr. Kenneth Young, Dr. Sylvia Gong, Mr. Tim Saunder, Mr. Gareth Jones, Mrs. Jessica Sagona, Mrs. Kunthi Pathmaraj, Ms. Bridget Chappell, and Mr. Jason Bradley for their crucial role in our ongoing research projects.

References

1. Masters, C. L., Cappai, R., Barnham, K. J., and Villemagne, V. L. (2006) Molecular mechanisms for Alzheimer's disease: implications for neuroimaging and therapeutics. *J. Neurochem.* **97**(6), 1700–25.
2. Bennett, D. A. (2000) Part I. Epidemiology and public health impact of Alzheimer's disease. *Dis. Mon.* **46**(10), 657–65.
3. Johnson, N., Davis, T., and Bosanquet, N. (2000) The epidemic of Alzheimer's disease. How can we manage the costs? *Pharmacoeconomics* **18**(3), 215–23.
4. Schneider, J., Murray, J., Banerjee, S., and Mann, A. (1999) EUROCARE: a cross-national study of co-resident spouse carers for people with Alzheimer's disease: I – Factors associated with carer burden. *Int. J. Geriatr. Psychiatry* **14**(8), 651–61.
5. Selkoe, D. J. (2002) Alzheimer's disease is a synaptic failure. *Science* **298**(5594), 789–91.
6. Masters, C. L. (2005) Neuropathology of Alzheimer's disease. In Dementia, Burns, A., O'Brien, J., and Ames, D., (Eds.), 3rd ed. Hodder Arnold, London, pp. 393–407.
7. Masters, C. L. and Beyreuther, K. (2005) The neuropathology of Alzheimer's disease in the year 2005. In Neurodegenerative diseases: neurobiology, pathogenesis and therapeutics, Beal, M. F., Lang, A. E., and Ludolph, A. C., (Eds.). Cambridge University Press, Cambridge, MA, pp. 433–40.
8. Jellinger, K. (1990) Morphology of Alzheimer disease and related disorders. In Alzheimer disease: epidemiology, neuropathology, neurochemistry, and clinics, Maurer, K., Riederer, P., and Beckmann, H., (Eds.). Springer, Berlin, pp. 61–77.
9. Michaelis, M. L., Dobrowsky, R. T., and Li, G. (2002) Tau neurofibrillary pathology and microtubule stability. *J. Mol. Neurosci.* **19**(3), 289–93.
10. Jellinger, K. A. and Bancher, C. (1998) Neuropathology of Alzheimer's disease: a critical update. *J. Neural. Transm. Suppl.* **54**, 77–95.
11. Masters, C. L., Simms, G., Weinman, N. A., Multhaup, G., McDonald, B. L., and Beyreuther, K. (1985) Amyloid plaque core protein in Alzheimer disease and down syndrome. *Proc. Natl. Acad. Sci. USA* **82**(12), 4245–9.
12. Cappai, R. and White, A. R. (1999) Amyloid beta. *Int. J. Biochem. Cell Biol.* **31**(9), 885–9.
13. Villemagne, V. L., Cappai, R., Barnham, K. J., Cherny, R., Opazo, C., Novakovic, K. E., Rowe, C. C., and Masters, C. L. (2006) The Abeta centric pathway of Alzheimer's disease. In Abeta peptide and Alzheimer's disease, Barrow, C. J. and Small, B. J., (Eds.). Springer, London, pp. 5–32.
14. McLean, C. A., Cherny, R. A., Fraser, F. W., Fuller, S. J., Smith, M. J., Beyreuther, K., Bush, A. I., and Masters, C. L. (1999) Soluble pool of Aß amyloid as a determinant of severity of neurodegeneration in Alzheimer's disease. *Ann. Neurol.* **46**(6), 860–6.
15. Naslund, J., Haroutunian, V., Mohs, R., Davis, K. L., Davies, P., Greengard, P., and Buxbaum, J. D. (2000) Correlation between elevated levels of amyloid beta-peptide in the brain and cognitive decline. *JAMA* **283**(12), 1571–7.
16. Lue, L. F., Kuo, Y. M., Roher, A. E., Brachova, L., Shen, Y., Sue, L., Beach, T., Kurth, J. H., Rydel, R. E., and Rogers, J. (1999) Soluble amyloid beta peptide concentration as a predictor of synaptic change in Alzheimer's disease. *Am. J. Pathol.* **155**(3), 853–62.
17. Wang, J., Dickson, D. W., Trojanowski, J. Q., and Lee, V. M. (1999) The levels of soluble versus insoluble brain Aß distinguish Alzheimer's disease from normal and pathologic aging. *Exp. Neurol.* **158**(2), 328–37.
18. Walsh, D. M., Klyubin, I., Shankar, G. M., Townsend, M., Fadeeva, J. V., Betts, V., Podlisny, M. B., Cleary, J. P., Ashe, K. H., Rowan, M. J., et al. (2005) The role of cell-derived oligomers of Abeta in Alzheimer's disease and avenues for therapeutic intervention. *Biochem. Soc. Trans.* **33**(Pt 5), 1087–90.
19. Walsh, D. M., Klyubin, I., Fadeeva, J. V., Cullen, W. K., Anwyl, R., Wolfe, M. S., Rowan, M. J., and Selkoe, D. J. (2002) Naturally secreted oligomers of amyloid beta protein potently inhibit hippocampal long-term potentiation in vivo. *Nature* **416**(6880), 535–9.
20. Petersen, R. C., Stevens, J. C., Ganguli, M., Tangalos, E. G., Cummings, J. L., and DeKosky, S. T. (2001) Practice parameter: early detection of dementia: mild cognitive impairment (an evidence-based review)-report of the Quality Standards Subcommittee of the American Academy of Neurology. *Neurology* **56**(9), 1133–42.
21. Petersen, R. C. (2000) Mild cognitive impairment: transition between aging and Alzheimer's disease. *Neurologia* **15**(3), 93–101.
22. Petersen, R. C. and Knopman, D. S. (2006) MCI is a clinically useful concept. *Int. Psychogeriatr.* **18**(3), 394–402; discussion 409–314.

23. Selkoe, D. J. (1991) The molecular pathology of Alzheimer's disease. *Neuron* **6**(4), 487–98.
24. Hardy, J. A. and Higgins, G. A. (1992) Alzheimer's disease: the amyloid cascade hypothesis. *Science* **256**(5054), 184–5.
25. Robinson, S. R. and Bishop, G. M. (2002) The search for an amyloid solution. *Science* **298**(5595), 962–4; author reply 962–964.
26. Hardy, J. (1997) Amyloid, the presenilins and Alzheimer's disease. *Trends Neurosci.* **20**(4), 154–9.
27. McKhann, G., Drachman, D., Folstein, M., Katzman, R., Price, D., and Stadlan, E. M. (1984) Clinical Diagnosis of Alzheimer's Disease: report of the NINCDS-ADRDA Work Group under the auspices of Department of Health and Human Services Task Force on Alzheimer's Disease. *Neurology* **34**, 939–44.
28. Masters, C. L. and Beyreuther, K. (2006) Alzheimer's centennial legacy: prospects for rational therapeutic intervention targeting the Abeta amyloid pathway. *Brain* **129** (Pt 11), 2823–39.
29. Schenk, D., Hagen, M., and Seubert, P. (2004) Current progress in beta-amyloid immunotherapy. *Curr. Opin. Immunol.* **16**(5), 599–606.
30. Dubois, B., Feldman, H. H., Jacova, C., Dekosky, S. T., Barberger-Gateau, P., Cummings, J., Delacourte, A., Galasko, D., Gauthier, S., Jicha, G., et al. (2007) Research criteria for the diagnosis of Alzheimer's disease: revising the NINCDS-ADRDA criteria. *Lancet Neurol.* **6**(8), 734–46.
31. Selkoe, D. J. (2000) The early diagnosis of Alzheimer's disease. In The pathophysiology of Alzheimer's disease, Scinto, L. F. M. and Daffner, K. R., (Eds.). Humana, Totowa, NJ, pp. 83–104.
32. Villemagne, V. L., Ng, S., Cappai, R., Barnham, K. J., Fodero-Tavoletti, M. T., Rowe, C. C., and Masters, C. L. (2006) La Lunga Attesa: towards a molecular approach to neuroimaging and therapeutics in alzheimer's disease. *Neuroradiol. J.* **19**, 51–75.
33. Mathis, C. A., Lopresti, B. J., and Klunk, W. E. (2007) Impact of amyloid imaging on drug development in Alzheimer's disease. *Nucl. Med. Biol.* **34**(7), 809–22.
34. Sair, H. I., Doraiswamy, P. M., and Petrella, J. R. (2004) In vivo amyloid imaging in Alzheimer's disease. *Neuroradiology* **46**(2), 93–104.
35. Villemagne, V. L., Rowe, C. C., Macfarlane, S., Novakovic, K. E., and Masters, C. L. (2005) Imaginem oblivionis: the prospects of neuroimaging for early detection of Alzheimer's disease. *J. Clin. Neurosci.* **12**(3), 221–30.
36. Ono, M., Wilson, A., Nobrega, J., Westaway, D., Verhoeff, P., Zhuang, Z. P., Kung, M. P., and Kung, H. F. (2003) 11C-labeled stilbene derivatives as Abeta-aggregate-specific PET imaging agents for Alzheimer's disease. *Nucl. Med. Biol.* **30**(6), 565–71.
37. Kung, M. P., Skovronsky, D. M., Hou, C., Zhuang, Z. P., Gur, T. L., Zhang, B., Trojanowski, J. Q., Lee, V. M., and Kung, H. F. (2003) Detection of amyloid plaques by radioligands for Abeta40 and Abeta42: potential imaging agents in Alzheimer's patients. *J. Mol. Neurosci.* **20**(1), 15–24.
38. Mathis, C. A., Bacskai, B. J., Kajdasz, S. T., McLellan, M. E., Frosch, M. P., Hyman, B. T., Holt, D. P., Wang, Y., Huang, G. F., Debnath, M. L., et al. (2002) A lipophilic thioflavin-T derivative for positron emission tomography (PET) imaging of amyloid in brain. *Bioorg. Med. Chem. Lett.* **12**(3), 295–8.
39. Zhang, W., Oya, S., Kung, M. P., Hou, C., Maier, D. L., and Kung, H. F. (2005) F-18 Polyethyleneglycol stilbenes as PET imaging agents targeting Abeta aggregates in the brain. *Nucl. Med. Biol.* **32**(8), 799–809.
40. Kudo, Y. (2006) Development of amyloid imaging PET probes for an early diagnosis of Alzheimer's disease. *Minim. Invasive Ther. Allied Technol.* **15**(4), 209–13.
41. Mathis, C. A., Wang, Y., Holt, D. P., Huang, G. F., Debnath, M. L., and Klunk, W. E. (2003) Synthesis and evaluation of 11C-labeled 6-substituted 2-arylbenzothiazoles as amyloid imaging agents. *J. Med. Chem.* **46**(13), 2740–54.
42. Klunk, W. E., Wang, Y., Huang, G. F., Debnath, M. L., Holt, D. P., Shao, L., Hamilton, R. L., Ikonomovic, M. D., DeKosky, S. T., and Mathis, C. A. (2003) The binding of 2-(4′-methylaminophenyl)benzothiazole to postmortem brain homogenates is dominated by the amyloid component. *J. Neurosci.* **23**(6), 2086–92.
43. Kung, M. P., Hou, C., Zhuang, Z. P., Skovronsky, D., and Kung, H. F. (2004) Binding of two potential imaging agents targeting amyloid plaques in postmortem brain tissues of patients with Alzheimer's disease. *Brain Res.* **1025**(1–2), 98–105.
44. Maezawa, I., Hong, H. S., Liu, R., Wu, C. Y., Cheng, R. H., Kung, M. P., Kung, H. F., Lam, K. S., Oddo, S., Laferla, F. M., et al. (2008) Congo red and thioflavin-T analogs detect Abeta oligomers. *J. Neurochem.* **104**(2), 457–68.

45. Agdeppa, E. D., Kepe, V., Petri, A., Satyamurthy, N., Liu, J., Huang, S. C., Small, G. W., Cole, G. M., and Barrio, J. R. (2003)In vitro detection of (S)-naproxen and ibuprofen binding to plaques in the Alzheimer's brain using the positron emission tomography molecular imaging probe 2-(1-[6-[(2-[(18)F]fluoroethyl)(methyl)amino]-2-naphthyl]ethylidene)malononitrile. *Neuroscience* **117**(3), 723–30.
46. Barrio, J. R., Huang, S. C., Cole, G., Satyamurthy, N., Petric, A., Phelps, M. E., and Small, G. (1999) PET imaging of tangles and plaques in Alzheimer disease with a highly lipophilic probe. *J. Label. Compd. Radiopharm.* **42**, S194–5.
47. Shoghi-Jadid, K., Small, G. W., Agdeppa, E. D., Kepe, V., Ercoli, L. M., Siddarth, P., Read, S., Satyamurthy, N., Petric, A., Huang, S. C., et al. (2002) Localisation of neurofibrillary tangles and ß-amyloid plaques in the brains of living patients with Alzheimer's disease. *Am. J. Geriatr. Psychiatry* **10**(1), 24–35.
48. Small, G. W., Agdeppa, E. D., Kepe, V., Satyamurthy, N., Huang, S. C., and Barrio, J. R. (2002) In vivo brain imaging of tangle burden in humans. *J. Mol. Neurosci.* **19**(3), 323–7.
49. Small, G. W., Kepe, V., Ercoli, L. M., Siddarth, P., Bookheimer, S. Y., Miller, K. J., Lavretsky, H., Burggren, A. C., Cole, G. M., Vinters, H. V., et al. (2006) PET of brain amyloid and tau in mild cognitive impairment. *N. Engl. J. Med.* **355**(25), 2652–63.
50. Lee, V. M. (2002) Related Amyloid binding ligands as Alzheimer's disease therapies. *Neurobiol. Aging* **23**(6), 1039–42.
51. Marshall, J. R., Stimson, E. R., Ghilardi, J. R., Vinters, H. V., Mantyh, P. W., and Maggio, J. E. (2002) Noninvasive imaging of peripherally injected Alzheimer's disease type synthetic A beta amyloid in vivo. *Bioconjug. Chem.* **13**(2), 276–84.
52. Walker, L. C., Price, D. L., Voytko, M. L., and Schenk, D. B. (1994) Labelling of cerebral amyloid in vivo with a monoclonal antibody. *J. Neuropathol. Exp. Neurol.* **53**(4), 377–83.
53. Poduslo, J. F., Ramakrishnan, M., Holasek, S. S., Ramirez-Alvarado, M., Kandimalla, K. K., Gilles, E. J., Curran, G. L., and Wengenack, T. M. (2007) In vivo targeting of antibody fragments to the nervous system for Alzheimer's disease immunotherapy and molecular imaging of amyloid plaques. *J. Neurochem.* **102**(2), 420–33.
54. Shi, J., Perry, G., Berridge, M. S., Aliev, G., Siedlak, S. L., Smith, M. A., LaManna, J. C., and Friedland, R. P. (2002) Labeling of cerebral amyloid beta deposits in vivo using intranasal basic fibroblast growth factor and serum amyloid P component in mice. *J. Nucl. Med.* **43**(8), 1044–51.
55. Klunk, W. E., Wang, Y., Huang, G. F., Debnath, M. L., Holt, D. P., and Mathis, C. A. (2001) Uncharged thioflavin-T derivatives bind to amyloid-beta protein with high affinity and readily enter the brain. *Life Sci.* **69**(13), 1471–84.
56. Mathis, C. A., Klunk, W. E., Price, J. C., and DeKosky, S. T. (2005) Imaging technology for neurodegenerative diseases: progress toward detection of specific pathologies. *Arch Neurol.* **62**(2), 196–200.
57. Ye, L., Morgenstern, J. L., Gee, A. D., Hong, G., Brown, J., and Lockhart, A. (2005) Delineation of positron emission tomography imaging agent binding sites on beta-amyloid peptide fibrils. *J. Biol. Chem.* **280**(25), 23599–604.
58. Lockhart, A., Ye, L., Judd, D. B., Merritt, A. T., Lowe, P. N., Morgenstern, J. L., Hong, G., Gee, A. D., and Brown, J. (2005) Evidence for the presence of three distinct binding sites for the thioflavin T class of Alzheimer's disease PET imaging agents on beta-amyloid peptide fibrils. *J. Biol. Chem.* **280**(9), 7677–84.
59. Klunk, W. E., Engler, H., Nordberg, A., Wang, Y., Blomqvist, G., Holt, D. P., Bergstrom, M., Savitcheva, I., Huang, G. F., Estrada, S., et al. (2004) Imaging brain amyloid in Alzheimer's disease with Pittsburgh Compound-B. *Ann. Neurol.* **55**(3), 306–19.
60. Price, J. C., Klunk, W. E., Lopresti, B. J., Lu, X., Hoge, J. A., Ziolko, S. K., Holt, D. P., Meltzer, C. C., DeKosky, S. T., and Mathis, C. A. (2005) Kinetic modeling of amyloid binding in humans using PET imaging and Pittsburgh Compound-B. *J. Cereb. Blood Flow Metab.* **25**(11), 1528–47.
61. Rowe, C. C., Ng, S., Ackermann, U., Gong, S. J., Pike, K., Savage, G., Cowie, T. F., Dickinson, K. L., Maruff, P., Darby, D., et al. (2007) Imaging beta-amyloid burden in aging and dementia. *Neurology* **68**(20), 1718–25.
62. Verhoeff, N. P., Wilson, A. A., Takeshita, S., Trop, L., Hussey, D., Singh, K., Kung, H. F., Kung, M. P., and Houle, S. (2004) In-vivo imaging of Alzheimer disease beta-amyloid with [11C]SB-13 PET. *Am. J. Geriatr. Psychiatry* **12**(6), 584–95.
63. Price, J. C., Klunk, W. E., Lopresti, B. J., Lu, X., Hoge, J. A., Ziolko, S. K., Holt, D. P., Meltzer, C. C., Dekosky, S. T., and

Mathis, C. A. (2005) Kinetic modeling of amyloid binding in humans using PET imaging and Pittsburgh Compound-B. *J. Cereb. Blood Flow Metab.* **25**, 1528–47.

64. Buckner, R. L., Snyder, A. Z., Shannon, B. J., LaRossa, G., Sachs, R., Fotenos, A. F., Sheline, Y. I., Klunk, W. E., Mathis, C. A., Morris, J. C., et al. (2005) Molecular, structural, and functional characterization of Alzheimer's disease: evidence for a relationship between default activity, amyloid, and memory. *J. Neurosci.* **25**(34), 7709–17.
65. Villemagne, V. L., Fodero-Tavoletti, M. T., Pike, K. E., Cappai, R., Masters, C. L., and Rowe, C. C. (2008) The ART of loss: Abeta imaging in the evaluation of Alzheimer's disease and other dementias. *Mol. Neurobiol.* DOI 10.1007/s12035-008-8019-y
66. Archer, H. A., Edison, P., Brooks, D. J., Barnes, J., Frost, C., Yeatman, T., Fox, N. C., and Rossor, M. N. (2006) Amyloid load and cerebral atrophy in Alzheimer's disease: an 11C-PIB positron emission tomography study. *Ann. Neurol.* **60**(1), 145–7.
67. Fagan, A. M., Mintun, M. A., Mach, R. H., Lee, S. Y., Dence, C. S., Shah, A. R., Larossa, G. N., Spinner, M. L., Klunk, W. E., Mathis, C. A., et al. (2006) Inverse relation between in vivo amyloid imaging load and cerebrospinal fluid Abeta(42) in humans. *Ann. Neurol.* **59**(3), 512–9.
68. Mintun, M. A., Larossa, G. N., Sheline, Y. I., Dence, C. S., Lee, S. Y., Mach, R. H., Klunk, W. E., Mathis, C. A., DeKosky, S. T., and Morris, J. C. (2006) [11C]PIB in a nondemented population: potential antecedent marker of Alzheimer disease. *Neurology* **67**(3), 446–52.
69. Price, J. L. and Morris, J. C. (1999) Tangles and plaques in nondemented aging and "preclinical" Alzheimer's disease. *Ann. Neurol.* **45**(3), 358–68.
70. Hulette, C. M., Welsh-Bohmer, K. A., Murray, M. G., Saunders, A. M., Mash, D. C., and McIntyre, L. M. (1998) Neuropathological and neuropsychological changes in "normal" aging: evidence for preclinical Alzheimer disease in cognitively normal individuals. *J. Neuropathol. Exp. Neurol.* **57**(12), 1168–74.
71. Morris, J. C. and Price, A. L. (2001) Pathologic correlates of nondemented aging, mild cognitive impairment, and early-stage Alzheimer's disease. *J. Mol. Neurosci.* **17**(2), 101–18.
72. Rabinovici, G. D., Furst, A. J., O'Neil, J. P., Racine, C. A., Mormino, E. C., Baker, S. L., Chetty, S., Patel, P., Pagliaro, T. A., Klunk, W. E., et al. (2007) 11C-PIB PET imaging in Alzheimer disease and frontotemporal lobar degeneration. *Neurology* **68**(15), 1205–12.
73. Engler, H., Santillo, A. F., Wang, S. X., Lindau, M., Savitcheva, I., Nordberg, A., Lannfelt, L., Langstrom, B., and Kilander, L. (2007) In vivo amyloid imaging with PET in frontotemporal dementia. *Eur. J. Nucl. Med. Mol. Imaging* **35**(1), 100–6.
74. Drzezga, A., Grimmer, T., Henriksen, G., Stangier, I., Perneczky, R., Diehl-Schmid, J., Mathis, C. A., Klunk, W. E., Price, J., DeKosky, S., et al. (2008) Imaging of amyloid plaques and cerebral glucose metabolism in semantic dementia and Alzheimer's disease. *Neuroimage* **39**(2), 619–33.
75. Yaffe, K., Petersen, R. C., Lindquist, K., Kramer, J., and Miller, B. (2006) Subtype of mild cognitive impairment and progression to dementia and death. *Dement. Geriatr. Cogn. Disord.* **22**(4), 312–9.
76. Pike, K. E., Savage, G., Villemagne, V. L., Ng, S., Moss, S. A., Maruff, P., Mathis, C. A., Klunk, W. E., Masters, C. L., and Rowe, C. C. (2007) {beta}-amyloid imaging and memory in non-demented individuals: evidence for preclinical Alzheimer's disease. *Brain* **130**(11), 2837–44.
77. Villemagne, V. L., Pike, K. E., Darby, D., Maruff, P., Savage, G., Ng, S., Ackermann, U., Cowie, T. F., Currie, J., Chan, S. G., et al. (2008) Abeta deposits in older non-demented individuals with cognitive decline are indicative of preclinical Alzheimer's disease. *Neuropsychologia* **46**(6), 1688–97.
78. Ng, S., Villemagne, V. L., Berlangieri, S., Lee, S. T., Cherk, M., Gong, S. J., Ackermann, U., Saunder, T., Tochon-Danguy, H., Jones, G., et al. (2007) Visual assessment versus quantitative assessment of 11C-PIB PET and 18F-FDG PET for detection of Alzheimer's disease. *J. Nucl. Med.* **48**(4), 547–52.
79. Rowe, C. C., Ackerman, U., Browne, W., Mulligan, R., Pike, K. L., O'Keefe, G., Tochon-Danguy, H., Chan, G., Berlangieri, S. U., Jones, G., et al. (2008) Imaging of amyloid beta in Alzheimer's disease with (18)F-BAY94-9172, a novel PET tracer: proof of mechanism. *Lancet Neurol.* 7(2), 129–35.
80. Friston, K. J., Frith, C. D., Liddle, P. F., and Frackowiak, R. S. (1991) Comparing functional (PET) images: The assessment of significant change. *J. Cereb. Blood Flow Metab.* **11**, 690–9.
81. Minoshima, S., Koeppe, R. A., Frey, K. A., Ishihara, M., and Kuhl, D. E. (1994)

Stereotactic PET atlas of the human brain: aid for visual interpretation of functional brain images. *J. Nucl. Med.* **35**(6), 949–54.
82. Tzourio-Mazoyer, N., Landeau, B., Papathanassiou, D., Crivello, F., Etard, O., Delcroix, N., Mazoyer, B., and Joliot, M. (2002) Automated anatomical labeling of activations in SPM using a macroscopic anatomical parcellation of the MNI MRI single-subject brain. *Neuroimage* **15**(1), 273–89.
83. McKeith, I. G., Galasko, D., Kosaka, K., Perry, E. K., Dickson, D. W., Hansen, L. A., Salmon, D. P., Lowe, J., Mirra, S. S., Byrne, E. J., et al. (1996) Consensus guidelines for the clinical and pathologic diagnosis of dementia with Lewy bodies (DLB): report of the consortium on DLB international workshop. *Neurology* **47**(5), 1113–24.
84. McKhann, G. M., Albert, M. S., Grossman, M., Miller, B., Dickson, D., and Trojanowski, J. Q. (2001) Clinical and pathological diagnosis of frontotemporal dementia: report of the Work Group on Frontotemporal Dementia and Pick's Disease. *Arch Neurol.* **58**(11), 1803–9.
85. Petersen, R. C., Smith, G. E., Waring, S. C., Ivnik, R. J., Tangalos, E. G., and Kokmen, E. (1999) Mild cognitive impairment: clinical characterization and outcome. *Arch Neurol.* **56**, 303–8.
86. Folstein, M. F., Folstein, S. E., and McHugh, P. R. (1975) "Mini-mental state". A practical method for grading the cognitive state of patients for the clinician. *J. Psychiatr. Res.* **12**(3), 189–98.
87. Morris, J. C. (1993) The Clinical Dementia Rating (CDR): current version and scoring rules. *Neurology* **43**(11), 2412–4.
88. Wilson, A. A., Garcia, A., Chestakova, A., Kung, H., and Houle, S. (2004) A rapid one-step radiosynthesis of the β-amyloid imaging radiotracer N-methyl-[11C]2(40-methylaminophenyl)-6-hydroxybenzothiazole ([11C]-6-OH-BTA-1). *J. Label. Compd. Radiopharm.* **47**, 679–82.
89. Lopresti, B. J., Klunk, W. E., Mathis, C. A., Hoge, J. A., Ziolko, S. K., Lu, X., Meltzer, C. C., Schimmel, K., Tsopelas, N. D., DeKosky, S. T., et al. (2005) Simplified quantification of Pittsburgh Compound B amyloid imaging PET studies: a comparative analysis. *J. Nucl. Med.* **46**(12), 1959–72.
90. Daube-Witherspoon, M. W., Matej, S., Karp, J. S., and Lewitt, R. M. (2001) Application of the 3D row action maximum likelihood algorithm to clinical PET imaging. *IEEE Trans. Nucl. Sci.* **48**(1), 24–30.
91. Logan, J., Fowler, J. S., Volkow, N. D., Wang, G. J., Ding, Y. S., and Alexoff, D. L. (1996) Distribution volume ratios without blood sampling from graphical analysis of PET data. *J. Cereb. Blood Flow Metab.* **16**, 834–40.
92. Mintun, M. A., Raichle, M. E., Kilbourn, M. R., Wooten, G. F., and Welch, M. J. (1984) A quantitative model for the in vivo assessment of drug binding sites with positron emission tomography. *Ann. Neurol.* **15**(3), 217–27.
93. Joachim, C. L., Morris, J. H., and Selkoe, D. J. (1989) Diffuse senile plaques occur commonly in the cerebellum in Alzheimer's disease. *Am. J. Pathol.* **135**(2), 309–19.
94. Mazziotta, J. C., Toga, A. W., Evans, A., Fox, P., and Lancaster, J. (1995) A probabilistic atlas of the human brain: theory and rationale for its development. The International Consortium for Brain Mapping (ICBM). *Neuroimage* **2**(2), 89–101.
95. Carson, R. E. (1996) Mathematical modeling and compartmental analysis. In Nuclear medicine, diagnosis and therapy, Harbert, J., Eckelman, W. C., and Neumann, R., (Eds.). Thieme Medical, New York, NY, pp. 167–94.
96. Logan, J., Fowler, J. S., Volkow, N. D., Wolf, A. P., Dewey, S. L., Schyler, D. J., Macgregor, R. R., Hitzemann, R., Bendriem, B., and Gatley, S. J. (1990) Graphical analysis of reversible radioligand binding from time-activity measurements applied to [N11C-methyl]-(-)-cocaine PET studies in human subjects. *J. Cereb. Blood Flow Metab.* **10**, 740–7.
97. Yaqub, M., Tolboom, N., Boellaard, R., van Berckel, B. N., van Tilburg, E. W., Luurtsema, G., Scheltens, P., and Lammertsma, A. A. (2008) Simplified parametric methods for [(11)C]PIB studies. *Neuroimage* **42**(1), 76–86.
98. Mueller, S. G., Weiner, M. W., Thal, L. J., Petersen, R. C., Jack, C. R., Jagust, W., Trojanowski, J. Q., Toga, A. W., and Beckett, L. (2005) Ways toward an early diagnosis in Alzheimer's disease: The Alzheimer's Disease Neuroimaging Initiative (ADNI). *Alzheimers Dement* **1**(1), 55–66.
99. Yee, S., Mathis, C., Klunk, W., Weissfeld, L., Lopresti, B., Bi, W., Ziolko, S., Berginc, M., DeKosky, S., and Price, J. (2007) Optimal time window for standardized uptake ratio as a simplified measure of PIB retension. *J. Nucl. Med.* **48**, 404p.
100. McNamee, R. L., Yee, S. H., Price, J. C., Klunk, W. E., Rosario, B., Weissfeld, L., Ziolko, S., Berginc, M., Lopresti, B.,

Dekosky, S., et al. (2009) Consideration of optimal time window for Pittsburgh compound B PET summed uptake measurements. *J. Nucl. Med.* **50**(3), 348–55.

101. Koivunen, J., Verkkoniemi, A., Aalto, S., Paetau, A., Ahonen, J. P., Viitanen, M., Nagren, K., Rokka, J., Haaparanta, M., Kalimo, H., et al. (2008) PET amyloid ligand [11C]PIB uptake shows predominantly striatal increase in variant Alzheimer's disease. *Brain* **131**(Pt 7), 1845–53.

Chapter 15

Molecular Imaging of Myocardial Remodeling After Infarction

Johan W.H. Verjans, Susanne W.M. van de Borne, Leonard Hofstra, and Jagat Narula

Abstract

Myocardial fibrosis after myocardial infarction plays a major role in cardiac remodeling, development of heart failure, and arrhythmias. Both replacement and interstitial fibrosis are determined by the extent of myofibroblastic proliferation and hence the extent of collagen deposition. It is logical to propose that a molecular imaging strategy that is able to determine the rate of myofibroblastic proliferation should be able to foretell the magnitude of myocardial remodeling and the likelihood of development of heart failure. Of various plausible targets on the proliferating myofibroblasts, receptors for neurohumoral agonists and overexpression of integrin moieties may offer best options for molecular imaging. In this chapter we describe the assessment of angiotensin II receptor and $\alpha v\beta 3$ integrin upregulation in a mouse model after myocardial infarction using real time in vivo fluorescence imaging and nuclear imaging.

Key words: Myocardial infarction, myocardial remodeling, myocardial fibrosis, myofibroblasts, angiotensin II receptor, integrins, molecular imaging.

1. Introduction

Myocardial fibrosis plays a major role in cardiac remodeling after MI. Replacement and interstitial collagen deposition during the process of remodeling is intimately associated with (myo)fibroblastic proliferation (1). On the one hand, the replacement fibrosis may prevent infarct expansion and aneurysm formation, and on the other hand interstitial fibrosis in areas remote from infarction may contribute to myocardial dysfunction (2). The expanding scars also contribute to development of ventricular arrhythmias and sudden death (3). The process of myocardial remodeling is causally linked to local upregulation of

K. Shah (ed.), *Molecular Imaging*, Methods in Molecular Biology 680,
DOI 10.1007/978-1-60761-901-7_15, © Springer Science+Business Media, LLC 2011

numerous neurohumoral factors after myocardial infarction (4), and the use of neurohumoral antagonists, including ACE inhibitors, angiotensin receptor blockers (ARB), selective aldosterone receptor antagonists have demonstrated to successfully prevent and reverse the remodeling process (5, 6).

Molecular imaging in myocardium has traditionally targeted the subcellular processes associated with myocellular death (7, 8). It is, however, expected that the window of opportunity for such an imaging may be rather short and may even interfere with the delivery of appropriate and timely intervention. It is also expected that targeting of the myocardial fibrosis may have more significant relationship with eventual development of irreversible and inexorable process of remodeling and hence evolution of heart failure (9). In addition, such strategy may also lend itself to serial assessment for demonstration of efficacy of numerous drugs aimed at prevention of myocardial remodeling and heart failure (10).

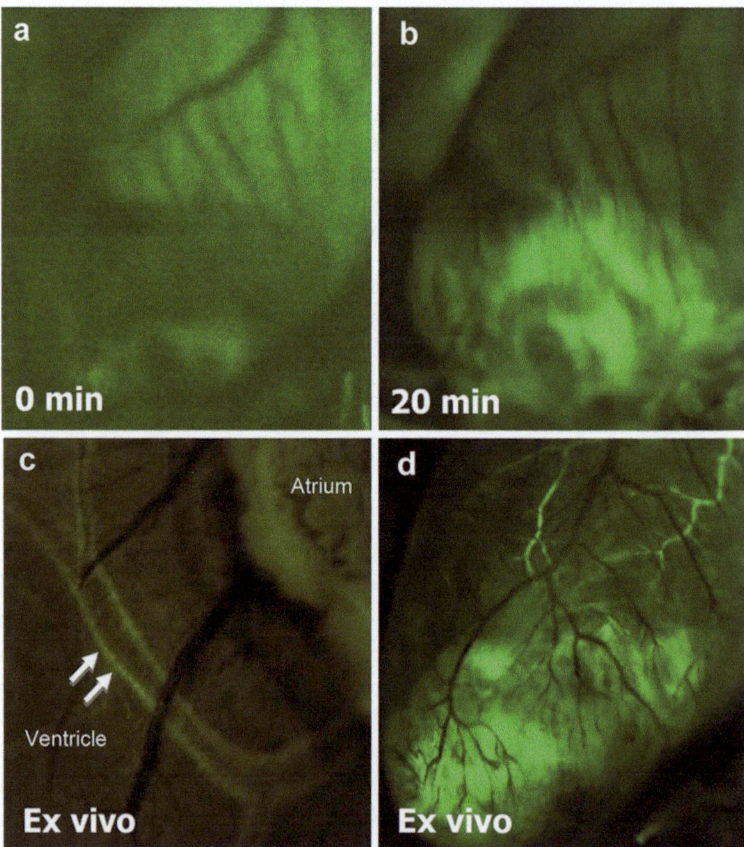

Fig. 15.1. **a** and **b** demonstrates the in vivo binding of green fluorescent APA in the infarct region 3 weeks after myocardial infarction at baseline before injection and after 20 min. **c** ex vivo image of the left coronary artery with APA uptake in the vessel wall. **d** is an example of an ex vivo image of a murine heart showing infarct and vascular uptake of green fluorescently labeled APA. (Reproduced with permission.)

We have recently focused on fluorescent and nuclear imaging of key targets expressed by the proliferating myofibroblasts, including angiotensin II receptors, using a novel fluorescein-labeled angiotensin-II-like peptide for fluorescence imaging and a radiolabeled angiotensin II type 1 receptor blocker for nuclear imaging (11). Subsequently, we focused on αvβ3 integrins, which is currently being evaluated in clinical trials (12). We first describe the protocol for in vivo intra vital imaging of angiotensin II receptors and integrin upregulation (**Figs. 15.1** and **15.2a**

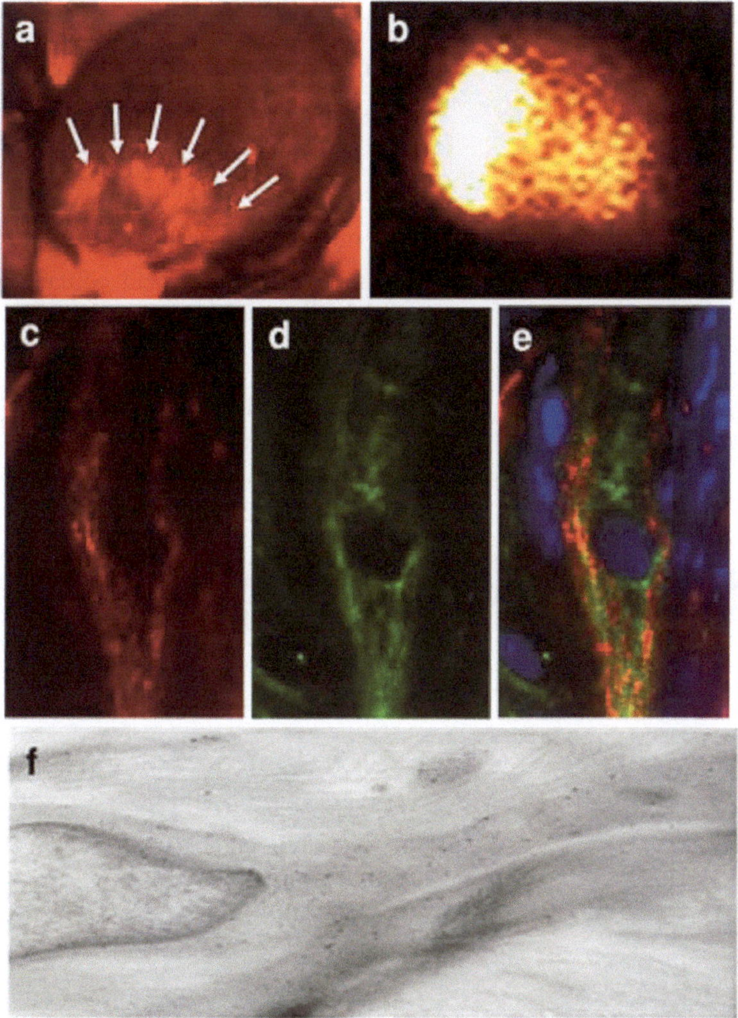

Fig. 15.2. CRIP imaging was performed 3.5 h after intravenous administration in 2-week post-MI animals. Cy5.5 fluorescence (*red*) was observed in the infarct zone (**a**, *arrows*). **b** shows ex vivo imaging of 99mTc labeled CRIP after MI. After sacrifice, images were taken of CRIP sections (*red*, **c**) after they were stained with anti-alpha smooth muscle actin (ASMA) antibody (*green*, **d**), along with colocalization image (**e**). CRIP was localized on ASMA positive myofibroblasts in the infarct area. For immunoelectron microscopy (**e**), intravenously administered CRIP was traced on myofibroblasts by gold-labeled anticyanine antibody (black immunogold particles, 10 nm). (Reproduced with permission.)

respectively), followed by nuclear imaging. Feasibility of distinct targeting and characterization of probe–target interaction was characterized by immunofluorescence and immunoelectron microscopic analyses (**Fig. 15.2b–e**).

2. Materials

2.1. Angiotensin II Peptide Analog (APA)

1. 23 mg of NH_2-CH_2CH_2-Gly-Arg-Val-Tyr-Ile-His-Pro-Ile-OH.
2. 16 mg of fluorescein NHS ester.
3. 12 μl of *N*-methylmorpholine and dimethylformamide.
4. 0.1 mmol Fmoc-Ile-Wang resin.
5. 0.5 mmol bromoacetic anhydride in dimethylformamide.
6. 0.5 mmol *N*-Boc-ethylenediamine in *N*-methylpyrrolidone.
7. 5 ml trifluoroacetic acid containing 2.5% triisopropylsilane and 2.5% water.

2.2. Cy5.5-RGD imaging peptide (CRIP)

The Cy5.5-RGD imaging peptide (CRIP) was kindly gifted by GE Healthcare (Oslo, Norway). The RGD peptide is a 2.5-kD bimodal 10-amino-acid peptide with an RGD motif and bicyclic structure conjugated to a fluorescent cyanine dye Cy5.5, and a chelate agent cPN216 for ^{99m}technetium labeling.

2.3. Radiolabeling of CRIP

1. 50 μg of tracer dissolved in 50 μl of methanol.
2. Freeze dried kit Cy5.5 RGD imaging peptide (GE healthcare, Oslo, Norway) and 1 ml of ^{99m}Technetium-O_4^-.
3. Standard instant thin-layer chromatography kit.

2.4. Surgery

1. Male Swiss Webster Mice (Charles River, Hollister, CA) at age 2–4 months and body weight ~40–50 g (**Note 1**).
2. For anesthesia, a dose of pentobarbital (75 mg/kg) and isoflurane gas (2.0–3.0%) is used.
3. A small animal heating pad is used (37.0–37.5) together with an ECG monitoring system.
4. Standard small animal surgery equipment.
5. Polyethylene tubing (PE-10) for jugular catheterization.

2.5. Real-Time Optical Imaging of Angiotensin II Receptors and $\alpha v\beta 3$ Integrins

1. For intravital fluorescence microscopy, a fluorescence stereomicroscope (Leica MZ16FA, Switzerland), equipped with a CCD camera (ORCA 285, Hamamatsu, Japan) and dye-specific excitation and emission filters.

2. APA imaging: A 470/50-nm band-pass excitation filter is used and emitted fluorescence is collected through a band-pass filter of 525/50 nm.
   - CRIP Integrin imaging: A 675/50-nm band-pass excitation filter is used and emitted fluorescence is collected through a band-pass filter of 700/50 nm.
3. Images are analyzed using SimplePCI software (Compix, Sewickley, PA).

2.6. Nuclear Imaging and Scintillation Counting

1. We use a micro SPECT/CT system (X-SPECT, Gamma Medica, Northridge, CA) with low-energy, high-resolution pinhole collimator for SPECT imaging with built-in software (**Note 2**).
2. Computed tomography imaging is performed using an X-ray tube (50 kVp and 0.6 mA).
3. Quantitative radiotracer uptake is measured with a gamma scintillation counter (1480 Wizard 3"; Wallac, USA).

2.7. Fluorescence Microsopy of the CRIP

1. Nikon Eclipse E-800 microscope.
2. Anti-α-smooth muscle actin antibody (Sigma, 1:2,000).
3. Donkey anti-mouse IgG FITC (Jackson Immunoresearch Europe, Newmarket, Suffolk, UK).

2.8. Electron Microscopy of Cyanine-5.5 Probe

1. Philips CM100 electron microscope (Eindhoven, the Netherlands).
2. Anti Cyanine antibody (Acris antibodies, Hiddenhausen, Germany).
3. Protein gold labeling.

3. Methods

The following experiments describe intravital fluorescence imaging of the myofibroblasts after myocardial infarction. Although a very good method for assess whether, how rapid, and where the probe is binding, which can be confirmed by ex vivo fluorescence microscopy, this method is not quantitative since it does not have tomographic capabilities (**Note 3**). Nuclear imaging is a tool without the high spatial and temporal resolution, but with (semi)quantitative and noninvasive imaging capacity. Therefore, the combination of in vivo and ex vivo optical imaging followed by validation using quantitative nuclear imaging of molecular and cellular processes is a very rapid and effective approach for screening and developing new imaging compounds in translational research.

3.1. Preparation of Fluorescein-APA

1. For preparation of the fluorescent peptide, 23 mg of NH_2-CH_2CH_2-Gly-Arg-Val-Tyr-Ile-His-Pro-Ile-OH, 16 mg of fluorescein NHS ester, and 12 μl of *N*-methylmorpholine were dissolved in dimethylformamide and the mixture stirred overnight.
2. The reaction product was purified by preparative RP-HPLC affording 19 mg pure fluorescein-APA.
3. The peptide sequence Arg-Val-Tyr-Ile-His-Pro-Ile was synthesized starting with 0.1 mmol Fmoc-Ile-Wang resin.
4. The N-terminus was bromoacetylated using 0.5 mmol bromoacetic anhydride in dimethylformamide for 30 min.
5. The bromoacetylated resin was treated with a solution of 0.5 mmol *N*-Boc-ethylenediamine in *N*-methylpyrrolidone for 30 min.
6. The simultaneous removal of side-chain protecting groups and cleavage of the peptide from the resin was carried out in 5-ml trifluoroacetic acid containing 2.5% triisopropylsilane and 2.5% water for 2 h.
7. Trifluoroacetic acid was removed in vacuo, diethyl ether added to the residue and the precipitated peptide washed with diethyl ether and air-dried, affording 120 mg of crude peptide.

3.2. Mouse Model of Post-MI Remodeling

1. Animals are anesthesized and put on a small animal heating pad (37.0–37.5°) in near-supine position (**Note 4**).
2. ECG recordings are monitored throughout the operation.
3. Thoracotomy is performed and heart is visualized. Pericardium is left intact (**Note 5**).
4. The left coronary is located and ligated on its second branching point using a 6-0 prolene suture (**Note 6**).
5. Thorax is closed using a 5-0 monocryl suture and the mouse is taken to a heated recovery room for 24 h.

3.3. Optical Imaging Using Fluorescent APA and CRIP

1. After anesthesizing the animal, a venous line (polyethylene, PE-10) is introduced into the left jugular vein for injection and fixated with a suture, after unilateral distal ligation of the vein.
2. APA or CRIP (50 μg bolus dissolved in PBS or saline) is injected intravenously into the internal jugular vein.
3. Real-time optical imaging is performed from baseline to desired time-point using a fluorescence stereomicroscope. Acquisition time for adequate in vivo images is 110 ms with current CCD camera (**Figs. 15.1a, b** and **15.2a**).

4. For ex vivo imaging, acquisition time is increased for improved images in a non-beating heart (**Fig. 15.1c, d**).

3.4. Radiolabeling of CRIP

1. For radiolabeling, 50 μg of tracer was dissolved in 50 μl of methanol and added to the freeze dried kit (GE healthcare, Oslo, Norway).
2. 1 ml of ^{99m}Technetium-O_4^- is added to this solution and left for 20–30 min (room temperature).
3. Radiolabeling radiopurity is tested using standard instant thin-layer chromatography (>90%).

3.5. Nuclear Imaging and Ex Vivo Quantitation of CRIP

1. After radiolabeling, the CRIP compound is injected intravenously into the tail vein.
2. Mice are anesthesized and put in the SPECT/CT isoflurane anesthesia system.
3. SPECT Images are acquired in 64 × 64 scaffold, 32 steps at 120 s/step on a 140 KeV photopeak of $^{99\,M}$Tc with 15% window (**Fig. 15.2b**).
4. CT images are acquired at 0.5 s per view (256 views in 360°).
5. Ex vivo images are acquired for 15 min in a 128 × 128 matrix.
6. Quantitative uptake is done with the scintillation counter, after cutting hearts into three bread-loaf slices (**Note 7**).
7. Similarly, biodistribution studies can be undertaken (e.g., lung, liver, spleen, kidney).

3.6. Fluorescence Microsopy of the Cy5.5 RGD Peptide

1. For localization of CRIP, non-radiolabeled compound is injected after myocardial infarction. Animals are sacrificed with pentobarbital (200 mg/kg) 3.5 h after injection of the compound.
2. The heart is put in OCT (Tissue-TEC), and frozen in liquid nitrogen.
3. Frozen sections are cut (5 μm) using a cryotome and stored at –20°C. rehydrated in PBS.
4. Sections are rehydrated in PBS and incubated for 2 h using anti-a-smooth muscle actin antibody (1:2,000) and is washed with PBS.
5. Secondary antibody is added for 1 h (donkey anti-mouse IgG FITC), in a dark chamber.
6. After washing in PBS one drop of Vectashield containing DAPI was added to each section.
7. Imaging is performed using fluorescence microscopy (**Fig. 15.2c, d**).

3.7. Immune Electron Microscopy

1. 8 weeks after myocardial infarction, mice are sacrificed and hearts are perfused with 0.2% glutaraldehyde/2% paraformaldehyde and 0.1 M phosphate buffer (pH 7.4).
2. Hearts are excised and stored in abovementioned buffer for at least 1 h.
3. Next, hearts moved to a 1% paraformaldehyde and 0.1 M phosphate buffer (pH 7.4, 4°C) for at least 24 h.
4. Tissue samples are stored at 2.3 M sucrose in 0.1 M phosphate buffer and are cut and moved to a grid-in methyl cellulose/2.3 M sucrose solution (1:1). Anti-cyanine was used (Acris antibodies, Hiddenhausen Germany) for labeling Cy5.5 in the specimens.
5. Finally, after protein A gold labeling sections are examined using an Philips CM100 electron microscope (**Fig. 15.2e**).

4. Notes

1. Mice are preferred to be same age/weight and at least 8 weeks. In our experience, mortality is lower in mice that are at least 8 weeks.
2. OsiriX is a free DICOM viewer which can also be used for reconstruction purposes of SPECT/CT images.
3. Optical tomography could overcome this problem, but still has problems with movement artifacts and interference of uptake at the thoracotomy site (this only applies to molecular imaging of processes that also occur at thoracotomy site, such as $\alpha v\beta 3$ integrin upregulation).
4. The mouse left foot is crossed over and fixed to the right side of the right foot. This causes the intercostal opening to give a more lateral view to the heart, with a better view on the left coronary tree, providing easier access for left coronary ligation.
5. Although coronary is less well visualized without pericardectomy, the physiological situation seems more adequately replicated leaving the pericardial sac intact with less post-operative adhesions.
6. The recognition and ligation technique requires practice as the coronary tree is small. The coronary tree of Swiss Webster is easier to visualize for ligation, when compared to C57Bl6 mice. However, this varies between different species and companies.
7. Infarct, peri-infarct, and remote regions are cut in slices using a mouse heart matrix (Zivic Laboratories, Inc).

Acknowledgments

We would like to thank GE healthcare for supplying the angiotensin II peptide and Cy5.5 RGD imaging peptide.

References

1. Swynghedauw, B. (1999) Molecular mechanisms of myocardial remodeling. *Physiol. Rev.* **79**, 215–62.
2. Spinale, F. G. (2007) Myocardial matrix remodeling and the matrix metalloproteinases: influence on cardiac form and function. *Physiol. Rev.* **87**, 1285–342.
3. Huikuri, H. V., et al. (2001) Sudden death due to cardiac arrhythmias. *N. Engl. J. Med.* **345**, 1473–82.
4. Sun, Y., et al. (2000) Infarct scar: a dynamic tissue. *Cardiovasc. Res.* **46**, 250–6.
5. Jessup, M., et al. (2003) Heart failure. *N. Engl. J. Med.* **348**, 2007–18.
6. Abraham, W. T., et al. (2008) Pharmacologic therapies across the continuum of left ventricular dysfunction. *Am. J. Cardiol.* **102**, 21G–28G.
7. Hofstra, L., et al. (2000) Visualisation of cell death in vivo in patients with acute myocardial infarction. *Lancet* **356**, 209–12.
8. Khaw, B. A., et al. (1995) Non-invasive detection of myocyte necrosis in myocarditis and dilated cardiomyopathy with radiolabelled antimyosin. *Eur. Heart J.* **16** (Suppl O), 119–23.
9. Jaffer, F. A., et al. (2007) Molecular imaging of cardiovascular disease. *Circulation* **116**, 1052–61.
10. Greenberg, B. (2008) Molecular Imaging of the remodeling heart: the next step forward. *J. Am. Coll. Cardiol. Imaging.* **1**, 363–5.
11. Verjans, J. W. H., et al. (2008) Noninvasive imaging of angiotensin receptors after myocardial infarction. *J. Am. Coll. Cardiol. Imaging.* **1**, 354–62.
12. van den Borne, S. W., et al. (2008) Molecular imaging of interstitial alterations in remodeling myocardium after myocardial infarction. *J. Am. Coll. Cardiol.* **52**, 2017–28.

Chapter 16

Dual-Radionuclide Brain SPECT for the Differential Diagnosis of Parkinsonism

Georges El Fakhri and Jinsong Ouyang

Abstract

Parkinsonism is a neurological syndrome characterized by tremor, bradykinesia, rigidity, and postural instability. The underlying causes of parkinsonism are numerous. It is of paramount importance to make clean distinction among these diseases. However, the differential diagnosis of parkinsonism is challenging. Simultaneous dual-radionuclide brain SPECT allows us to assess both blood perfusion and dopamine transporter function under the identical physiological conditions. This approach has been proven to improve the differential diagnosis of parkinsonism. The simultaneous ^{99m}Tc-ECD/^{123}I-FP-CIT brain SPECT protocols, which are used for the differential diagnosis of idiopathic Parkinson's disease and multiple system atrophy as well as corticobasal degeneration and progressive supranuclear palsy, are presented.

Key words: Parkinsonism, IPD, MSA, CBD, PSP, SPECT, dual-radionuclide, perfusion, neurotransmission, ANN, MC-JOSEM.

1. Introduction

Parkinsonism is a neurological syndrome characterized by tremor, bradykinesia, rigidity, and postural instability. The underlying causes of parkinsonism are numerous. Idiopathic Parkinson's disease (IPD) is the most prevalent cause, but about a third of the patients with parkinsonian symptoms have other diseases instead, which include but are not limited to multiple system atrophy (MSA), corticobasal degeneration (CBD), and progressive supranuclear palsy (PSP). It is of paramount importance to

K. Shah (ed.), *Molecular Imaging*, Methods in Molecular Biology 680,
DOI 10.1007/978-1-60761-901-7_16,

make clean distinction among these diseases. For example, distinction IPD from other neurological disorders will allow the physician to avoid certain medications such as classic neuroleptics (e.g., haloperidol, fluphenazine, or thioridazine) for non-PD patients, which, even at low doses, can have life-threatening side effects (1). However, the differential diagnosis of parkinsonism continues to be challenging with high misdiagnosis rate because parkinsonian diseases have similar symptoms. It is reported that at least 10–25% of patients, who are initially diagnosed as having IPD, actually have another disorder when reviewed pathologically (2, 3).

Imaging techniques may provide crucial information for the differential diagnosis of parkinsonism. Single photon emission computed tomography (SPECT) is one of the promising functional imaging techniques that can be used by physicians to differentially diagnose parkinsonism and gauge disease progression and effectiveness of treatment.

Simultaneous dual-radionuclide SPECT not only ensures perfect registration of the two tracers under identical physiological conditions, but also reduces acquisition time. This is particularly important when imaging parkinsonian patients who typically have movement disorders. One of the dual-radionuclide SPECT approaches is to assess brain perfusion and neurotransmission simultaneously. It would yield valuable insight into the conditions of the brain and allow us to relate the measures of uptake to quantitative measures of motor and cognitive function. For example, blood perfusion and dopamine transporter (DAT) function can be assessed using simultaneous ^{99m}Tc-ECD/^{123}I-FP-CIT. However, simultaneous ^{99m}Tc/^{123}I SPECT is particularly challenging because the emission energies of ^{99m}Tc (140 keV) and ^{123}I (159 keV) are very close; not only are down-scattered ^{123}I photons detected in the ^{99m}Tc window, but, equally importantly, primary photons of each radionuclide are detected in the wrong window (cross talk), making the discrimination between them on the basis of energy challenging. Several approaches, which compensate for scatter, cross talk, and high-energy septal penetration in simultaneous ^{99m}Tc/^{123}I imaging, have been proposed and successfully tested in Monte Carlo simulation, phantom, and clinical studies (4–8).

Using dual-radionuclide brain SPECT for the differential diagnosis of parkinsonism has been published (9–11). In this article, the protocol for the following clinical applications will be presented. The details about the methods and results can be found in the original publications (8, 10).

1. The differential diagnosis of IPD and MSA.
2. The differential diagnosis of CBD and PSP.

2. Materials

2.1. Brain SPECT Camera and Radiotracers

1. Triple-head SPECT camera equipped with low-energy, high resolution (LEHR) parallel-hole collimator.
2. ^{99m}Tc-ECD (^{99m}Tc-Ethylcysteinate dimer) is a commercially available perfusion radiotracer.
3. ^{123}I-FP-CIT[^{123}I-*N*-ω-fluoropropyl-2ß-carboxymethoxy-3ß-(4-iodophenyl) nortropane] is a commercially available neurotransmission radiotracer.

2.2. Artificial Neural Network

The artificial neural network (ANN) devised for simultaneous scatter and cross-talk corrections is a multilayer perceptron (MP) using a back-propagation algorithm as a learning tool (4). It is made of partly connected artificial neurons organized in multiple layers. Each neuron has several inputs and one output. Inputs can be external data as well as outputs of other neurons. The effect of each input is regulated through a specific weight derived from the learning phase. A weighted sum of the inputs is used to calculate the internal state of the neuron using an activation function. This activation value, weighted by links, is propagated to the following neurons. Data are used as input to the first layer ("input layer"). The last layer is the "output layer." These two layers are separated by "hidden layers." Each neuron of each layer is connected with each neuron of the next layer. The MP was composed of an input layer (26 neurons), a hidden layer (13 neurons) and an output layer comprising two neurons.

1. The energy spectrum in each pixel was sampled in 26 energy channels of 4 keV each between 79 and 183 keV.
2. Normalized spectral values (ratio of photon counts in each channel to total photon count) were used as inputs. The two output neurons yielded the ratio of estimated primary to total photon counts of ^{99m}Tc or ^{123}I in each pixel.
3. The learning phase consisted of submitting to the network typical spectral images together with the true expected value of the primary/total photon ratio of each radionuclide. A phantom study, independent of the brain studies, based on Monte Carlo simulation of both ^{99m}Tc and ^{123}I, was performed to obtain learning samples.

2.3. Fast Monte Carlo Based Joint Ordered-Subset Expectation-Maximization

The fast Monte Carlo based joint ordered-subset expectation-maximization (MC-JOSEM) is a reconstruction algorithm that incorporates accurate scatter and cross-talk corrections, which are obtained by a fast Monte Carlo simulation, into a joint

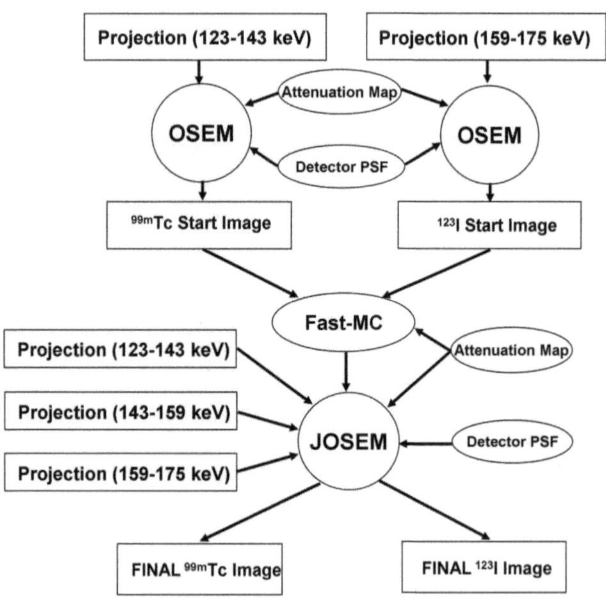

Fig. 16.1. Flow chart of MC-JOSEM.

iterative reconstruction process. MC-JOSEM algorithm for the reconstruction of ^{99m}Tc/^{123}I is illustrated in **Fig. 16.1** (5).

1. Two photopeak projections at two detector energy windows, 129–151 keV and 159–175 keV, were used to reconstruct ^{99m}Tc and ^{123}I images, respectively, using standard OSEM, while modeling the attenuation map and the detector point spread function (PSF) in both the projector and backprojector. Each reconstruction process used one detector energy window associated with one radionuclide.

2. The scatter and cross-talk contributions to all energy windows were estimated using a fast MC algorithm while using the reconstructed ^{99m}Tc and ^{123}I images at the fifth iteration as starting images. Ten million photon histories were generated, and each event underwent a number of interactions before exiting the imaging volume. Scatter maps were simulated at each projection angle for many energy windows throughout the entire energy spectrum for all the primary and scattered photons that have non-negligible probability of being detected in the two detected energy windows used by the scanner. These scatter maps were then blurred by the PSFs to form the projection for each detector energy window to obtain the scatter and cross-talk estimates.

3. A joint OSEM incorporating two radionuclides and three detector energy windows (129–151, 151–159, and 159–175 keV) was performed. All the image volumes and projection sets, and therefore all the radionuclides and energy

windows, contribute to the iterative reconstruction process. For JOSEM, each forward projection has contributions from all the radionuclides, while each backprojection has contributions from all the energy windows. This is different from conventional OSEM, where only one radionuclide and one energy window are involved in the reconstruction process. The same scatter estimate was included in the forward projection for each iteration of JOSEM. Instead of subtracting the low-noise estimate of the scatter and cross-talk contributions directly from the measured projections, the estimate was included when forward projecting to preserve the Poisson statistics.

2.4. Statistical Parametric Mapping Software

The Statistical Parametric mapping (SPM) is a suite of MATLAB functions and subroutines with some externally compiled C routines. SPM was written to organize and interpret the functional neuroimaging data. SPM2 is a major update to the SPM software, containing substantial theoretical, algorithmic, structural, and interface enhancements over previous versions.

3. Methods

Section 3.1 (**Section 3.2**) describes the methods for the differential diagnosis of IPD and MSA (CBD and PSP). Although either ANN-based OSEM or MC-JOSEM can be used for both studies and MC-JOSEM is expected to be superior to ANN-based OSEM, only the method used in the original publication is presented for each application.

3.1. Differential Diagnosis of IPD and MSA

1. Thirty-four patients were included in the study, all of whom provided informed consent according to institutional guidelines.
2. Five patients (four males, one female) were clinically assessed as having IPD. Five patients (two males, three females) were clinically assessed as having MSA. The mean UPDRS motor score and Heohn and Yahr stage were, respectively, 16 ± 6.1 and 1.8 ± 0.6 for the IPD group, and 16.4 ± 5.3 and 2.6 ± 0.5 for the MSA group. Available clinical data at the time of SPECT examination included medication (levodopa agonists and other medications), UPDRS motor scores, and results from other tests (MRI, neuropsychological tests).
3. Nine patients (five males, four females) were healthy volunteers. They were screened for normalcy by physical

and paraclinical examinations as well as the complete patient history. High spatial resolution T2 and 3D-SPGR-T1 MRI scan results were normal.

4. Each patient was injected with 185 MBq ^{123}I-FP-CIT. Two hours later, the patient was injected with 740 MBq ^{99m}Tc-ECD.
5. Three hours after the injection of ^{123}I-FP-CIT and 1 h after the injection of ^{99m}Tc-ECD, data were acquired in eight energy windows in 79–179 keV using the triple-head SPECT camera equipped with LEHR parallel-hole collimator.
6. Projection data were corrected for scatter, cross-talk, and ^{123}I high-energy penetration using ANNs (4, 12).
7. ANN-corrected projections were first reconstructed with no compensations to yield the contour of the scalp, which was drawn individually on each study, and the "narrow beam geometry" uniform attenuation map ($\mu = 0.15$ cm^{-1} for ^{99m}Tc and 0.12 cm^{-1} for ^{123}I).
8. The primary ^{99m}Tc and ^{123}I projections estimated with ANNs were reconstructed using OSEM a second time with patient-specific attenuation yielding perfusion and neurotransmission studies for each subject.
9. Perfusion and DAT function were assessed using voxel-based SPM2 as well as volume of interest quantitation in brain regions identified by SPM2 as significantly different between pairs of the three subject groups.
10. Discrimination between different subject groups based on perfusion and DAT binding potential (BP) was assessed by discriminant analysis, which yielded for each subject a likelihood ratio of belonging to a group and used to compute the area under the receiver operating characteristic (ROC) curve.

3.2. Differential Diagnosis of CBD and PSP

1. Nineteen patients were included in the study, all of whom provided informed consent according to institutional guidelines.
2. Twenty patients were clinically assessed as having CBD. Fourteen patients were clinically assessed as having MSA.
3. Nine patients (five males, four females) were healthy volunteers. They were screened for normalcy by physical and paraclinical examinations as well as the complete patient history. High spatial resolution T2 and 3D-SPGR-T1 MRI scan results were normal.
4. Each patient was injected with 185 MBq ^{123}I-FP-CIT. Two hours later, the patient was injected with 740 MBq ^{99m}Tc-ECD.

5. Three hours after the injection of ^{123}I-FP-CIT and 1 h after the injection of ^{99m}Tc-ECD, data were acquired using the triple-head SPECT camera equipped with LEHR parallel-hole collimator.
6. Photopeak projections at detector energy window 129–151 keV were used to reconstruct to yield the contour of the scalp, which was drawn individually on each study, and the "narrow beam geometry" uniform attenuation map ($\mu = 0.15\ \text{cm}^{-1}$ for ^{99m}Tc and $0.12\ \text{cm}^{-1}$ for ^{123}I).
7. Two photopeak projections at two detector energy windows, 129–151 and 159–175 keV, were used to reconstruct ^{99m}Tc and ^{123}I images, respectively, using standard OSEM, while modeling the attenuation map and the detector point spread function (PSF) in both the projector and backprojector. Each reconstruction process used one detector energy window associated with one radionuclide.
8. The scatter and cross-talk contributions to all energy windows were estimated using a fast MC algorithm while using the reconstructed ^{99m}Tc and ^{123}I images at the fifth iteration as starting images.
9. A joint OSEM incorporating two radionuclides and three detector energy windows (129–151, 151–159, and 159–175 keV) was performed.
10. Same as number 9 in **Section 3.1**.
11. Same as number 10 in **Section 3.2**.

4. Notes

1. A triple-head SPECT camera, such as Picker Prism 3000XP (Marconi Medical Systems, Cleveland, OH) and Trionix Triad (Twinsburg, OH), uses three flat detectors to surround the brain. CeraSPECT (Digitalscintigraphics Inc., Waltham, MA) is another type of dedicated brain SPECT, which has high sensitivity (13, 14). It uses a single continuous cylindrical sodium-iodide (NaI(Tl)) annular crystal and a three-segment parallel-hole collimator. The crystal is stationary; the collimator rotates within it. At a given angular position, three parallel-hole projections, at 120° intervals, are acquired simultaneously. The sensitivity for such annular camera can be further enhanced using special designed annular variable focusing collimator (15, 16).

2. ^{99m}Tc-HMPAO is another useful ^{99m}Tc-labeled perfusion radiotracer in addition to ^{99m}Tc-ECD. In addition to ^{123}I-FP-CIT, other useful ^{123}I-labeled neurotransmission radiotracers to image DAT include ^{123}I-altropane, ^{123}I-ßCIT, ^{123}I-IBZM, and ^{123}I-epidepride.
3. For ANN method, projections must be acquired for many energy windows. This is, however, not always possible because the number of energy windows that can be used during a data acquisition is usually very limited for most SPECT systems. If the list-mode is available, the solution is to acquire data using list-mode and then rebin the data into all the energy windows.
4. SimSET (17) and GATE (18) are two Monte Carlo simulation toolkits that can be used to generate phantom learning samples for ANN method.
5. In April 2009, SPM8, which contains major enhancements over previous versions, was released.
6. The clinical diagnoses of IPD and MSA were, respectively, based on the UKPDSBB criteria (2) and on consensus statement on the diagnosis of MSA (19).
7. The clinical diagnoses of CBD and PSP, were based on the CBDMCCS (20) and NINDS criteria (21), respectively.
8. **Figure 16.2** shows transaxial slices of ^{123}I-FP-CIT at the striatal level and the corresponding ^{99m}Tc-ECD from representative IPD and MSA patients and a normal control.
9. A significant decrease in striatal FP-CIT was found in the SPM2 analysis ($p < 0.05$, corrected) in IPD and MSA compared to normal subjects, and in IPD compared to

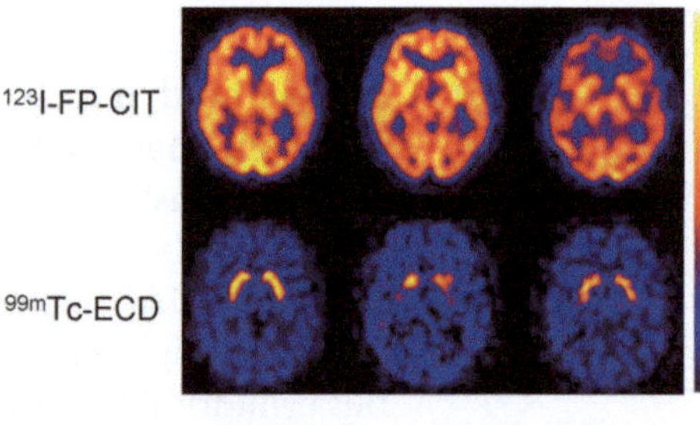

Fig. 16.2. Transaxial slices of the ^{123}I-FP-CIT study at the striatal level and of the corresponding ^{99m}Tc-ECD study from representative IPD and MSA patients and a normal control. Images were spatially normalized in the same anatomical referential with SPM2.

MSA. Furthermore, it shows that perfusion was significantly decreased in the left and right caudate nucleus and nucleus lentiformis (putamen + globus pallidus) in MSA compared to controls and with IPD ($p < 0.05$, corrected). Striatal BP was lower in IPD (55%) and MSA (23%) compared to normal controls, and in IPD compared to MSA ($p < 0.05$).

10. The asymmetry index is defined as: $AI = (A_l - A_r)/(A_l + A_r)$, where A_l and A_r are the mean activity concentration within the left and right structures, respectively. AI was significantly greater ($p < 0.05$) for IPD than MSA and normal controls in both the caudate nucleus (1.9 and 4.4 times, respectively) and the putamen (2.4 and 3.6 times, respectively).
11. No significant regional perfusion differences between IPD and normal subjects. Perfusion was significantly reduced by 28% ($p < 0.01$) and 18% ($p < 0.05$) in caudate nucleus and nucleus lentiformis, respectively, in MSA as compared to normal subjects. Perfusion was also reduced by 8 and 14% in the right and left caudate nucleus and by 14 and 17% in the left and right nucleus lentiformis, respectively, in MSA as compared to IPD.
12. **Figure 16.3** shows a comparison of reconstructed images using ANN-OSEM and MC-JOSEM.
13. MC-JOSEM demonstrated the expected decrease in perfusion in left (21%) and right (14%) parietal cortex in CBD versus PSP ($p < 0.05$ corrected), as compared to ANN (only right parietal cortex, 10%, $p < 0.01$). MC-JOSEM yielded significantly greater discrimination power between PSP and CBD than did ANN.

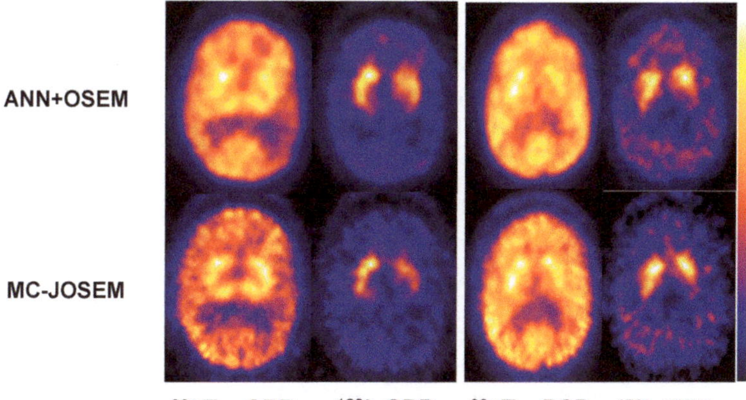

Fig. 16.3. Comparison of reconstructed images using ANN-OSEM and MC-JOSEM.

References

1. Turjanski, N. and Lloyd, G. G. (2005) Psychiatric side-effects of medications: recent developments. *Adv. Psychiatr. Treat.* **11**, 58–70.
2. Hughes, A. J., Daniel, S. E., Kilford, L., and Lees, A. J. (1992) Accuracy of clinical diagnosis of idiopathic Parkinson's disease: a clinico-pathological study of 100 cases. *J. Neurol. Neurosurg. Psychiatry* **55**, 181–4.
3. Hughes, A. J., Daniel, S. E., and Lees, A. J. (2001) Improved accuracy of clinical diagnosis of Lewy body Parkinson's disease. *Neurology* **57**, 1497–9.
4. El Fakhri, G., Maksud, P., Kijewski, M. F., Habert, M. O., Todd-Pokropek, A., Aurengo, A., and Moore, S. C. (2000) Scatter and cross-talk corrections in simultaneous Tc-99m/I-123 brain SPECT using constrained factor analysis and artificial neural networks. *IEEE Trans. Nucl. Sci.* **47**, 1573–80.
5. Moore, S. C., Ouyang, J., Park, M. A., and El Fakhri, G. (2006) Monte Carlo based compensation for patient scatter, detector scatter, and cross talk contamination in In-111 SPECT imaging. *Nucl. Instrum. Methods Phys. Res. A* **569**, 472–6.
6. Ouyang, J., El Fakhri, G., and Moore, S. C. (2007) Fast Monte Carlo based joint iterative reconstruction for simultaneous $^{99m}Tc/^{123}I$ SPECT imaging. *Med. Phys.* **34**, 263–3272.
7. Du, Y., Tsui, B. M. W., and Frey, E. C. (2007) Model-based crosstalk compensation for simultaneous $^{99m}Tc/^{123}I$ dual-isotope brain SPECT imaging. *Med. Phys.* **34**, 3530–43.
8. Du, Y. and Frey, E. C. (2009) Quantitative evaluation of simultaneous reconstruction with model-based crosstalk compensation for $^{99m}Tc/^{123}I$ dual-isotope simultaneous acquisition brain SPECT. *Med. Phys.* **36**, 2021–33.
9. El Fakhri, G., Habert, M. O., Maksud, P., Kas, A., Malek, Z., and Kijewski, M. F. (2006) Quantitative simultaneous $^{99m}Tc/^{123}I$-Fp-CIT SPECT in Parkinson's disease and multiple system atrophy. *Eur. J. Nucl. Med.* **33**, 87–92.
10. Laere, K. V., Casteels, C., Ceuninck, L. D., Vanbilloen, B., Maes, A., Mortelmans, L., Vandenberghe, W., Verbruggen, A., and Dom, R. (2006) Dual-tracer dopamine transporter and perfusion SPECT in differential diagnosis of parkinsonism using template-based discriminant analysis. *J. Nucl. Med.* **47**, 384–92.
11. El Fakhri, G., Ouyang, J., Maksud, P., Trott, C., and Habert, M. O. (2008) Improved discrimination between parkinsonian syndromes using Monte Carlo joint iterative reconstruction (MC-JOSEM). *J. Nucl. Med.* **49**, 152p.
12. El Fakhri, G., Moore, S. C., Maksud, P., Aurengo, A., and Kijewski, M. F. (2001) Absolute activity quantitation in simultaneous $^{123}I/^{99m}Tc$ brain SPECT. *J. Nucl. Med.* **42**, 300–8.
13. Genna, S. and Smith, A. P. (1988) The development of ASPECT, an annular single crystal brain camera for high efficiency SPECT. *IEEE Trans. Nucl. Sci.* **35**, 654–8.
14. Smith, A. P. and Genna, S. (1988) Acquisition and calibration principles for ASPECT—A SPECT camera using digital position analysis. *IEEE Trans. Nucl. Sci.* **35**, 740–3.
15. El Fakhri, G., Ouyang, J., Zimmerman, R. E., Fischman, A. J., and Kijewski, M. F. (2006) Performance of a novel collimator for high-sensitivity brain SPECT. *Med. Phys.* **33**, 209–15.
16. Ouyang, J., El Fakhri, G., Xia, W., Kijewski, M. F., and Genna, S. (2006) The design and manufacture of an annular variable-focusing collimator for high-sensitivity brain SPECT. *IEEE Trans. Nucl. Sci.* **53**, 2613–8.
17. Harrison, R. L., Haynor, D. R., Gillispie, S. B., Vannoy, S. D., Kaplan, M. S., and Lewellen, T. K. (1993) A public-domain simulation system for emission tomography—Photon tracking through heterogeneous attenuation using importance sampling. *J. Nucl. Med.* **34**, P60.
18. Jan, S., et al. (2004) GATE: a simulation toolkit for PET and SPECT. *Phys. Med. Biol.* **49**, 4543–61.
19. Gilman, S., Low, P. A., Quinn, N., Albanese, A., Ben-Shlomo, Y., Fowler, C. J., etal (1999) Consensus statement on the diagnosis of multiple system atrophy. *J. Neurol. Sci.* **163**, 94–8.
20. Lang, A. E., Riley, D. E., and Bergeron, C. (1994) Cortical-basal ganglionic degeneration. In Neurodegenerative disease, Calne D. B., (Ed.). Saunders, Philadelphia, PA, 877–94.
21. Litvan, I., Agid, Y., Calne, D., et al. (1996) Clinical research criteria for the diagnosis of progressive supranuclear palsy (Steele-Richardson-Olszewski syndrome): report of the NINDS-SPSP international workshop. *Neurology* **47**, 1–9.

INDEX

K. Shah (ed.), *Molecular Imaging*, Methods in Molecular Biology 680,
DOI 10.1007/978-1-60761-901-7, © Springer Science+Business Media, LLC 2011

E

F

G

H

I

J

K

L

M

N

O

P

Q

R

S

T

U

V

MIX
Papier aus verantwortungsvollen Quellen
Paper from responsible sources
FSC® C105338

If you have any concerns about our products, you can contact us on
ProductSafety@springernature.com

In case Publisher is established outside the EU, the EU authorized representative is:
Springer Nature Customer Service Center GmbH
Europaplatz 3, 69115 Heidelberg, Germany

Printed by Libri Plureos GmbH
in Hamburg, Germany